Therapeutic Targets of the TNF Superfamily

ADVANCES IN EXPERIMENTAL MEDICINE AND BIOLOGY

Therapeutic Targets of the TNF Superfamily

Edited by

Iqbal S. Grewal, PhD

Department of Preclinical Therapeutics, Seattle Genetics, Inc., Bothell, Washington, USA

Springer Science+Business Media, LLC
Landes Bioscience

Springer Science+Business Media, LLC
Landes Bioscience

Printed in the USA.

Springer Science+Business Media, LLC, 233 Spring Street, New York, New York 10013, USA
http://www.springer.com

Please address all inquiries to the publishers:
Landes Bioscience, 1002 West Avenue, Austin, Texas 78701, USA
Phone: 512/ 637 6050; FAX: 512/ 637 6079
http://www.landesbioscience.com

Therapeutic Targets of the TNF Superfamily, edited by Iqbal S. Grewal, Landes Bioscience / Springer
Science+Business Media, LLC dual imprint / Springer series: Advances in Experimental Medicine and
Biology

ISBN: 978-0-387-89519-2

While the authors, editors and publisher believe that drug selection and dosage and the specifications and
usage of equipment and devices, as set forth in this book, are in accord with current recommendations
and practice at the time of publication, they make no warranty, expressed or implied, with respect to
material described in this book. In view of the ongoing research, equipment development, changes in
governmental regulations and the rapid accumulation of information relating to the biomedical sciences,
the reader is urged to carefully review and evaluate the information provided herein.

Library of Congress Cataloging-in-Publication Data

Therapeutic targets of the TNF superfamily / edited by Iqbal S. Grewal.
    p. ; cm. -- (Advances in experimental medicine and biology ; v. 647)
  Includes bibliographical references and index.
  ISBN 978-0-387-89519-2
  1. Tumor necrosis factor. 2. Tumor necrosis factor--Agonists--Therapeutic use. I. Grewal, Iqbal S.
II. Series.
  [DNLM: 1. Tumor Necrosis Factors--therapeutic use. 2. Autoimmune Diseases--drug therapy. 3.
Inflammation--drug therapy. 4. Neoplasms--drug therapy. 5. Receptors, Tumor Necrosis Factor--
therapeutic use. W1 AD559 v.647 2009 / QW 568 T3985 2009]
  QR185.8.T84.T44 2009
  616.07'9--dc22
                            2008047209

PREFACE

Tumor necrosis factor (TNF) superfamily is a rapidly growing family of cytokines that interacts with a corresponding superfamily of receptors. Ligand-receptor interactions of this superfamily are involved in numerous biological processes ranging from hematopoiesis to pleiotropic cellular responses, including activation, proliferation, differentiation, and apoptosis. The particular response depends on the receptor, the cell type, and the concurrent signals received by the cell. Worldwide interest in the TNF field surged dramatically early in 1984 with the cloning and defining of the profound cellular effects of the first member of this family, TNFα. Subsequently, the major influence of TNFα on the development and functioning of the immune system was established. Today, over 20 human TNF ligands and their more than 30 corresponding receptors have been identified. Few receptors still remain orphans. What has emerged over the years is that most TNF ligands bind to one distinct receptor and some of the TNF ligands are able to bind to multiple TNF receptors, explaining to some extent the apparent disparity in the number of TNF receptors and ligands. Yet, in spite of some redundancy in TNF ligand/receptor interactions, it is clear that in vivo spatial, temporal, and indeed cell- and tissue-specific expression of both ligands and their receptors are important factors in determining the precise nature of cellular, physiological and pathological processes they control.

TNF superfamily has been the most highly investigated area of basic medical research for over two decades. These investigations have benefited from the enormous growth in our understanding of the principal functions of the immune system and the explosion in the knowledge involved in regulation of normal and pathological immune response. In addition, much has been learned about the molecular mechanisms of programmed cell death and the escape of tumor cells from apoptotic demise and from discovery of the key role played by TNF ligands in this process. As the functioning of these superfamily members is very complex, understanding TNF ligands and their receptor biology requires a mélange of research activities in many different disciplines including organ development, molecular biology, experimental pathology, and immunology. As a consequence of intensive studies in multiple areas over many years, much has been learned. A key role of members of this superfamily in normal functioning of the immune system, autoimmunity, and other fundamental cellular process by which tumor cells develop has been established. Many novel mechanisms involving TNF superfamily members in the disease development process have been defined, and a unified concept and new perspectives have also emerged. For example, abrasions in the innate immune system, not always considered critical in autoimmunity, have come under increasing attention. Additionaly, TNF-directed and not antigen- directed therapy has emerged as the most impressive therapeutic advance in managing autoimmunity in humans. These findings provide a foundation for novel drug design efforts that are poised to utilize newly acquired knowledge. Several of these strategies have already materialized into successful therapeutics such as use of TNF for cancers and anti-TNFα antibodies and TNFR-Fc for autoimmune diseases, and many have advanced to human clinical trials, while many more are still being tested in preclinical settings.

As in other rapidly evolving fields, these advances are not necessarily congruent and are often difficult to organize into a cogent whole. The aim of *Therapeutic Targets of the TNF Superfamily* is to make readily available the major research important in the exploitation of this family for developing therapeutic strategies for human diseases, in a single volume. Under the auspices of Landes Bioscience, I have undertaken the task to concisely consolidate current knowledge of key TNF superfamily members focusing on both basic aspects and their clinical application. In this volume, a number of leading scientists in the field cover many aspects of biology of TNF superfamily members, ranging from the cloning and characterization of TNF ligands and their receptors, through the use of animal models to study their functions in vivo and their exploitation for human therapeutic use. Each chapter also includes relevant background information and provides useful bibliography for a more detailed analysis, making the study of TNF ligands/receptors accessible at all levels of expertise.

I would like to express my sincere thanks to all of my contributors for their excellent effort and undertaking this project with such enthusiasm, to Cynthia Conomos and Ronald G. Landes for commissioning me to edit this volume, and Megan Klein and the staff of Landes Bioscience for help with publication coordination. This volume presents the state-of-the art account on the role of TNF superfamily members in the pathogenesis and their use in current intervention of cancers and autoimmune disease. This text will be highly valuable for investigators to understand the disease processes regulated by TNF superfamily members and to develop effective therapeutics. A view into the future, inspired by the comprehensive work presented in this volume, predicts that researchers studying TNF superfamily members will continue to make rapid progress in identifying relevant components to the disease process and new therapeutic strategies to target many human diseases including cancers, autoimmune disease, and others.

Iqbal S. Grewal, PhD

ABOUT THE EDITOR...

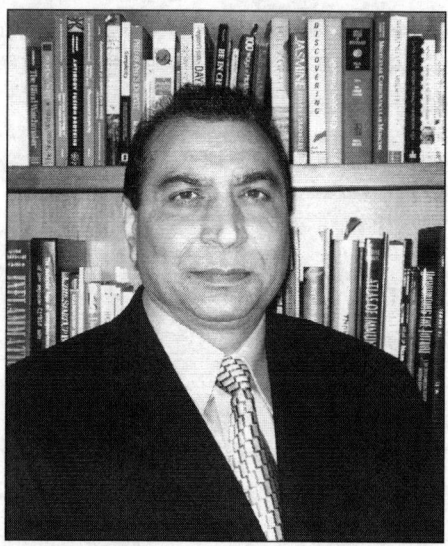

IQBAL S. GREWAL, PhD. is well-known in the field of T-cell co-stimulation and autoimmunity and has extensively investigated several members of the TNF superfamily and molecules important for lymphocyte co-stimulation. His research has focused on the basic molecular and cellular processes to determine the biological roles of these molecules in normal physiology and immunity and their potential utility as agents or targets for the treatment of autoimmune diseases and cancers. His experience in discovering and developing innovative protein-based biotherapeutics in many disease areas has translated some of his findings into key drug candidates for the treatment of autoimmune disease and cancers.

Dr Grewal currently holds the position of Vice President of Preclinical Therapeutics at Seattle Genetics, Inc. in Bothell, Washington. He is responsible for preclinical translational research functions in support of the development of monoclonal antibodies and antibody-drug conjugates as therapeutics in the areas of autoimmunity and oncology. Before joining Seattle Genetics, Inc. Dr Grewal performed drug discovery research and preclinical development at Genentech in South San Francisco, California, where he identified and validated several novel molecules as therapeutic candidates in oncology and autoimmune disease. Prior to Genentech, Dr Grewal worked at Yale University School of Medicine. Before that, he held various research positions at the University of California, Los Angeles (UCLA). Dr Grewal has presented his work at both national and international meetings, as well as published over 100 scientific publications, 75 abstracts, 60 patent applications. He is a fellow of the Royal College of Pathologists, London and member of several distinguished societies. Dr Grewal holds a PhD in Immunology from UCLA and completed his post-doctoral fellowship at Howard Hughes Medical Institute at Yale University School of Medicine.

PARTICIPANTS

Bharat B. Aggarwal
Cytokine Research Laboratory
Department of Experimental
  Therapeutics
The University of Texas
  MD Anderson Cancer Center
Houston, Texas
USA

Robert Benschop
Lilly Research Laboratories
Eli Lilly and Co.
Indianapolis, Indiana
USA

Tamar Boursalian
Department of Preclinical
  Therapeutics
Seattle Genetics, Inc.
Bothell, Washington
USA

Michael Croft
Molecular Immunology
La Jolla Institute for Allergy
  and Immunology
La Jolla, California
USA

Martin Ehrenschwender
Department of Molecular Internal
  Medicine
Medical Clinic and Polyclinic II
University of Wuerzburg
Wuerzburg
Germany

Christina Falschlehner
Department of Immunology
Division of Medicine
Imperial College London
London
UK

Tom M. Ganten
Internal Medicine
University of Heidelberg
Heidelberg
Germany

Hans Peter Gerber
Department of Preclinical
  Therapeutics
Seattle Genetics, Inc.
Bothell, Washington
USA

Michael J. Gough
Robert W. Franz Cancer Center
Earle A. Chiles Research Institute
Providence Portland Medical Center
Portland, Oregon
USA

Iqbal S. Grewal
Department of Preclinical
   Therapeutics
Seattle Genetics, Inc.
Bothell, Washington
USA

Ronald Koschny
Internal Medicine
University of Heidelberg
Heidelberg
Germany

Ajaikumar B. Kunnumakkara
Cytokine Research Laboratory
Department of Experimental
   Therapeutics
The University of Texas
   MD Anderson Cancer Center
Houston, Texas
USA

Che-Leung Law
Department of Preclinical
   Therapeutics
Seattle Genetics, Inc.
Bothell, Washington
USA

Seung-Woo Lee
Molecular Immunology
La Jolla Institute for Allergy
   and Immunology
La Jolla, California
USA

Andreas Leibbrandt
Institute of Molecular
   Biotechnology of the Austrian
   Academy of Sciences
Vienna
Austria

Julie McEarchern
Department of Preclinical
   Therapeutics
Seattle Genetics, Inc.
Bothell, Washington
USA

Songqing Na
Lilly Research Laboratories
Eli Lilly and Co.
Indianapolis, Indiana
USA

Giuseppe Nocentini
Dipartimento di Medicina
   Clinica e Sperimentale
Sezione di Farmacologia
   Tossicologia e Chemioterapia
Università di Perugia; IBiT
   Foundation, Perugia
Polo Scientifico e Didattico di Terni
Perugia
Italy

Ezogelin Oflazoglu
Department of Preclinical
   Therapeutics
Seattle Genetics, Inc.
Bothell, Washington
USA

Josef M. Penninger
Institute of Molecular
   Biotechnology of the Austrian
   Academy of Sciences
Vienna
Austria

Carlo Riccardi
Dipartimento di Medicina Clinica
  e Sperimentale
Sezione di Farmacologia, Tossicologia
  e Chemioterapia
Università di Perugia; IBiT
  Foundation, Perugia
Polo Scientifico e Didattico di Terni
Perugia
Italy

Maureen C. Ryan
Seattle Genetics, Inc.
Bothell, Washington
USA

Uta Schaefer
Division of Apoptosis Regulation
German Cancer Research Center
Heidelberg
Germany

Gautam Sethi
Cytokine Research Laboratory
Department of Experimental
  Therapeutics
The University of Texas
  MD Anderson Cancer Center
Houston, Texas
USA

Bokyung Sung
Cytokine Research Laboratory
Department of Experimental
  Therapeutics
The University of Texas
  MD Anderson Cancer Center
Houston, Texas
USA

Harald Wajant
Department of Molecular Internal
  Medicine
Medical Clinic and Polyclinic II
University of Wuerzburg
Wuerzburg
Germany

Henning Walczak
Department of Immunology
Division of Medicine
Imperial College London
London
UK

Carl F. Ware
Division of Molecular Immunology
La Jolla Institute for Allergy
  and Immunology
La Jolla, California
USA

Tao Wei
Lilly Research Laboratories
Eli Lilly and Co.
Indianapolis, Indiana
USA

Andrew D. Weinberg
Robert W. Franz Cancer Center
Earle A. Chiles Research Institute
Providence Portland Medical Center
Portland, Oregon
USA

CONTENTS

7. TARGETING CD70 FOR HUMAN THERAPEUTIC USE.................... 108

Tamar Boursalian, Julie McEarchern, Che-Leung Law and Iqbal S. Grewal

8. 4-1BB AS A THERAPEUTIC TARGET FOR HUMAN DISEASE........ 120

Seung-Woo Lee and Michael Croft

9. RANK(L) AS A KEY TARGET FOR CONTROLLING BONE LOSS.....130

Andreas Leibbrandt and Josef M. Penninger

10. TARGETING THE LIGHT-HVEM PATHWAY 146

Carl F. Ware

14. TRAIL AND OTHER TRAIL RECEPTOR AGONISTS AS NOVEL CANCER THERAPEUTICS

Christina Falschlehner, Tom M. Ganten, Ronald Koschny, Uta Schaefer
and Henning Walczak

15. THERAPEUTIC POTENTIAL OF VEGI/TL1A IN AUTOIMMUNITY AND CANCER

Gautam Sethi, Bokyung Sung and Bharat B. Aggarwal

CHAPTER 1

Overview of TNF Superfamily:
A Chest Full of Potential Therapeutic Targets

Iqbal S. Grewal*

Abstract

Since the discovery of tumor necrosis factor TNFα about 25 years ago, TNF superfamily has grown to a large family of related proteins consisting of over 20 members that signal through over 30 receptors. Members of this superfamily have wide tissue distribution and play important roles ranging from regulation of the normal biological processes such as immune responses, hematopoiesis and morphogenesis to their role in tumorigenesis, transplant rejection, septic shock, viral replication, bone resorption and autoimmunity. Thus, many approaches to harness the potency of TNF superfamily members to treat human diseases have been developed. Indeed, TNF and TNF agonistic molecules have been approved for human use in the United States and other countries. Many other TNF family members show promise for several therapeutic applications, including cancer, infectious disease, transplantation and autoimmunity. This chapter will give overview of TNF superfamily for exploitation for therapeutic use in humans.

Introduction

In middle of the nineteenth century, a surprising observation was made that in some cancer patients spontaneous regression of their tumors occurred if they were infected with bacterial infections.[1] This landmark discovery led to the idea of existence of a tumor necrotizing molecule and use of Coley's toxins (bacterial extracts) for the treatment of human cancers.[2] A century later, a factor from bacterial extracts, lipopolysaccharide (LPS), was isolated that was identified to be responsible for anti-tumor effects.[3] This effect of LPS on tumor regression was later shown to be due to induction of a factor in the serum. This factor was named as tumor-necrotizing factor[4] and later designated as tumor-necrosis factor (TNF).[5] Subsequently TNF was isolated[6] and its gene was cloned[7] and TNF became the prototype of a rapidly growing family of related proteins now called the TNF superfamily.

The TNF superfamily is now composed of over 20 TNF-related ligands all sharing many key structural features. A majority of these ligands are synthesized as type II transmembrane proteins. These ligands contain a relatively long extracellular domain and a short cytoplasmic region.[8] Their extracellular domains can be cleaved by specific metalloproteinases to generate a soluble molecule. In general, cleaved and noncleaved ligands are active as noncovalent homotrimers, although some members can also exist as heterotrimers. Both membrane-bound and secreted ligands are expressed by a variety of normal and malignant cell types.[9] Since most of TNF-superfamily members are expressed as transmembrane cell surface proteins, it is believed they are acting at a local level. Key members of this family include APRIL, BAFF, 4-1BBL, CD30L, CD40L, CD70, CD95L, OX40L, LTα, LTβ, RANKL, NGF, TNFα and TRAIL (Fig. 1). More than 30 receptors for the TNF ligands belonging to the TNF receptor (TNFR) superfamily have been identified in

*Iqbal S. Grewal—Seattle Genetics, Inc., 21823 30th Drive SE, Bothell, WA 98021, USA.
 Email: igrewal@seagen.com

Therapeutic Targets of the TNF Superfamily, edited by Iqbal S. Grewal.
©2009 Landes Bioscience and Springer Science+Business Media.

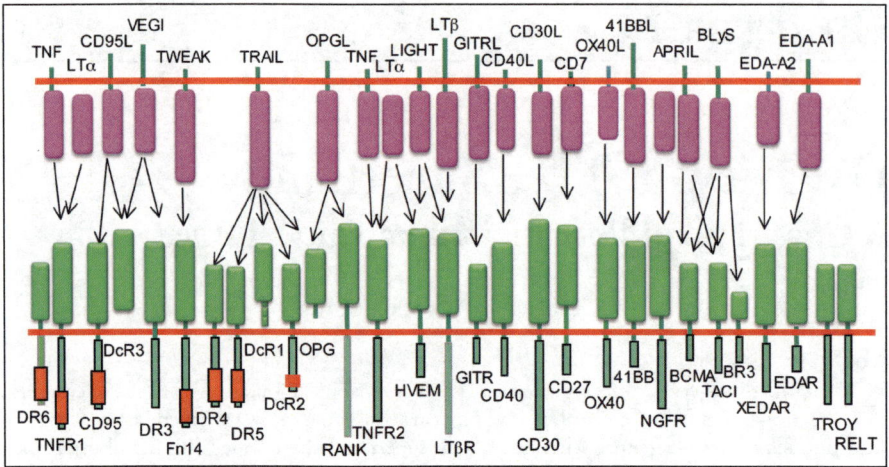

Figure 1. TNF superfamily ligands and their known receptors. Ligands and their receptors are shown in a diagramatic form. Many ligands bind to more than one receptor as indicated by arrows. Ligands for DR6, TROY and RELT have not yet been discovered. Red boxes shown in the cytoplasmic part of the receptors indicate presence of a death domain. A color version of this image is available at www.eurekah.com

humans and in mice. These receptors are type I membrane proteins characterized by the presence of a distinctive cystein-rich domain in their extra-cellular portion.[9] Most of TNF ligands bind to a single receptor, but few of them bind to more than one receptor. For example, TRAIL is known to bind five receptors (DR4, DR5, DcR1, DcR2 and OPG). TNF receptors exert their cellular responses through signaling sequences in their cytoplasmic regions.

Based upon these cytoplasmic sequences and signaling properties, the TNF receptors can be classified into three major groups.[10] The first group includes receptors that contain a death domain (DD) in their cytoplasmic tail. These receptors include CD95, TNFR1, DR3, DR4, DR5 and DR6. Binding of TNF superfamily ligands to their DD containing receptors causes complex signaling through adaptor proteins, such as tumor necrosis factor receptor—associated death domain (TRADD), resulting in activation of the caspase cascade and apoptosis of the cell.[11] The second groups of receptors contain one or more TNF receptor-associated factors (TRAF) interacting motifs (TIM) in their cytoplasmic tails. This group includes TNFR2, CD40, CD30, CD27, LT-βR, OX40, 4-1BB, BAFFR, BCMA, TACI, RANK, NGFR, HVEM, GITR, TROY, EDAR, XEDAR, RELT and Fn14.[12] Ligand binding to TIM containing TNF receptors induces recruitment of TRAF family members and activation of cellular signaling pathways including activation of a nuclear factor-κB (NF-κB), Jun N-terminal kinase (JNK), p38, extracellular signal regulated kinase (ERK) and phosphoinisitide-3 kinase.[12] The third group of TNF receptor family members does not contain functional intracellular signaling domains or motifs. These receptors include DcR1, DcR2, DcR3 and OPG. Although this group of receptors lacks the ability to provide intracellular signaling, they can effectively act as decoys to compete for ligand binding and block the signaling through other two groups of receptors.[13]

Signaling events induced by TNFR superfamily members regulate a very broad array of developmental processes and play pivotal roles in numerous biological events in mammals including induction of apoptosis, survival, differentiation and proliferation of cells. The majority of TNF superfamily ligands are predominantly expressed on cells involved in the immune system including B-cells, T-cells, NK cells, monocytes and dendritic cells. In contrast, TNF receptors are expressed by a wide variety of cells that have both hematopoetic and nonhematopoeitic origins. Thus, numerous activities are assigned to TNF superfamily members, in particular, their profound role in regulation of both normal and pathogenic immune responses.

The strong role played by TNF superfamily members in normal development is illustrated by the identification of disease causing mutations in both ligands and receptors. Humans with mutations in TNFR1, CD95, CD95L, RANK, EDA and CD40L manifest profound abnormalities. For example, mutations in TNFR1 are linked to periodic fever syndromes called TNFR1-associated periodic syndromes, which is manifested as unexplained episodes of fever and severe localized inflammation.[14] Individuals who have mutations in CD95 and CD95L manifest autoimmune lymphoproliferative syndrome (ALPS),[15] a phenotype that is similar to those of lpr and gld mice, which also have mutations in CD95 and CD95L respectively.[16] Because of lack of CD95 signals, ALPS patients have defective lymphocyte apoptosis and have an increased risk of developing T- and B-cell lymphomas.[15] Humans with mutations in CD40L gene, an X-linked hyper-IgM syndrome, have severe defects in immunoglobulin isotype switching mechanisms. This is illustrated by the accumulation of large amounts of IgM in the serum of patients with the CD40L gene mutation and their susceptibility to opportunistic infections.[17] Two mutations in RANK gene are linked to familial expansile osteolysis, a rare autosomal dominant bone disorder which is characterized by focal areas of increased bone remodeling. In this disease, an increased activity of osteoblasts and osteoclasts causes the osteolytic lesions to develop in the long bones during early adulthood. Both of these mutations have been linked to an increase in RANK-mediated NF-κB signaling in vitro, consistent with observed phenotype in vivo in humans.[18] Mutations in EDA results in hypohydrotic ectodermal dysplasia, both in humans and mice, which is characterized by the loss of hair, sweat glands and teeth.[19] A similar phenotype is also seen with mutations in receptor for EDA. EDA regulates the initiation and morphogenesis of hair and teeth by activating NF-κB in the ectoderm. Additionally, mutations in death receptors such as CD95 and DR4 have been linked to various carcinomas and lymphomas.[22,21] A critical in vivo role for BR3 (receptor for BAFF) in B-cell ontogeny is also illustrated by the finding of severe deficiency in B-cell development in mice with mutations in *br3* gene.[22]

Therapeutic Potential of TNF Superfamily for Anticancer Treatment

As mentioned earlier, a group of TNF superfamily receptors are death receptors and have the unique ability to transmit an intracellular death signal and TNF ligands such as TNF, CD95L and TRAIL are capable of inducing apoptosis in tumor cells. Because TNF receptors are expressed on many tumor cells, TNF was exploited for its antitumor effects. Its use as an anti-cancer agent, however, is limited because of its systemic toxicity.[23] Many approaches are being considered to improve its toxicity profile. For example, inhibition of matrix metalloproteinases has been documented to reduce the toxicity induced by TNF.[24] Furthermore, TNF has been successfully used to treat limb soft-tissue sarcomas and other large tumors when administered locally by isolated limb perfusion to avoid its systemic effects.[25] Similar to the use of TNF, in vivo use of CD95L is also limited by its lethal hepatotoxicity resulting from massive hepatocyte apoptosis. This led to testing of other TNF ligands that may selectively affect tumor survival in humans without significant toxicity. When TRAIL was investigated in this context, it was discovered that TRAIL can specifically kill tumor cells without harming normal cells, suggesting it could be used for the treatment of cancer. This is supported by a myriad of animal studies investigating the anticancer potential of TRAIL where very promising results have been seen.[26,27] In addition to TRAIL, agonistic antibodies specific for its receptors DR4[28] and DR5[29] are also being explored for their antitumor effects and are now in clinical testing. Since a number of other TNF family members such as, CD30, CD40, CD70, BR3, BCMA are also expressed on tumor cells, antibody based therapies are being developed to target these molecules and are currently undergoing clinical trials. In addition, some of these molecules are also being exploited as targets for antibody-drug conjugates (CD30 and CD70) and for radioimmunotherapy (BLyS receptors TACI and BR3).[30]

As TNF superfamily members play a profound role in the activation of immune response, therapeutic approaches to target TNF superfamily members to boost anti-tumor host responses have also been developed. Use of agonistic molecules to target TNF receptors for some members of the family are being tested in the clinic. These include, agonistic anti-CD40 antibodies, soluble CD40L and OX40L.[31,32] In cases, such as CD40, where the target is also expressed on tumor cells, rationally designed antibody-based therapies combining the induction of tumor cell apoptosis and activation of tumor-specific adaptive immunity can be considered. This will enable promotion of antitumor host immune response and could help to eradicate large established and heterogeneous tumors without requiring expression of tumor-specific antigens on all tumor cells.

Therapeutic Potential of TNF Superfamily for Autoimmune and Inflammatory Disease

It is clear now that the immune system is regulated not only by cell proliferation and differentiation but also by apoptosis and TNF superfamily members control and orchestrate the immune response at multiple levels.[33] Thus, TNF superfamily members have been implicated in both innate and adaptive immune responses such as defense against pathogens, inflammatory response and autoimmunity, as well as the normal development of the immune system.[33,34] TNF superfamily members such as TNF, LTα, LTβ and RANKL provide crucial role in the development of secondary lymphoid organs. CD95 is important for the regulation of immune system for both the development of T-cells in thymus and for the induction of apoptosis of activated T-cells important for the downregulation the immune response.[35] TNF superfamily members, such as TNF, CD95L and TRAIL, also contribute to the cytotoxic effector cell response in the recognition and elimination of virus-infected cells. Some members of the family are also important for the integrity of the host tissues. For example, the eye is maintained as an immune-privileged site by the expression of CD95L by the corneal cells. CD95L kills the inflammatory cells and protects the eye from inflammatory attack.[36] Similarly, TRAIL has also been shown to have an important role in regulation of lymphocyte functions in the periphery by inhibiting cell-cycle progression by T-cells.[37]

Since most of the TNF ligands are expressed by the cells of the immune systems, their crucial role in regulation and proliferation of B-cells, T-cells and monocytes as well as in homeostasis has been well documented.[38] Thus, importance of CD95L in peripheral T-cell homeostasis and crucial role of 4-1BBL, CD27, CD30L, OX40 and CD40L in costimulation T-cells has been well described.[34] As CD30, CD40 and receptors for TNF, LT, APRIL, BAFF and CD70 are expressed on B-cells these family members are implicated in the control of maturation and survival of B-cells.[11,39] Many TNF superfamily members are also important for the activation and development of effector cells such as CD40L for B-cells; 4-1BBL, OX40L and CD70 for T-cells; and CD40 and RANKL for dendritic cells.[38] In addition, several TNF ligands such as BAFF, CD30L, CD40L, OX40L, 4-1BBL and CD70 have been implicated in the development of autoimmunity.[38] A potential role of TRAIL and other members of the TNF superfamily in organ transplantation has also been documented.[40] A profound role of TNF superfamily members such as CD40L and TNFα has been described for protective Th1-type host response against infection with bacteria. TNFα has been also implicated in LPS-mediated septic shock. In addition to their profound role in autoimmune and inflammatory response, members of the TNF superfamily have also been implicated in chronic heart failure, bone resorption, AIDS, Alzheimer's disease, transplant rejection and atherosolerosis.[9]

Accordingly, approaches to target many of TNF superfamily receptors and ligands for treatment of autoimmunity and other inflammatory diseases are being exploited. Indeed, a number of biologic TNF blocking therapies including humanized monoclonal antibodies (e.g., infliximab or adalimumab) or recombinant fusion proteins of IgG and soluble receptors (e.g., etanercept) have been developed and are being used in humans now to inhibit the inflammation associated with Crohn's disease and rheumatoid arthritis.[41] TNF receptor fusion proteins are also in development for heart disease. In addition number of other therapies targeting TNF superfamily including TACI-FC, BR3-Fc, anti-BLyS, anti-CD70, anti-OX40L and anti-CD40L are currently in clinical testing.

Challenges for Targeting TNF Superfamily Members

Although soluble TNF and anti-TNF agents have been approved for human therapies and are being successfully used in human patients, there are number of toxicities associated with these therapies. At the time of the discovery of TNF, the main role attributed to this cytokine was in tumor killing, however, it is now evident that TNF can also play a much broader role in tumorigenesis. The molecular mechanism of action of TNF is mediated through the activation of NF-κB, which is known to regulate various molecules involved in invasion and metastasis of the tumors. In addition, TNF use in humans leads to direct toxicity of the liver resulting in damage of hepatocytes. Similar to the use of TNF, CD95L use also results in hepatotoxicity, suggesting a similar mechanism of action of CD95L. The continued examination of signal transduction of TNF superfamily members is needed to develop approaches for tissue specific interventions, which could allow targeted therapies to have fewer side effects.

Three different antibodies against CD40L were tested in clinical trials for potential therapies for autoimmune and inflammatory disease. However, thromboembolic complications were associated with all three antibodies, which led to a complete stop in clinical testing of these antibodies.[42] Mechanism underlying anti-CD40L antibody induced thromboembolism remains to be elucidated. This issue is discussed in detail in reference 31, where alternative approaches to target CD40L are being considered.

Increased risk of development of tuberculosis and lymphoma is also seen with anti-TNF therapies.[43] This is consistent with the important role of TNF in regulation of many cellular processes and in activation of macrophages which are key players in killing *Mycobacterium tuberculosis*. Several of the harmful effects of TNF and its superfamily members are thought to be mediated through the activation of NF-κB. As all TNF superfamily members have potential to activate NF-κB and induce large numbers of genes, it is not surprising that their products are implicated in a wide variety of toxicities. Thus the beneficial role of therapies targeting TNF family members and their potential immunosuppressive or toxic effects must be critically examined in both animal studies and in human trials.

Summary and Conclusions

It is clear that over 20 members of the TNF superfamily and their receptors have been identified and these molecules have a wide-ranging role in many cellular and physiological functions. The key mechanism of the action of these molecules includes activation of NF-κB, JNK, p38 MAPK and ERK1/ERK2. Signals stemming from TNF-superfamily members promote multiple cellular events including apoptosis, proliferation, survival and differentiation. These molecules are also shown to mediate hematopoiesis, immune surveillance, tumor growth and protection from infection. In addition TNF superfamily members are also implicated in inflammatory immune response, autoimmunity, septic shock and osteoporosis. Based on the profound role the TNF superfamily plays in multiple cellular events it is no surprise that many approaches to target this family for therapeutic use are being developed. Indeed, TNF and its inhibitors have been approved as therapeutics. These include TNF for human use in the treatment of sarcomas and melanomas,[25,44] anti-TNF antibodies for rheumatoid arthritis and Crohn's disease,[45] Anti-TNF therapy using soluble TNFR2 for rheumatoid arthritis.[41] A number of new molecules targeting TNF superfamily are also being exploited for the treatment of cancers and various autoimmune diseases. How several members of the TNF superfamily are exploited for the therapeutic use is discussed in detail in the following chapters.

References

1. Bruns P. Die heilwirkung des erysipels auf geschwulste. Beitr Klin Chir 1868; 3:443–446.
2. Coley WB. Contribution to the knowledge of sarcoma. Ann Surg 1891; 14:199–220.
3. Shear MJ, Turner FC. Chemical treatment of tumors. V. Isolation of the hemorrhage-producing fraction from serratia marcescens (bacillus prodigiosus) culture filtrate. J Natl Cancer Inst 1943; 4:81–97.

4. O'Malley WE, Achinstein B, Shear MJ. Action of bacterial polysaccharide on tumors. II. Damage of sarcoma 37 by serum of mice treated with serratia marcescens polysaccharide and induced tolerance. J Natl Cancer Inst 1962; 29:1169–1175.

5. Carswell EA, Old LJ, Kassel RL et al. An endotoxin-induced serum factor that causes necrosis of tumors. Proc Natl Acad Sci USA 1975; 72:3666-3670.

6. Aggarwal BB, Kohr WJ, Hass PE et al. Human tumor necrosis factor. Production, purification and characterization. J Biol Chem 1985; 260:2345-2354.

7. Pennica D, Nedwin GE, Hayflick JS et al. Human tumour necrosis factor: precursor structure, expression and homology to lymphotoxin. Nature 1984; 312:724-729.

8. Gruss HJ, Dower SK. Tumor necrosis factor ligand superfamily: involvement in the pathology of malignant lymphomas. Blood 1995; 85:3378-3404.

9. Aggarwal BB. Signaling pathways of the TNF superfamily: a double-edged sword. Nat Rev Immunol 2003; 3:745-756.

10. Dempsey PW, Doyle SE, He JQ et al. The signaling adaptors and pathways activated by TNF superfamily. Cytokine Growth Factor Rev 2003; 14:193-209.

11. Kischkel FC, Lawrence DA, Chuntharapai A et al. Apo2L/TRAIL-dependent recruitment of endogenous FADD and caspase-8 to death receptors 4 and 5. Immunity 2000; 12:611-620.

12. Darnay BG, Ni J, Moore PA et al. Activation of NF-kappaB by RANK requires tumor necrosis factor receptor-associated factor (TRAF) 6 and NF-kappaB-inducing kinase. Identification of a novel TRAF6 interaction motif. J Biol Chem 1999; 274:7724-7731.

13. Gibson SB, Oyer R, Spalding AC et al. Increased expression of death receptors 4 and 5 synergizes the apoptosis response to combined treatment with etoposide and TRAIL. Mol Cell Biol 2000; 20:205-212.

14. McDermott MF, Aksentijevich I, Galon J et al. Germline mutations in the extracellular domains of the 55 kDa TNF receptor, TNFR1, define a family of dominantly inherited autoinflammatory syndromes. Cell 1999; 97:133-144.

15. Straus SE, Jaffe ES, Puck JM et al. The development of lymphomas in families with autoimmune lymphoproliferative syndrome with germline Fas mutations and defective lymphocyte apoptosis. Blood 2001; 98:194-200.

16. Nagata S. Human autoimmune lymphoproliferative syndrome, a defect in the apoptosis-inducing Fas receptor: a lesson from the mouse model. J Hum Genet 1998; 43:2-8.

17. Ramesh N, Seki M, Notarangelo LD et al. The hyper-IgM (HIM) syndrome. Springer Semin Immunopathol 1998; 19:383-399.

18. Hughes AE, Ralston SH, Marken J et al. Mutations in TNFRSF11A, affecting the signal peptide of RANK, cause familial expansile osteolysis. Nat Genet 2000; 24:45-48.

19. Botchkarev VA, Fessing MY. EDAR signaling in the control of hair follicle development. J Investig Dermatol Symp Proc 2005; 10:247-51.

20. Takayama H, Takakuwa T, Tsujimoto Y et al. Frequent Fas gene mutations in testicular germ cell tumors. Am J Pathol 2002; 161:635-641.

21. Takayama H, Takakuwa T, Dong Z et al. Fas gene mutations in prostatic intraepithelial neoplasia and concurrent carcinoma: analysis of laser capture microdissected specimens. Lab Invest 2001; 81:283-288.

22. Yan M, Brady JR, Chan B et al. Identification of a novel receptor for B lymphocyte stimulator that is mutated in a mouse strain with severe B-cell deficiency. Curr Biol 2001; 11:1547-1552.

23. Feinberg B, Kurzrock R, Talpaz M et al. A phase I trial of intravenously-administered recombinant tumor necrosis factor-alpha in cancer patients. J Clin Oncol 1988; 6:1328-1334.

24. Wielockx B, Lannoy K, Shapiro SD et al. Inhibition of matrix metalloproteinases blocks lethal hepatitis and apoptosis induced by tumor necrosis factor and allows safe antitumor therapy. Nat Med 2001; 7:1202-1208.

25. Eggermont AM, de Wilt JH, ten Hagen TL. Current uses of isolated limb perfusion in the clinic and a model system for new strategies. Lancet Oncol 2003; 4:429-437.

26. Ashkenazi A. Targeting death and decoy receptors of the tumour-necrosis factor superfamily. Nat Rev Cancer 2002; 2:420-430.

27. Kelley SK, Ashkenazi A. Targeting death receptors in cancer with Apo2L/TRAIL. Curr Opin Pharmacol 2004; 4:333-339.

28. Chuntharapai A, Dodge K, Grimmer K et al. Isotype-dependent inhibition of tumor growth in vivo by monoclonal antibodies to death receptor 4. J Immunol 2001; 166:4891-4898.

29. Ichikawa K, Liu W, Zhao L et al. Tumoricidal activity of a novel anti-human DR5 monoclonal antibody without hepatocyte cytotoxicity. Nat Med 2001; 7:954-960.

30. Buchsbaum DJ, LoBuglio AF. Targeting of 125I-labeled B-lymphocyte stimulator. J Nucl Med 2003; 44:434-436.

31. Law CL, Grewal IS. Therapeutic interventions targeting CD40L (CD154) and CD40: The opportunities and challenges. In: Grewal IS, ed. Therapeutic Targets of the TNF Superfamily. Austin: Landes Bioscience, 2008; 8-36.
32. Seshasayee D, Lee WP, Zhou M et al. In vivo blockade of OX40 ligand inhibits thymic stromal lymphopoietin driven atopic inflammation. J Clin Invest 2007; 117:3868-78.
33. Locksley RM, Killeen N, Lenardo MJ. The TNF and TNF receptor superfamilies: integrating mammalian biology. Cell 2001; 104:487-501.
34. Smith CA, Farrah T, Goodwin RG. The TNF receptor superfamily of cellular and viral proteins: activation, costimulation and death. Cell 1994; 76:959-62.
35. Nagata S. Fas ligand-induced apoptosis. Annu Rev Genet 1999; 33:29-55.
36. Griffith TS, Brunner T, Fletcher SM et al. Fas ligand-induced apoptosis as a mechanism of immune privilege. Science 1995; 270:1189-92.
37. Song K, Chen Y, Göke R et al. Tumor necrosis factor-related apoptosis-inducing ligand (TRAIL) is an inhibitor of autoimmune inflammation and cell cycle progression. J Exp Med 2000; 191:1095-104.
38. Watts TH. TNF/TNFR family members in costimulation of T-cell responses. Annu Rev Immunol 2005; 23:23-68.
39. Mackay F, Silveira PA, Brink R. B-cells and the BAFF/APRIL axis: fast-forward on autoimmunity and signaling. Curr Opin Immunol 2007; 19:327-36.
40. Adams AB, Larsen CP, Pearson TC et al. The role of TNF receptor and TNF superfamily molecules in organ transplantation. Am J Transplant 2002; 2:12-8.
41. Shealy DJ, Visvanathan S. Anti-TNF antibodies: lessons from the past, roadmap for the future. Handb Exp Pharmacol 2008; 181:101-29.
42. Sidiropoulos PI, Boumpas DT. Lessons learned from anti-CD40L treatment in systemic lupus erythematosus patients. Lupus 2004; 13:391-7.
43. Gardam MA, Keystone EC, Menzies R et al. Anti-tumour necrosis factor agents and tuberculosis risk: mechanisms of action and clinical management. Lancet Infect Dis 2003; 3:148-55.
44. Lans TE, Bartlett DL, Libutti SK. Role of tumor necrosis factor on toxicity and cytokine production after isolated hepatic perfusion. Clin Cancer Res 2001; 7:784-90.
45. Mitoma H, Horiuchi T, Tsukamoto H et al. Mechanisms for cytotoxic effects of anti-tumor necrosis factor agents on transmembrane tumor necrosis factor alpha-expressing cells: Comparison among infliximab, etanercept and adalimumab. Arthritis Rheum 2008; 58:1248-1257.

Therapeutic Interventions Targeting CD40L (CD154) and CD40:
The Opportunities and Challenges

Che-Leung Law* and Iqbal S. Grewal

Abstract

CD40 was originally identified as a receptor on B-cells that delivers contact-dependent T helper signals to B-cells through interaction with CD40 ligand (CD40L, CD154). The pivotal role played by CD40-CD40L interaction is illustrated by the defects in B-lineage cell development and the altered structures of secondary lymphoid tissues in patients and engineered mice deficient in CD40 or CD40L. CD40 signaling also provides critical functions in stimulating antigen presentation, priming of helper and cytotoxic T-cells and a variety of inflammatory reactions. As such, dysregulations in the CD40-CD40L costimulation pathway are prominently featured in human diseases ranging from inflammatory conditions to systemic autoimmunity and tissue-specific autoimmune diseases. Moreover, studies in CD40-expressing cancers have provided convincing evidence that the CD40-CD40L pathway regulates survival of neoplastic cells as well as presentation of tumor-associated antigens to the immune system. Extensive research has been devoted to explore CD40 and CD40L as drug targets. A number of anti-CD40L and anti-CD40 antibodies with diverse biological effects are in clinical development for treatment of cancer and autoimmune diseases. This chapter reviews the role of CD40-CD40L costimulation in disease pathogenesis, the characteristics of therapeutic agents targeting this pathway and status of their clinical development.

Introduction

CD40 (TNFRSF5), a member of the tumor necrosis factor (TNF) receptor superfamily, is a signaling cell surface receptor. Sequence motifs involved in CD40-mediated signal transduction have been identified in the CD40 cytoplasmic tail that interact with the TNFR-associated factors (TRAFs) to trigger downstream signal cascades that in turn modulate the transcriptional activities of a variety of survival and growth-related genes.[1-3] CD40 is expressed on B-cells at multiple stages of differentiation, monocytes, macrophages, platelets, follicular dendritic cells, dendritic cells (DCs), eosinophils and activated CD8+ T-cells.[4-6] In non-hematopoietic tissues, CD40 is expressed on thymus and kidney epithelial cells, keratinocytes, synovial membrane and dermal fibroblasts and activated endothelium.[7-9] The endogenous ligand for CD40 is CD40L (CD154, TNFSF5).[4,5,7,10] Expression of CD40L on T-cells is tightly regulated; it is only transiently expressed on activated CD4+, CD8+ and γδ T-cells.[11] Besides activated T-cells, CD40L is expressed by monocytes, activated B-cells, epithelial and vascular endothelial cells, smooth muscle cells and DCs. The functional relevance of CD40L expression on these cell types remains to be

*Corresponding Author: Che-Leung Law—Department of Preclinical Therapeutics, Seattle Genetics Inc., 21823 30th Drive SE, Bothell, Washington 98021, USA.
Email: claw@seagen.com

Therapeutic Targets of the TNF Superfamily, edited by Iqbal S. Grewal.
©2009 Landes Bioscience and Springer Science+Business Media.

fully understood.[5] However, expression of CD40L on activated platelets may participate in the pathogenesis of thrombotic diseases.[6,12,13]

The best characterized function of the CD40-CD40L interaction is in contact-dependent reciprocal interaction between antigen-presenting cells (APCs) and T-cells.[10,14] On resting B-cells, binding of CD40L to CD40 promotes B-cell survival and activation, drives rapid expansion of antigen-activated B-cells and facilitates plasma cells and memory B-cell differentiation. CD40 signaling is required for germinal center formation, immunoglobulin (Ig) gene somatic hypermutation, affinity maturation and isotype switching. The physiological importance of CD40 signaling is illustrated by patients suffering from the X-linked hyper-IgM (XHIGM) syndrome.[15] In this primary immunodeficiency, mutations in the CD40L locus abolish functional CD40-CD40L interaction. Disease manifestations include over-representation of circulating IgM and the inability to produce IgG, IgA and IgE. Consequently, patients have profoundly suppressed secondary humoral immune responses, increased susceptibility to recurrent infections and a higher frequency of developing cancer.[16-20]

Genetic deletion of either the *Cd40* or *Cd40l* locus in mice reproduces the major defects seen in XHIGM patients. The most prominent defect seen in the CD40[-/-] mice is the failure to form germinal centers. Thymus-independent IgG and IgM responses remain relatively normal in these mice, but antibody responses to thymus-dependent antigens and antibody class-switching are suppressed.[21,22] Similar to the CD40[-/-] mice, the primary defects in CD40L[-/-] mice also reside in the B-cell compartment.[23-27] Ineffective priming of T-cells to the immunizing protein antigen appears to be the major culprit behind the reduced humoral response in the CD40L[-/-] mice.[28]

In the T-cell compartment, functional differentiation of CD4 and CD8 cells have different requirements for CD40-CD40L costimulation compared to B-lineage cells. Helper Th-cell-mediated functions including local inflammatory reactions to lymphocytic choriomeningitis virus (LCMV) infection and ability to clear secondary viral infection are minimally affected in CD40[-/-] or CD40L[-/-] mice.[29] Likewise, CD40L[-/-] mice can mount potent, primary virus-specific CD8 T-cell responses against LCMV, Pichinde virus and vesicular stomatitis virus.[27,29-31] In contrast, the memory Cytolic T-Lymphocyte (CTL) response in CD40L[-/-] mice is much less efficient than in wild-type mice even though memory CTL activity is detectable in CD40L[-/-] mice.[27,32] Inadequate Th cell priming in these CD40L[-/-] mice is believed to be the main reason behind their diminished memory CTL responses.[27,31,32] Functional T-cell-macrophage interaction in CD40L[-/-] mice is also hampered, resulting in altered macrophage-mediated inflammatory responses, heightened susceptibility to infection by *Leishmania amazonensis* and failure to generate a protective secondary immune response against the parasite.[33]

CD40 signaling to DCs is probably the most important requirement in T-cell priming. CD40 ligation on DCs up-regulates MHC class II antigens, the costimulatory molecules CD80, CD86 and CD70 and adhesion molecules including CD54, thereby promoting antigen presentation, inducing DC maturation and enhancing their costimulatory activity.[5,10] Mature DCs stimulate activated T-cells to increase IL-2 production that facilitates Th and CTL expansion.[28,34,35] CD40-stimulated DCs also secrete IL-12, TNFα, IL-8 and MIP-1α that favor Th1 cell differentiation and promote Th cell migration to sites of inflammation.[36-38] In addition, CD40-activated DC cells presenting antigens in the context of MHC class I molecules are potent stimulators of CTL precursors, a process known as cross-priming, which is critical for cell-mediated immunity against viral infection and transformed cells expressing tumor-associated antigens.[39,40] The importance of CD40 in CTL cross-priming is confirmed by the observation that administration of agonistic monoclonal antibodies (mAbs) against CD40 is sufficient to substitute the need of Th-cells for the generation of robust CTL responses.[41]

In the reticuloendothelial system, CD40 ligation provides a pro-inflammatory signal. Triggering CD40 up-regulates the adhesion molecules CD54, E-selectin and VCAM-1 on monocytes, fibroblasts, keratinocytes, smooth muscle cells and activated endothelial cells.[8,10,36,42] At the same time, the pro-inflammatory cytokines IL-1, IL-6, IL-12, IFNγ and TNFα are secreted by these

CD40-activated cells.[8,10,36,42] This activation ultimately contributes to cellular infiltrates into the inflamed sites through extravasation and chemotaxis.

CD40L Expression in Autoimmune and Inflammatory Conditions

Increased serum or plasma levels of soluble CD40L (sCD40L) is found in patients suffering from systemic lupus erythematosus (SLE),[43-45] Sjögren's syndrome (SS),[44] inflammatory bowel disease (IBD)[46] and cardiovascular disease.[47,48] Plasma levels of sCD40L correlates with anti-dsDNA titers[49] and disease severity in lupus patients.[45,49] In patients with cardiovascular disease increased sCD40L indicates an increased risk of cardiovascular events[47] and susceptibility for vascular damage.[48] Besides being a biomarker, sCD40L may directly promote disease progression. Soluble CD40L at biologically active concentrations has been detected in lupus patients.[43,45,49] Indeed, serum from lupus patients, but not normal donors, augment the expression of CD95 and ICAM-1 on B-cells,[45,49] suggesting that sCD40L in these patients may contribute to disease development through non-specific activation of innocent, bystander CD40+ cells.

CD40L+ T-cells are also over-represented in patients suffering from autoimmune diseases, including peripheral blood mononuclear cells (PBMCs) of SLE patients,[50,51] rheumatoid arthritis (RA) joints[52] and synovial tissues.[53-55] In multiple sclerosis (MS) patients, CD40 and CD40L transcripts are detected in PBMCs[56] while CD40L+ Th cells colocalize with CD40+ macrophages and microglial cells in active lesions in brain tissues derived from these patients.[57] Parallel with the increased propensity to express CD40L, intrinsic functional defects, manifested as hyper-reactivity, are detectable in T-cells derived from autoimmune patients. The polyclonal mitogens phorbol ester and ionomycin induce higher levels of CD40L on T-cells derived from lupus and RA patients over a longer period of time than those from normal donors.[50-52] Similar hyper-responsiveness has been demonstrated in T-cells from psoriasis[58] IBD patients.[59]

Aberrant CD40L expression on non-T-lineage cells such as epithelial tissues of the salivary gland and salivary duct of SS patients[60] and on B-cells[50,61] and monocytes[62,63] of SLE patients has also been observed. These CD40L+ non-T-lineage cells may provide the signal required for auto-antigen presentation and inflammatory reactions. The accumulation of CD40+ B-cells and tissue macrophages with CD40L+ T-cells in ileal lesions of Crohn's disease patients,[64,65] the organization of B and T-cells into follicular structures in RA synovium[55] and the expression of CD40 and CD40L on the mononuclear cells infiltrating the salivary glands of SS patients[60] substantiate this idea.

CD40-Mediated Inflammatory Reaction

In SLE, ex vivo production of pathogenic anti-nuclear autoantibody production by patient lymphocytes can be completely blocked by a neutralizing anti-CD40L.[50] Activated T-cells from lupus patients are more active in stimulating B-cells to express the costimulatory molecule CD80 compared to those from normal donors.[51] In RA synovial tissues, CD40 is expressed by monocytes and synovial cells, both are excellent sources of the inflammatory mediators TNFα and IL-12. Ligation of CD40 on RA synovial tissue cells increased the production of TNFα,[54] while anti-CD40L reduces spontaneous ex vivo IL-12 production by RA synovial cells,[66] suggesting that CD40 signaling can stimulate inflammatory cytokines secretion in RA synovium. Moreover, freshly isolated peripheral blood and synovial T-cells express CD40L and they can stimulate B-cells to secrete IgG and dendritic cells to secrete IL-12 in a CD40L-dependent manner.[53]

In inflammatory reactions, CD40-CD40L interaction is involved in atherosclerosis plaque formation. In emerging atheroma CD40L+ T-cells accumulate early on and persist as lesions advance.[13,67] Ligation of CD40 on atheroma-associated cells in vitro promotes expression of proinflammatory cytokines, matrix metalloproteinases and adhesion molecules which may enhance atherogenesis and plaque destabilization.[13,67,68] Activated T-cells[69] and CD40L+ platelets[12] can stimulate endothelial cells to express MCP-1α, IL-8, IL-6 and adhesion molecules while CD40L-mediated microglial cell activation results in IL-12 secretion[70]—all of these favor Th1 inflammatory responses and atherosclerosis.

Immune-mediated neovascularization enables, at least in part, recruitment of inflammatory infiltrates into sites of tissue damage. The angiogenic cytokine vascular endothelial growth factor (VEGF) is produced by endothelial cells, fibroblast-like synovial (FLS) cells and intestinal fibroblasts. Stimulation of FLS cells with CD40L⁺ L cells or CD40L⁺CD4⁺ T-cells increases VEGF production.[71] As TNFα induces VEGF production by FLS cells,[71] CD40L can also indirectly stimulate FLS cells to secrete VEGF through induction of TNFα secretion by synoviocytes.[54] CD40 signaling in human intestinal fibroblasts promotes IL-8, VEGF and hepatocyte growth factor (HGF) secretion, which can in turn facilitate the migration and tubular formation of human intestinal microvascular endothelial cells.[72] As lamina propria T-cells can be a source of CD40L in situ,[72] CD40-CD40L interaction may partially be responsible for gut inflammation-driven angiogenesis in IBD. Moreover, in endothelial cells CD40 signaling stimulates VEGF secretion, potentially constituting an autocrine loop for angiogenesis.[73]

Genetic Evidence for the Contribution of CD40-CD40L Interaction in Experimental Autoimmune and Inflammatory Diseases

Experiments in mice deficient in either CD40 or CD40L expression have provided strong evidence that the CD40-CD40L pathway is involved in priming, the effector and inflammatory phases of multiple diseases. CD40L$^{-/-}$ allogeneic CD4⁺ T-cells are much less effective in inducing graft versus host disease (GVHD) than wild type T-cells.[74] In a dextran sulfate sodium (DSS)-induced colitis model, DSS is administered to mice to induce intestinal mucosal injury and inflammation, recruitment and activation of macrophages and T-cells, followed by the secretion of Th1 and Th2 cytokines and inflammatory mediators, resulting in severe colitis. CD40$^{-/-}$ and CD40L$^{-/-}$ mice are protected from DSS-induced colitis. Histopathological analysis reveals diminished inflammatory infiltrates, tissue damage and angiogenesis.[72] Similarly, CD40L$^{-/-}$CD45RB^{high}CD4⁺ T-cells induce a milder form of colitis than wild-type CD45RB^{high}CD4⁺ T-cells when they are used to reconstitute histocompatible B6 Rag1$^{-/-}$ hosts.[75] In a model of HgCl$_2$-induced autoimmunity similar to idiopathic lupus, CD40L$^{-/-}$ mice do not respond to HgCl$_2$ challenge. Serum Ig, anti-nucleolar, or anti-chromatin antibody titers, C3 complex deposition in kidney glomeruli and spleens are profoundly reduced. HgCl$_2$ also fails to up-regulate the activation markers CD44 and CTLA-4 on CD40L$^{-/-}$ T-cells.[76]

CD40L$^{-/-}$ mice have been back-crossed onto different mouse strains that are predisposed to autoimmunity. In an experimental autoimmune encephalomyelitis (EAE) model, mice carrying a transgenic T-cell receptor specific for myelin basic protein (MBP) in a CD40L-deficient genetic background fail to develop EAE when challenged with MBP. Co-administration with mature CD86⁺ APCs restores disease development, suggesting that CD40L-induced in vivo maturation of APCs is required for successful T-cell priming and to evoke autoimmunity.[77] Back-crossing CD40L$^{-/-}$ mice onto the apolipoprotein E-deficient (ApoE$^{-/-}$) mice that are predisposed to hypercholesterolemia and formation of atherosclerotic lesions markedly reduce atherogenesis.[78] Although the onset of atherosclerotic plaque development is not affected in CD40L$^{-/-}$ApoE$^{-/-}$ mice, the plaque areas are much smaller than those found in CD40L$^{+/+}$ApoE$^{-/-}$ mice. Advanced plaques are stabilized with increased collagen and reduced lipid contents. Inflammatory infiltrates of T-cells and macrophages are also diminished in the CD40L$^{-/-}$ApoE$^{-/-}$ mice.[68] Likewise, mice resulted from back-crossing of CD40L$^{-/-}$ mice onto the Fas-deficient MRL/Mpr-lpr/lpr mice, a model for human SLE, demonstrate suppressed lupus symptoms, including the lack of histological signs of glomerulonephritis. Although antibody against small nuclear ribonucleoproteins is still detectable in these mice, they do not produce anti-dsDNA antibodies or IgG rheumatoid factors.[79]

Mice harboring a CD40L transgene under the control of a V$_H$ promoter spontaneously develop severe transmural intestinal inflammation in the colon and ileum that is associated with the generation of autoantibodies against colon tissues and elevated IFNγ secretion from lamina propria T-cells.[80] Interestingly, these CD40L transgenic mice also produce anti-nuclear, anti-DNA and anti-histone autoantibodies and demonstrate immune-complex-mediated glomerulonephritis typical of SLE.[81] Back-crossing CD40L transgenic mice onto CD40$^{-/-}$ mice completely reverses colitis development.[80] In a different transgenic mouse strain, the human keratin-14 promoter was used to target CD40L expression to epidermal basal keratinocytes.[82] Mice heterozygous for this CD40L transgene develop spontaneous dermatitis. Adoptive transfer of T-cells from CD40L transgenic mice induces development of dermatis, suggesting priming and effector T-cell development in the transgenic environment. Although ectopic expression of CD40L is restricted to keratinocytes, transgenic mice develop systemic lesions similar to SLE.[82] Collectively, heightened CD40 signaling appears to be responsible for wide-spread systematic and tissue-associated inflammatory reactions, possibly by breaking immune tolerance.

Therapeutic Targeting of CD40L: Proof of Concept Preclinical Animal Models of Autoimmunity and Inflammation

Transplantation

Anti-CD40L suppresses both acute GVHD (aGVHD) and chronic GVHD (cGVHD). In aGVHD, disease development is dependent on the interaction between CD40L+ allo-reactive T-cells and CD40+ recipient APCs[74] and can be induced even in the absence of the CD28 signals.[83] Treatment with anti-CD40L suppresses onset of aGVHD,[74,83,84] accompanied by reduced frequency of host-reactive Th cells[74] and CTL.[84] Anti-CD40L blockade in vivo specifically prevents the priming of Th1 cells through the inhibition of IL-12 secretion[85] and is manifested through a decrease in the frequency of effector cells expressing IL-2, IL-12 p40, IFNγ and perforin transcripts.[74] In cGVHD, the interaction between allo-reactive Th cells and host B-cells results in production of anti-DNA antibodies, splenomegaly, proteinuria and immune complex-mediated renal lesions. Anti-CD40L treatment alleviates these symptoms.[84,86] In order to achieve maximal therapeutic efficacy anti-CD40L treatment needs to begin at disease induction. Delaying treatment until disease onset renders anti-CD40L completely non-efficacious, strongly arguing that CD40L is crucial for disease priming.[86]

Rejection of solid allografts is associated with strong transcriptional activation and protein expression of CD40 and CD40L genes.[87] Like its activity observed in GVHD, anti-CD40L prolongs the survival of fully disparate murine cardiac allografts,[87] allogeneic hepatocytes,[88] islet allografts[89] and limb allografts.[90] Again, prolonged allograft survival can be achievable only when anti-CD40L is administered simultaneously at the time of allograft implantation. Delays in administration invariably lead to graft rejection,[87] confirming once again that anti-CD40L treatment preferentially interferes with the priming phase of alloantigen recognition. Even if anti-CD40L administration begins at time of transplant neither permanent protection against rejection nor tolerance induction can be achieved.

Simultaneous blockade of the CD40-CD40L and CD80/CD86-CD28 pathways is a promising approach to enhance the efficacy of anti-CD40L. Synergism between anti-CD40L and murine CTLA4-Ig to induce indefinite allograft survival has been observed for cardiac and skin allografts.[91,92] More interestingly, combined anti-CD40L and CTLA4-Ig treatment is efficacious even in cardiac and skin xenografts.[93] Combined CD40-CD40L and CD80/CD86-CD28 blockade profoundly inhibits proliferation of reactive T-cells,[91,92] while induces apoptosis in T-cells that have already entered cell division cycle.[92] In contrast to anti-CD40L monotherapy, anti-CD40L mAb plus CTLA-4-Ig almost completely abrogate graft-induced expression of Th1 and Th2 cytokines at the transcript and protein levels in allografts.[91,93] Induction of CD80/B7-1 transcripts is also reduced when compared to anti-CD40L mAb or CTLA-4-Ig monotherapy.[91] In the xeno-transplant models, xenoantibody titers in mice receiving both anti-CD40L and CTLA4-Ig are much lower.[93] These results suggest that blockade targeting simultaneously the CD40 and CD28 costimulatory pathways may promote graft survival by interfering with priming as well as effector phases of the rejection process.

A second approach to improve the therapeutic activity of anti-CD40L is by donor-specific transfusion in which the hosts are treated with donor cells in the presence of anti-CD40L mAbs before allograft implantation. Mechanistically, this is very similar to the classical example of peripheral tolerance induction. In the absence of CD40L signal due to blockade by anti-CD40L mAbs, allogeneic APCs within the transfused donor cell population fail to up-regulate CD80 and CD86. In this situation, host allo-reactive T-cells only receive the signal from allo-antigens on donor cells without costimulatory signals. As a result, allo-reactive T-cells are either anergized or deleted, rendering the host tolerant to future allografts derived from the same donor. This approach enables long-term survival of islet allografts[94] and skin allografts[95] beyond that allowed by anti-CD40L monotherapy.

Experimental Rheumatoid Arthritis

In the collagen-induced arthritis mouse model, administration of anti-CD40L following immunization with type II collagen effectively blocks arthritis development as reflected by diminished joint inflammation, anti-collagen antibody titers, recruitment of inflammatory infiltrates into joint tissues, bone and cartilage erosion.[96] The KRN transgenic mouse (K/BxN) is a spontaneous arthritis model in which autoreactive T-cells expressing a transgenic T-cell receptor specific for glucose-6-phosphate isomerase (G6PI) induce the production of arthritogenic autoantibodies against. Although an anti-CD40L fails to alleviate disease symptoms when given in a therapeutic setting, it prevents arthritis development and arthritogenic antibody production when administered prophylactically before disease onset.[97] In AB29 transgenic mice, deletion of rheumatoid factor-expressing B-cells induced by human IgG can be rescued in the presence of Th-cell activity.[98-100] Anti-CD40L, but not antibodies against IL-15 or IL-4, can reverse the Th-cell effect, leading to deletion of rheumatoid factor-expressing B-cells and ablation of rheumatoid factor production[100]

Systemic Lupus Erythematosus

In the lupus prone (NZW x NZB)F1 and (SWR x NZB)F1 (SNF1) strains of mice, treatment with anti-CD40L mAb can control disease development at multiple stages. Treatment before disease delays onset, reduces the incidence of immune complex-mediated glomerulonephritis and provides survival benefits.[101,102] Although the frequency of auto-reactive T-cells appears to remain unchanged, anti-DNA autoantibody production is profoundly suppressed, suggesting that anti-CD40L likely acts through T-B-cell costimulation blockade.[101,102] Importantly, the effects of anti-CD40L appear to be reversible in that mice are capable of responding to challenge of a neo-antigen after completion of anti-CD40L treatment, suggesting that temporary CD40-CD40L blockade may not lead to major changes in the immune repertoire.[102] In the (NZW x NZB)F1 mice delay in disease onset can be observed even if treatment started when mice are 20-26 weeks old.[103]

Administration of anti-CD40L in a therapeutic setting when lupus nephritis has been establish in the SNF1 mice can still reduce proteinuria and diminishes inflammation, sclerosis/fibrosis and vasculitis in the kidneys.[104] However, long-term anti-CD40L dosing in nephritic mice is required to maintain survival and inhibit mediators of renal fibrosis.[105] To circumvent long-term general immunosuppression, combined costimulatory blockade of CD28-CD80/86 and CD40-CD40L has been studied. In (NZB x NZW)F1 mice, a brief simultaneous blockade of the CD28 and CD40 costimulation by CTLA4-Ig and anti-CD40L at disease onset can produce long lasting benefits even after treatment has been terminated.[106,107] It is encouraging that a majority of mice developing proteinuria after receiving CTLA4-Ig and anti-CD40L treatment can still benefit from a second course of treatment,[107] providing further evidence that combined CD28 and CD40 costimulation blockade given in an intermittent basis may be able to provide long term therapeutic benefits with limited general immunosuppression.

Multiple Sclerosis

In EAE models, treatment with anti-CD40L is efficacious in preventing disease onset,[57,108] pathologic development of ongoing disease[57] and relapse of established disease.[109] While inhibition of T-cell priming is the most probable mechanism that prevents disease onset,[57,77] the therapeutic activity of anti-CD40L in the relapsing setting is likely exerted through blockade of Th1 effector function differentiation.[109] In mice treated with anti-CD40L at the peak of EAE or during remission IFNγ production, delayed-type hypersensitivity response against the immunizing myelin peptide, and the frequency of encephalitogenic effector T-cells are all profoundly reduced. Anti-CD40L also alleviates clinical symptom development in mice adoptively implanted with encephalitogenic T-cells, suggesting that CD40-CD40L blockade may prevent effector T-cell migration into the CNS and/or down-modulate the ability of effector T-cells to activate macrophages and microglial in the CNS.[109] Moreover, co-administration of anti-CD40L and CTLA4-Ig provides additive therapeutic effects in EAE as supported by a complete absence of mononuclear infiltrates into the CNS and significant proliferation of primed, peripheral T-cells.[110]

Inflammatory Bowel Disease

Colitis can be induced in mice by the hapten (2,4,6,-trinitrobenzene sulfonic acid, TNBS). Anti-CD40L treatment in this model affects T-cell priming, since anti-CD40L mAb can completely prevent disease development when administered during the disease induction phase while it is relatively inert if administered after disease establishment.[85] Anti-CD40L demonstrates reciprocal effects on the Th1 and Th2 cytokine profiles. While alleviation of disease symptom and pathology is accompanied by a reduction of IFNγ production by lamina propria T-cells, production of the Th2 cytokine IL-4 is enhanced.[85]

Another commonly used approach to induce IBD in mice is by adoptive transfer of naïve CD45RB^{high}CD4$^+$ T-cells from BALB/c mice into histocompatible SCID mice.[111] A second comparable model involves reconstitution of B6 Rag1$^{-/-}$ mice with histocompatible naïve CD45RB^{high}CD4$^+$ T-cells.[75] The third model utilizes CD4$^+$ T-cell lines established from C3H/HeJBir mice that are highly susceptible to colitis due to their hypersensitivity toward intestinal commensal enteric bacteria-derived antigens.[112] Reconstitution of SCID mice with these histocompatible CD4$^+$ T-cell lines induces colitis in the hosts, typical of Th1 responses, with increased production of IL-12 and IFNγ[112] and the ability of T-cell lines to induce disease is directly correlated to the level of CD40L expressed on their cell surface.[113] In all 3 disease models, disease onset can be completely abrogated by anti-CD40L mAb treatment at the time of T-cell reconstitution.[75,111,113] Similar to the TNBS-induced colitis model, anti-CD40L treatment eliminated symptoms of wasting and is accompanied with prevention of intestinal inflammation, reduced levels of the cytokines INFγ, TNFα, IL-10 and IL-12, as well as reduced mucosal leukocyte infiltration and decreased CD54 expression.[75,111] Interestingly, delaying anti-CD40L treatment until disease onset in the CD45RB^{high}CD4$^+$ histocompatible T-cell adoptive transfer models can still lead to significant clinical and histological improvements and down-regulated cytokine expression, suggesting once again that CD40-CD40L blockade can affect the effector phase of certain pathologic immune responses.[75,111]

Atherosclerosis

The efficacy of CD40-CD40L blockade in treating experimental atherosclerosis has been evaluated in the low density lipoprotein receptor-deficient (LDLR$^{-/-}$) mice. Markedly higher serum levels of low and intermediate density lipoproteins are observed in LDLR$^{-/-}$ mice on a diet with moderately elevated cholesterol contents, leading to atherosclerotic lesions similar to those found in the CD40L$^{-/-}$ApoE$^{-/-}$ mice.[78] Treatment of LDLR$^{-/-}$ with antibody against mouse CD40L concomitant with the beginning of a 12-week high cholesterol diet significantly inhibits atherosclerosis development as measured by multiple parameters. Thus, in treated mice atherosclerotic lesions are much reduced in sizes and lipid content while infiltration of macrophages and T-cells into atheroma and VCAM-1 expression in atheroma is also markedly decreased.[13] These results are in line with a role of CD40-CD40L interaction in the initiation of atherogenesis. In a therapeutic setting when anti-CD40L treatment administered during the last 13 weeks of a 26-week high cholesterol diet in LDLR$^{-/-}$ mice further pathologic progression of established atherosclerotic lesions is prevented. In addition, the composition of atheroma is altered in favor of improving plaque stabilization, as indicated by the decreased recruitment of macrophages and reduced lipid content that were accompanied by increased collagen and smooth muscle cells.[114]

Clinical Experience with Anti-CD40L

The mAb 5c8 is the first anti-human CD40L reported in the literature.[115] Functional characterization of 5c8 conclusively confirmed the role of the CD40-CD40L pathway in regulating human lymphocyte functions.[116-119] As 5c8 recognizes non-human primate (NHP) CD40L, treatment with 5c8 and/or CTLA4-Ig has been tested in rhesus monkey receiving MHC Class I and II disparate renal allografts. While control animals reject the allografts in 5-8 days, CTLA4-Ig or 5c8 alone prolongs rejection-free survival to 20-98 days. Combining CTLA4-Ig and 5c8 results in two of four animals experienced extended (>150 days) rejection-free allograft survival without the need of additional chronic immunosuppressive treatments.[120] With these exciting preclinical data several anti-CD40L mAbs have been developed for clinical testing in humans (Table 1).

Ruplizumab (BG9588, hu5c8)

Humanized 5c8 (ruplizumab, hu5c8, or BG9588) contains a human IgG1 backbone. In a pharmacokinetics and pharmacodynamics study, ruplizumab produced a dose-dependent reduction in anti-tetanus toxoid antibody titers; both primary and recall immune responses were suppressed.[121] Ruplizumab effectively prevents acute rejection of MHC-mismatched renal allografts in rhesus monkeys.[122] Graft survival of longer than 500 days can be achieved in some ruplizumab-treated animals. Rhesus renal allograft recipients under conventional immunosuppressive regimens of steroid, cyclosporine and mycophenolate mofetil have been successfully converted to ruplizumab maintenance monotherapy, showing graft survival of over 300 days.[123] Ruplizumab is also effective in rescuing grafts undergoing acute rejection after completion of induction therapy.[124] Besides renal allografts, ruplizumab has demonstrated efficacy in intrahepatic islet allografts in rhesus monkeys[125] and baboons,[126] cardiac allografts in cynomolgus monkeys[127] and skin allografts in rhesus monkeys.[128] Due to its cross-reactivity to canine CD40, ruplizumab has also been shown to reduce the radiation dose needed to establish bone marrow mixed chimerism in a canine model of donor-specific transfusions in DLA-identical marrow transplantation.[129]

The strong preclinical data on ruplizumab propelled its evaluation in transplantation and SLE patients in phase I and II clinical trials. In the phase II trial in lupus nephritis in which the study was terminated prematurely due to the development of thromboses in some of the patients, efficacy of ruplizumab was supported by the reduced symptoms associated with lupus nephritis. Reductions in proteinuria, anti-double-stranded DNA antibodies and hematuria were observed in some of the patients.[130,131] Ruplizumab treatment was also correlated to a decrease in the frequency of B-lymphocytes spontaneously secreting immunoglobulin[130] as well as IgD+CD38+ germinal center B-lymphocytes and CD38^{high} plasmacytes.[132]

Table 1. Therapeutic antibodies targeting CD40L

Drug Name	Molecular Characteristics	Mechanism(s) of Action	Clinical Development Status
Ruplizumab, hu5c8, BG9588, Antova	Humanized IgG1	• Costimulatory blockade • T-cell depletion	• Phase II trial SLE • Phase II trial in kidney transplantation
Toralizumab, hu24-31, IDEC-131	Humanized IgG1	• Costimulatory blockade	• Refractory immune thrombocytopenic purpura • SLE
ABI793	Fully human IgG1	• Costimulatory blockade	• Preclinical

Toralizumab (IDEC-131, hu24-31)

The humanized anti-CD40L antibody, toralizumab (also known as IDEC-131) of IgG1 isotype, was derived from the murine anti-CD40L hybridoma 24-31.[133] It blocks CD40L binding to CD40 and inhibits T-cell-dependent B-cell proliferation and differentiation, similar to ruplizumab. As the Fab' fragment of toralizumab shows activity similar to the intact IgG molecule, it is believed that CD40-CD40L blockade is the principal behind the therapeutic activity seen in this antibody.[133]

Toralizumab inhibits both primary and secondary antibody responses in cynomolgus monkeys challenged with ovalbumin[133] or influenza vaccine.[134] In a MHC-mismatched rhesus skin allograft model, toralizumab prolonged graft survival when administered with rapamycin.[135] Similar to skin allograft transplantation, toralizumab prolonged heterotopic cardiac allografts in cynomolgus monkeys, which was improved by co-treatment with anti-thymocyte globulin, but without establising tolerance.[136] In contrast, in rhesus renal allograft transplant, toralizumab has can facilitate tolerance when administered in combination with cyclosporine and donor-specific transfusion, suggesting that tissue-specific factors may determine whether tolerance can be achieved by CD40-CD40L blockade.[137]

In a phase I, dose-escalating trial of toralizumab in patients with refractory immune thrombocytopenic purpura, patients were given a single infusion of toralizumab. Increase in platelet count was observed in a subset of patients treated at 10 mg/kg. The frequency of B-cells producing anti-GPIIb/IIIa antibodies, GPIIb/IIIa-induced T-cell proliferation and anti-GPIIb/IIIa antibody production by antigen-dependent T-B-cell collaboration was all suppressed, while T-cell response to irrelevant antigen was not affected.[138] One of the patients was reported to potentially achieved tolerance after toralizumab treatment.[139] In the phase I trial in SLE patients, a single dose of toralizumab up to 15 mg/kg was found to be well-tolerated and no treatment related lymphocyte depletion was observed.[140] A subsequent randomized, double-blinded, placebo-controlled phase II study was conducted in SLE patients. Although toralizumab was found to be safe and well-tolerated, no statistical significant improvement was observed in the treatment versus the placebo group.[141] Multiple phase I and II trials were planned for toralizumab. Unfortunately, all clinical trials on toralizumab were stopped due to a thromboembolic event in a Crohn's disease patient.

ABI793

The third anti-CD40L developed is ABI793, a human IgG1 derived from the HuMAb mice (Medarex Inc., Annandale, NJ).[142] ABI793 has similar properties to both ruplizumab and toralizumab with respect to blockade of CD40-CD40L-mediated costimulation and cross-reactivity with NHP CD40, but it binds to an epitope on CD40L distinct from the one recognized by ruplizumab and toralizumab.[142] ABI-793 has demonstrated activity in prolonging renal allograft survival in cynomolgus and rhesus monkeys.[142,143] In a pig-to-baboon xenotransplantation model involving the heart or hematopoietic progenitor cells ABI-793 was found to be effective in suppressing antibody production by the recipients against the xenografts.[144] Regrettably, thromboembolism was also observed in both the cynomolgus and rhesus renal transplant models leading the conclusion that thromboembolic complications may be a class effect of anti-CD40L antibodies unrelated to epitope specificity.

Mechanism(s) of Action of Anti-CD40L mAbs: Toxicity versus Efficacy

The thromboembolic complications observed in preclinical and clinical settings from three different anti-CD40L mAbs have led to a complete halt in clinical development of anti-CD40L mAbs antibodies.[145,146] The mechanism underlying anti-CD40L-induced thromboembolism, however, remains to be elucidated. A plausible reason may be the co-expression of CD40L and the low affinity activating Fc receptor FcγRIIA on platelets. Upon binding to CD40L on platelets the Fc domains of anti-CD40L may interact with FcγRIIA expressed on the same platelet or neighboring platelets leading to FcγRIIA cross-linking, which is a potent signal for platelet activation. Hence, anti-CD40L has been hypothesized to induce platelet aggregation and thromboembolism through

FcγRIIA-mediated platelet activation.[147] It is noteworthy that mice do not express an FcγRIIA ortholog.[147] This could offer a reason why thromboembolism has never been observed in mouse models when the efficacy of anti-CD40L mAbs is examined. In addition to Fc-FcγRIIA interaction, a role of serum calcium may also contribute to anti-CD40L-induced thromboembolism.[148] Consistent with this hypothesis of anti-CD40L-mediated platelet activation, a combination of the anti-coagulant heparin, prostaglandin E1 and the cyclooxygenase inhibitor ketorolac can reduce the incidence of thromboembolism in cynomolgus renal allograft recipients receiving anti-CD40L treatment.[149]

With respect to the mechanism through which anti-CD40L mAbs achieve in vivo suppression of cell-mediated immune responses, anti-CD40L costimulation blockade only exerts modest inhibition of T-cell responses in mixed lymphocyte reaction.[91,120] The primary defects in CD40L knockout mice reside mainly in the B-cell compartment in germinal center formation and memory B-cell differentiation [23-25] while T-cell-mediated responses are by and large normal in these mice.[30] Acute islet allograft rejection in mice still occurs even though the CD40-CD40L pathway has been eliminated as demonstrated in CD40 knockout graft recipients.[150] Taken together, CD40-CD40L costimulation blockade may not be the sole in vivo mechanism of action for anti-CD40L.

Recent reports support a role for Fc-mediated depletion of CD40+ activated T-cells, through complement fixation and interaction with FcγR expressed on immune effector cells in the therapeutic efficacy of anti-CD40L. Depletion activity of anti-CD40L mAbs appear to be especially important in transplantation settings. In mice, anti-CD40L mAb did not prolong skin and islet allograft survival in recipients defective in the complement activation cascade, e.g., in C3−/−, cobra venom factor-treated, or C5-deficient DBA/2 recipients.[150,151] Anti-CD40L mAbs also failed to prevent skin allograft rejection in recipients deficient in FcγRI and FcγRIII expression.[151] Moreover, an aglycoslyated form of the anti-CD40L hu5c8, having reduced activity in complement fixation and FcγR interaction, is ineffective in prolonging the survival of rhesus renal and islet allografts.[152] These results strongly support the notion that therapeutic efficacy of anti-CD40L in transplantation settings critically depends on antibody effector functions and involves the depletion of reactive, activated CD40L+ T-cells.[153] On the other hand, evidence is available to demonstrate that anti-CD40L mAbs devoid of any effector function are still therapeutically active in modulating certain immune responses. An effector function-deficient, aglycosylated form of an anti-CD40L mAb was efficacious in reducing pathogenic autoantibody production in murine models of SLE[152] and EAE.[154] Similarly, aglycosylated hu5c8 has retained its ability to suppress both primary and secondary antibody responses against tetanus toxoid in cynomolgus monkeys, despite losing its ability to prolong renal and islet allograft survival in rhesus monkeys.[152] These observations strongly argue that both depletion of CD40+ activated T-cells and CD40-CD40L costimulation blockade are important mechanisms underlying the therapeutic effects of anti-CD40L treatment.

Potential Alternative Therapeutic Approaches Targeting CD40L

If platelet activation through binding of anti-CD40L Fc domains to FcγRIIA is proven to be the culprit behind thromboembolism complications in anti-CD40L therapies, engineered antibodies to eliminate Fc-mediated functions may yield therapeutics fully capable of blocking CD40-CD40L costimulation. These molecules may not be active in transplantation settings, but they may retain sufficient efficacy in autoimmune diseases including SLE and MS, as predicted by murine models.[152,154] To this end, a non-complement-activating human IgG4 derivative of ABI793, AFN746, has been developed.[155] Since human IgG4 does not bind FcγRIIA,[156] AFN746 may have reduced capacity to activate platelets. Remarkably, in the 12th International Congress of Immunology Abstract # 3117 reported that AFN746-treated animals did not show thromboembolic vascular lesions, reduction in platelet counts and acute renal tubular necrosis previously reported for other anti-CD40L mAb. Treatment with AFN746 prolonged renal allograft survival in cynomolgus monkeys, albeit inferior to its parent ABI793.[157] The reduced activity of AFN746 to delay allograft rejection is consistent with studies in both mice[150,151] and NHP[152] demonstrating a critical requirement of anti-CD40L-mediated activated T-cell depletion in transplant settings. It will be of particular interest to evaluate the efficacy of AFN746 in non-transplant experimental models to further define its utility in costimulation blockade. It is possible that other IgG modifications to selectively disable Fc-mediated effector functions may result in anti-CD40L antibodies with the desired therapeutic efficacy but not the propensity for inducing thromboembolism.[158,159]

Other alternatives to IgG engineering can also be conceived to leverage CD40-CD40L costimulation blockade in treatment of autoimmunity without invoking the side effects of thromboembolism. These include high affinity Fab' or F(ab')$_2$ fragments derived from anti-CD40L mAb or recombinant CD40. Such molecules may suffer from the disadvantage of accelerated clearance from serum compared to typical IgG molecules, but with the appropriate formulatioin including the use of pegylation technologies it is likely that the serum half lives of these molecules can be increased to the extent that they can exert meaningful therapeutic effects.[160-162] Other custom designed molecules, in particular peptidomimetics, are being developed to block costimulation pathways mediated by CD80/86-CD28 or CD40-CD40L interactions.[163] The feasibility of this approach is supported by studies reporting synthetic peptides that either mimick the biological activity of trimeric CD40L[164] or block the binding of CD40L to CD40.[163,165] The binding affinity of these peptides is relatively low[163] and huge quantities are required to block binding in vitro.[165] Clearly, more efforts are needed to improve the binding affinity, in vivo pharmacokinetic properties, as well as stability against serum proteases and peptidases of these peptidomimetics before they become suitable for clinical development. A class of non-agonistic anti-CD40 mAb has been generated with the unique properties to block the binding of CD40L to CD40, as will be discussed later on. They may provide yet another approach to circumvent issues associated with anti-CD40L-mediated thromboembolism. At least two of these non-agonistic anti-CD40 mAb have entered clinical trials.

Finally, the therapeutic efficacy of anti-CD40L in transplantation settings may involve the depletion of reactive, activated T-cells.[153] It is therefore possible that depleting antibodies against other T-cell activation markers co-expressed with CD40L, e.g., CD30, CD70, CD134/OX-40 and CD137/4-1BB, can eliminate at least a subset of CD40L$^+$ T-cells and may achieve the therapeutic efficacy seen with anti-CD40L in transplantation settings.[166] A chimeric anti-CD70 mAb has recently been reported to exert its antitumor activity in xenografts modeling lymphoma and multiple myeloma through antibody effector functions of antibody dependent cellular cytotoxicity ADCC, phagocytosis and complement fixation.[167] It will be of interest to evaluate the potential of such antibody in activated T-cell depletion therapy. Alternatively, arming of antibodies with cytotoxic drugs is a widely used approach for cancer treatment.[168] The antibody drug conjugate gemtuzumab ozogamicin[169] and the IL-2 toxin denileukin diftitox[170] are approved drugs for acute myelogenous leukemia and cutaneous T-cell lymphoma, respectively. The utility of antibody drug conjugates against other lymphocyte activation markers such as CD30[171] and CD70[172] in depletion of CD40L$^+$ activated T-cells and hence their potential to down-modulate immune responses warrant further investigation.

CD40 Signaling in Transformed Cells

Characteristic of the TNFR superfamily members, the physiologic consequences of CD40 signaling are highly pleiotropic, depending on the cell types involved, their differentiation and activation status, as well as the nature of the signaling ligand. In contrast to normal B-cells in which CD40 signaling usually promotes survival and stimulates proliferation, CD40 ligation induces apoptosis in many types of transformed cells.[173,174] Murine lymphoma B-cell lines respond to anti-CD40 mAb treatment to undergo growth arrest.[175-177] Similarly, CD40-mediated proliferation inhibitory effect is observed in lymphoma cell lines derived from patients with aggressive, high grade B-cell lymphoma.[178-181] Furthermore, anti-CD40 treatment can suppress the in vivo growth of xenografts established from these transformed cell lines,[178-181] leading to the hypothesis that CD40 may be a potential therapeutic target for lymphoma treatment.

The exact mechanism that accounts for sensitivity of high grade lymphoma B-cells to CD40-mediated cell death is unknown. Certain transformed B-cells may be arrested at specific maturational stage(s) that are predisposed to CD40-induced apoptosis. Indeed, CD40 ligation on normal resting B-cells readily induces Fas expression. As a result, CD40-activated B-cells become sensitive to Fas-mediated apoptosis.[182-184] B-cells from patients with acute lymphoblastic leukemia, chronic lymphocytic leukemia (CLL) and non-Hodgkin's lymphoma (NHL) have been reported to undergo CD40-dependent Fas induction, predisposing them to Fas-mediated apoptosis.[185,186] Besides Fas, CD40 triggering induces transcripts encoding FLICE, FADD and TRADD.[187] Similarly, anti-CD40- or CD40L-mediated apoptosis of Burkitt's lymphoma cell lines can be correlated to the upregulation of Bax transcripts and protein.[181] In addition, hydrolysis of sphinogmyelin and formation of the pro-apoptotic metabolite ceramide[188] as well as activation of the MAPK pathway[189] have also been implicated to play a role in transducing the apoptotic signal mediated by CD40 ligation. Interestingly, CD40 ligation can overcome p53 mutations in some lymphoma B-cell lines to induce apoptosis.[190] The induction of p73, a member of the p53 family, is a potential mechanism through which CD40 signaling restores the capability of stress-induced cell cycle arrest.[191]

Different from high grade lymphoma, CD40 signaling in low grade lymphoma B-cells, exemplified by follicular lymphoma and CLL cells, usually promotes cellular activation and survival.[192-196] The anti-CD40 antibody G28-5 reduces fludarabine-induced apoptosis of B-CLL cells through an NFκB/Rel-dependent pathway.[197] Concomitant with survival enhancement, costimulatory molecules including CD80, CD86 and ICAM-1/CD54 are induced which can enhance the immuno-stimulatory effects of these lymphoma B-cells.[174,198,199] As such, significant interest has been generated to explore the potential of CD40 signaling in promoting immune surveillance against B-CLL. Viral transduction of the CD40L gene into autologous B-CLL cells to boost their costimulatory activities of B-CLL has been clinically tested.[200,201] Unexpectedly, in these clinical trials rapid reduction in circulating leukemia cell counts and lymph node size incompatible with the kinetics of an adaptive immune response was observed,[200,201] suggesting alternative mechanism(s) for leukemic cell clearance. While induction of pro-survival Bcl-x(L), A1 and Mcl-1 genes can be readily detectable in B-CLL cells stimulated by CD40L and IL-4,[202] Bcl-2 has been shown to be down-regulated in the same cells upon CD40 signaling.[202,203] Interestingly, this is paralleled by up-regulation of pro-apoptotic proteins including Bid, Noxa and Bcl-x(S).[202,204] CD40 ligation on B-CLL cells also upregulates members of the TNFR members, e.g., Fas, death receptor 5 (DR5), TNFRI and TNFRII.[203,204] Co-culture with CD4+ cytotoxic lymphocytes or transfectants expressing both the DR5 ligand TRAIL and Fas ligand effectively induces caspase-dependent apoptosis of CD40-stimulated B-CLL cells.[204] The addition of an inhibitor against the apoptosis suppressing protein XIAP,[205] autocrine production of TNFα and IFNγ,[203] and IL-21 treatment[206] all sensitize CD40L-activated B-CLL cells toward apoptosis. Unlike culturing B-CLL cells simultaneously with fludarabine and anti-CD40,[197] pretreatment with CD40L-expressing transfectants actually sensitizes B-CLL cells toward subsequent fludarabine-induced apoptosis.[203] Induction of p73, a transcription factor related to p53, is correlated to the CD40-mediated sensitization of B-CLL cells toward fludarabine.[191] Thus, the fate of B-CLL cells subsequent to CD40 triggering likely depends on a multitude of factors that can tip the balance toward either survival or cell death. Strategies in CD40 pre-activation combined with subsequent chemotherapy regimens may be clinically beneficial to B-CLL patients.

In multiple myeloma (MM), the anti-CD40 mAb G28-5 increases the clonogenicity of freshly isolated MM cells[207] and stimulates proliferation of MM cell lines.[207,208] In contrast, other anti-CD40 mAbs including 5C11[209] and B-B$_{20}$[210,211] induce cell cycle arrest and apoptosis in the IL-6-dependent MM cell line XG2. A direct cytotoxic effect of CD40 signaling to MM cells has not been clearly established. Nevertheless, the protein synthesis inhibitor cycloheximide[212] and the immuno-modulatory drug lenalidomide[213] can sensitize MM cells toward CD40-mediated apoptosis. At the same time, CD40-signaling can disrupt the IL-6 paracrine loop required by MM cells for survival by down-regulating the p85 subunit of the IL-6 receptor.[212] Thus, the response of MM cells to CD40 signaling may be dependent both on the maturational stage of the myeloma cells in question as well as the epitopes on which anti-CD40 mAbs bind to.

In contrast to malignant B-lineage cells, carcinoma cells exhibit more uniform response toward CD40 stimulation. CD40L or anti-CD40 treatment of CD40⁺ carcinoma cell lines derived from bladder, pancreatic, ovarian, breast, cervical and skin carcinomas generally results in weak inhibition of proliferation.[9,214-217] CD40 ligation on carcinoma cell lines also enhances apoptosis induced by agents including the cytotoxic drug cisplatin, TNFα, anti-Fas and ceramide,[218-222] suggesting the potential utility of using anti-CD40 mAbs in combination with chemotherapeutic drugs in the treatment of carcinomas.

CD40 and Cancer Immune Surveillance

Promoting immune surveillance may contribute to the antitumor activity of CD40 signaling. The immuno-stimulatory effects of in vivo CD40 ligation by CD40L or anti-CD40 have been correlated with immune responses against histocompatible tumors.[41,223,224] A deficient immune response against tumor cells may result from a combination of factors such as decreased expression of MHC, poor expression of tumor-associated antigens, appropriate adhesion or costimulatory molecules and the production of immunosuppressive proteins like TGFβ by the tumor cells.[225] CD40 ligation on transformed cells up-regulates adhesion proteins (e.g., CD54), costimulatory molecules (e.g., CD86), MHC antigens, cytokines (e.g., IL-6, TNFα), as well as chemokines (IL-8, MCP-1, RANTES), thereby enhancing the immunogenicity through augmented presentation of tumor-associated antigens by the tumors and/or increasing recruitment of immune cells into tumor sites.[198,216,226-228] CD40 signaling is required for DC maturation and mature DCs are responsible for presenting tumor-derived antigens to CD8⁺ CTL precursors through cross-priming.[39,40,229] Activation and differentiation of CTL precursors by mature DCs into tumor-specific effectors CTLs may enhance cell-mediated immune responses against tumor cells. Finally, the presence of CD40 on the surface of carcinoma cell lines is also required for the generation of tumor-specific T-cell responses.[216]

Characteristics of Anti-CD40 Antibodies

Anti-CD40 mAbs differ significantly from each other with respect to their binding affinity to CD40, ability to block interaction between CD40L and CD40 and biological activities. Deletional analysis on the extracellular domain of CD40 has suggested that the amino-terminus constitutes the epitopes recognized by CD40L as well as anti-CD40 mAbs.[230] Cross-blocking experiments demonstrate the possibility of at least three CD40 epitopes.[230-233] Antibodies against the first can completely inhibit CD40L-CD40 binding while those against the second one are partial inhibitors.[230-233] Antibody against the third, surprisingly, can promote binding between CD40L and CD40.[232]

Anti-CD40 mAbs also elicit distinct functional outcomes with respect to homotypic adhesion,[232] B-cell proliferation and apoptosis,[230-232,234] CD23 induction[235] and IgE synthesis.[236] In general, a direct correlation between the ability of anti-CD40 mAb to activate B-cells and their affinity[230] or the location of CD40 epitope[230-232] does not seem to exist. For example, whereas the blocking mAb G28-5 activates resting B-cells and potently costimulates with anti-IgM to drive B-cell proliferation,[175,230,232] a second blocking mAb 5D12 is a much weaker activator and does not costimulate with anti-IgM.[230,234] The most intriguing aspect of CD40 epitopes is probably the functional interplay observed when different epitopes are ligated by combining different anti-CD40 mAbs or anti-CD40 mAbs with CD40L. Several anti-CD40 mAbs whose epitopes are mapped outside of the CD40L binding site costimulate DNA synthesis with CD40L in resting B-cells, although alone by themselves these mAbs only moderately activate resting B-cells.[231,232,236] Similarly, strong costimulation of resting B-cells can be elicited by combining two non-cross-blocking anti-CD40 mAb.[231] Cooperativity between CD40 epitopes is observed in the induction of growth arrest and cell death in transformed B-cells.[180] Distinct epitopes on CD40 relative to CD40L binding have also been defined on mouse CD40[41,229,237,238] and functional cooperativity between anti-mCD40 mAb recognizing distinct epitopes similar to the situation with human CD40 has been detected.[238] Collectively, the biological effects resulting from CD40 ligation by CD40L or anti-CD40 mAb are likely contributed by both simple receptor cross-linking as well as conformational changes imposed onto CD40 upon ligand binding.

The pleiotropic effects of CD40 signaling combined with the availability of different CD40 targeting molecules have provided a multitude of possibilities for therapeutic interventions (Table 2). In CD40[+] transformed cells a strong agonistic signaling ligand in the form of recombinant CD40L or a fully agonistic antibody can directly induce apoptosis and activate presentation of tumor-associated antigens to both helper and cytotoxic T-cells. On the opposite end of the spectrum, antibodies that block CD40L binding to CD40 but do not activate any signaling cascade may have significant therapeutic values in suppressing autoimmune and inflammatory responses.

Clinical Experience in Therapeutic Targeting of CD40

Recombinant CD40L

A trimeric form of recombinant human CD40L (rhuCD40L),[239] using an isoleucine zipper as the trimerization motif, enhances the expression of costimulatory molecules and proinflammatory cytokines, delivers proliferation inhibitory signals to transformed cell lines and demonstrates antitumor activity in ovarian carcinoma xenograft models.[214-216,218] A phase I trial using rhuCD40L was conducted in patients with solid tumors and intermediate or high grade NHL.[240] The maximum tolerated dose (MTD) was reached at a modest dose of 0.1 mg/kg/day for 5 daily doses. Partial responses and stable disease have been observed in this clinical trial.[240] The ability of CD40L to induce immune response against leukemia cells has been tested in a patient with plasma cell leukemia (PCL). Leukemia cells from this patient were activated ex vivo by IL-4 plus CD40L-expressing transfectants and used to stimulate autologous tumor-specific T-cells. This patient then received autologous tumor-specific T-cells and vaccination with irradiated CD40-activated PCL cells. A temporary decrease of PCL cells was observed after the first cycle of adoptive T-cell transfer.[241] In a separate clinical trial in CLL patients, autologous B-CLL cells were transduced with a replication-defective adenovirus expressing CD40L. Re-infusion of CD40L[+] autologous B-CLL cells was associated with in vivo expression of costimulatory molecules on bystander, non-infected CLL cells, increased plasma levels of IL-12 and IFNγ and increased blood CD4[+] counts containing leukemia-specific T-cells.[242] Concerns have been raised to the possibility of selective survival of CD40-mediated lymphoma cells,[243] but clinical data support the hypothesis that CD40 signaling may be therapeutically efficacious.

SGN-40

SGN-40 is an IgG1 humanized form of S2C6 generated using a human bladder carcinoma cell line as the immunogen.[244-246] S2C6 exerts minimal stimulatory effects on normal B-cells but has the unique activity to promote CD40L- and IL-4-stimulated B-cell proliferation.[231] It also reduces the viability of lymphoma B-cell lines in vitro and prolongs the survival of mice harboring human lymphoma xenografts.[180,181] As murine IgG1 antibodies are devoid of effector functions, the in vivo antitumor activity of S2C6 is likely a result of cytotoxic signaling. In the renal cell carcinoma (RCC) line ACHN, S2C6 induces MCP-1, IL-8 and GM-CSF.[247] Pulmonary metastases subsequent to ACHN implantation can be substantially reduced by S2C6 treatment, suggesting that S2C6-mediated release of chemokines and cytokines from the ACHN cells may augment host innate antitumor immune responses.[247]

Humanization of S2C6 to contain the human IgG1 backbone yielded SGN-40. SGN-40 mediates ADCC against transformed cell lines derived from NHL, Hodgkin's lymphoma (HL), (MM) and RCC.[248-250] It also mediates phagocytosis of CD40[+] tumor cells by monocyte-derived macrophages.[250] In addition to antibody effector functions, SGN-40 induces apoptosis in lymphoma B-cells.[181,249] Both apoptotic signaling and antibody effector functions are important for the antitumor activity of SGN-40 against lymphoma B-cells.[249] Unlike NHL B-cells, MM cells are not sensitive toward SGN-40-mediated cytotoxicity.[212] Instead, signals delivered by SGN-40 to MM cells down-regulate the gp80 subunit of the IL-6 receptor that can suppress IL-6 driven autocrine growth in MM cells.[212] Pretreatment with the immunomodulatory drug lenalidomide, however,

Table 2. Biologics targeting CD40

Drug Name	Molecular Characteristics	Mechanism(s) of Action	Clinical Development Status
Recombinant CD40L	Trimerized by an isoleucine motif	• Binds CD40 • Delivers agonistic signals • Activates antigen presentation and immune surveillance against neoplastic cells	• Solid tumors and immediate or high grade lymphoma • Gene therapy of over-expressing CD40L in CLL
SGN-40	Humanized IgG1	• Antibody effector functions (ADCC, ADCP) • Partial agonist • Apoptosis induction in lymphoma B-cells • Down-regulates IL-6 receptor p85 expression	• Phase I trials in NHL, MM and CLL
HCD122, Chir-12.12	Fully human IgG1	• Antibody effector functions (ADCC, ADCP) • Antagonist • Blocks CD40L-mediated signaling • Inhibits CD40L-mediated signal transduction, cell proliferation and cytokine secretion	• Phase I trials in MM and CLL
ch5D12	Chimeric IgG4	• Antagonist • Blocks CD40L-mediated proliferation in normal B-cells • Non-depleting	• Phase I/IIa trial in moderate to severe Crohn's disease
CP-870,893	Fully human IgG2	• Agonist • Delivers agonistic signals • Activates antigen presentation and immune surveillance against neoplastic cells	• Phase I trial in advanced solid tumors
Teneliximab, Chi220, BMS-224819	Chimeric IgG1	• Partial agonist • Blocks CD40L binding • B-cell depleting • Inhibits primary and secondary antibody response	• Preclinical
Chi Lob7/4	Chimeric	• Inhibits proliferation of CD40⁺ transformed epithelial and B-lineage cells • Mediates antibody effector functions (ADCC, CDC)	• Preclinical

can sensitize MM cells against SGN-40-mediated cytotoxicity.[213] In addition, lenalidomide also enhances SGN-40-mediated ADCC of CD40[+] target MM cells.[213] In the Ramos Burkitt's lymphoma xenograft model, a combination of SGN-40 with CHOP (cyclophosphamide, adriamycin, vincristine, prednisone) is significantly more active than either SGN-40 or CHOP alone,[251] suggesting potential utility of combining SGN-40 with chemotherapeutics in clinical settings.

A single-arm phase I trial of SGN-40 in MM patients has been conducted.[252] Pharmacokinetics analysis revealed dose-dependent changes in Cmax and AUC similar to what have been reported in NHPs.[253] In an interim summary, SGN-40 was found to be well-tolerated and MTD was not reached at the dose of 8 mg/kg. Although objective responses were not detected in this study, several patients demonstrated either stable disease or reduction in their serum M-protein. Another phase I study of SGN-40 was conducted in NHL patients with diffuse large B-cell (DLBCL), follicular (FL), mantle cell (MCL), marginal zone (MZL) or small lymphocytic (SLL) lymphoma.[254] Similar to the phase I MM trial, SGN-40 was found to be well-tolerated at doses up to 8 mg/kg. Objective responses have been observed in DLBCL, MCL and MZL patients in this trial.[254] These phase I clinical trials have provided encouraging data and the rationale for further clinical evaluation of SGN-40 in NHL and MM.

HCD122 (Chir-12.12)

HCD122, formerly known as Chir-12.12, is a fully human anti-CD40 IgG1 mAb generated from the XenoMouse® mice (Abgenix Inc.). HCD122 is characterized as an antagonist based on its ability to block CD40-CD40L binding and compete off bound CD40L.[255] As a consequence, HCD122 inhibits CD40L-mediated signaling events[256,257] as well as CD40L-mediated proliferation of normal B-cells.[258] In line with its antagonistic nature, this antibody alone does not initiate biochemical pathways typical of CD40 ligation,[255] stimulate proliferation in normal B-cells[258] or primary lymphoma B-cells.[259]

In ex vivo experimental systems, HCD122 blocks the pro-survival signal delivered by CD40L to CLL and FL B-cells in a dose-dependent manner.[258,259] In a MM and bone marrow stromal cell (BMSC) coculture system, CD40L promotes the secretion of IL-6 and VEGF as well as enhances the adhesion of MM cells to fibronectin and BMSC. HCD122 inhibited these CD40L-mediated responses.[256] Besides blocking CD40L functions, HCD122 also engages Fc-dependent antibody effector functions including ADCC and antibody-dependent cellular phagocytosis (ADCP).[255,256] Single and multiple dose toxicological studies on HCD122 have been conducted in cynomolgus monkeys.[260,261] Consistent with its B-cell depletion activity, reductions of B-cells in the peripheral blood and germinal centers in spleen and lymph node has been observed in HCD122-treated monkeys.[260,261]

Phase I clinical trials of HCD122 in CLL[262] and MM[263] patients have been initiated. Transient decline in leukemic cell counts after HCD122 infusion has been reported in the CLL trial[262] and one partial response has been recorded in the MM trial.[263] Dose escalation is underway for both of these trials.[262,263]

Chimeric 5D12 (ch5D12)

A second antagonistic anti-CD40 mAb is 5D12.[264] 5D12 demonstrates weak but detectable activity to stimulate DNA synthesis in resting tonsillar B-cells,[230] but it does not costimulate normal B-cell proliferation with anti-IgM, even in the presence of IL-2.[234] On the other hand, 5D12 inhibits CD40L-mediated proliferation of normal B-cells[234] and contact-dependent, activated T-cell-mediated immunoglobulin secretion by B-cells.[265] Because of its cross-reactivity to the marmoset CD40 ortholog, 5D12 was tested for its ability to intervene disease development in a chronic demyelinating EAE model in outbred marmoset monkeys.[266] 5D12 delayed disease onset when administered at time of disease initiation and suppressed disease progression even when it was administered after T-cell priming had taken place.[266] A chimeric 5D12 (ch5D12) with human IgG4 isotype has been generated for clinical testing.[267-269] Repeat experiments using the marmoset EAE model confirmed that ch5D12 had retain the therapeutic activity of its parent.[268,269] Consistent with the lack of Fc-FcγR-mediated functions with human IgG4, ch5D12 did not impart any significant changes to the frequency of circulating B-cells.[267] Instead, a marked reduction in the number of germinal centers in lymph node associated with increased number of apoptotic cells was observed in monkeys receiving 25 mg/kg of ch5D12,[270] supporting CD40-CD40L costimulation blockade to be the main action exerted by ch5D12.

A phase I/IIa study on ch5D12 was conducted in Crohn's disease patients. Overall response and remission rates were reported to be 72 and 22%, respectively. Intensity of the lamina propria cell infiltrate was reduced with no evidence of global changes in the relative composition of circulating T and B-cells.[271] These data suggest that antagonizing CD40-CD40L interaction using a non-depleting anti-CD40 mAb may be beneficial in some autoimmune and inflammatory disease settings. Ch5D12 is currently under humanization for further clinical studies.

CP-870,893

Agonistic anti-CD40 mAbs are expected to deliver stronger cytotoxic signals to transformed cells. They should also promote immune surveillance against cancer cells through enhanced expression of key costimulatory molecules and inflammatory mediators, leading to tumor-associated antigen presentation and ultimately reversal of tumor-induced immune tolerance. It is therefore possible that agonistic anti-CD40 mAbs will be efficacious even against tumors that do not express CD40. CP-870,893 is a human IgG2 mAb has been generated in the Abgenix XenoMouse and characterized as a potent agonist. Since human IgG2 does not have significant Fc-mediated antibody effector functions, CP-870,893 is probably a non-depleting mAb. Instead, agonistic signaling through CD40 to mediate direct tumor cell killing or enhancement of immune surveillance are the likely mechanisms of action for CP-870,893.[272] Consistent with its agonistic nature, treatment of monocyte-derived DCs with CP-870,893 up-regulates CD80, CD86, CD83 and MHC class II expression as well as secretion of IL-12 and MIP1α.[272]

A phase I clinical trial has been conducted to evaluate the safety of CP-870,893 in patients with advanced solid tumors. Pharmacodynamic observations indicative of agonistic CD40 signaling included transient induction of the costimulatory molecule CD86 on circulating B-cells as well as increases in circulating levels of IL-6 and TNFα. Side effects included elevations in serum liver transaminases similar to previously observed with recombinant CD40L[240] and in mice treated with agonistic anti-mouse CD40 mAbs.[273,274] Objective partial responses in melanoma patients were observed, suggesting that agonistic signaling by CD40 may indeed activate antitumor immune responses.

Teneliximab (Chi220, BMS-224819)

Teneliximab, also known as Chi220 or BMS-224819, is a chimeric antibody of IgG1 isotype. This antibody blocks the CD40-CD40L interaction, but is characterized as a partial agonist as it can costimulate with anti-IgM to induce low levels of normal B-cell proliferation.[275] Teneliximab depletes peripheral blood B-cells in NHPs,[275,276] inhibits primary and secondary antibody responses against T-cell-dependent antigens.[275] Teneliximab alone prolonged renal allograft survival in cynomolgus monkeys.[276] In islet allotransplantation, teneliximab alone only gave short term, transient graft survival benefit; a combination of teneliximab and CTLA4-Ig, however, resulted in long-term graft survival.[275] Mechanistically, CD40-CD40L costimulation blockade rather than B-cell depletion might be the key mechanism for teneliximab, as the potent B-cell depleting agent rituximab did not provide the allograft survival benefit seen with teneliximab.[275] Clinical development plan for teneliximab has not yet been disclosed.

Chi Lob7/4

Chi Lob7/4 is the latest chimeric anti-CD40 mAb reported in the literature. Chi Lob7/4 inhibits the proliferation of malignant epithelial and NHL cell lines. It also exhibits ADCC activity; however, in contrast to SGN-40 and HCD122, Chi Lob7/4 also mediates CDC against NHL cell line targets.[277] Clinical development plan for Chi Lob7/4 also has not yet been disclosed.

Considerations for Therapeutics Targeting CD40

As multiple clinical trials on various CD40 targeting molecules are still currently ongoing, it is not possible to conclude what mechanism(s) will provide the most beneficial therapeutic effects. At the same time, the molecular design necessary to maximally harness the potential clinical benefits of targeting CD40 remains to be established. It is possible that multiple biologics targeting CD40 will be developed, each exploiting different facets of the CD40 biology to achieve certain desired therapeutic activities.

Fully agonistic anti-CD40 mAb and recombinant CD40L may be most suitable as adjuvants to boost immune surveillance and reverse tumor-induced tolerance. This approach is very attractive since it may be applicable even to CD40⁻ cancers. Unfortunately, since CD40 is widely expressed in normal tissues, strong agonists against CD40 may cause considerable inflammatory side effects as observed in mice receiving agonistic anti-CD40 mAb.[278] This has been mirrored at least in part by clinical findings obtained with recombinant CD40L[240] and the agonistic anti-CD40 mAb CP-870,893.[278] Further clinical studies with these molecules will require optimization in dosing and administration schedules to maximize their immuno-stimulatory effects while minimizing their toxic side effects. Co-administration with anti-inflammatory agents may mitigate some of the side effects, but it is important to understand how this may negatively impact the immuno-stimulatory activity of CD40 agonists. Localized administration could be another avenue to limit side effects resulted from systemic delivery.

Conversely, antagonistic anti-CD40 mAb are not expected to elicit the same side effects as the agonists. The safety profiles established for the antagonists HCD122 and ch5D12 by and large agree with this prediction. Both antibodies can be administered at higher doses and more frequently than CP-870,893.[262,263,271] The non-depleting, IgG4 mAb ch5D12 is particularly interesting,[267] since it may provide a therapeutics with a mechanism of action similar to anti-CD40L but without its side effect of causing thromboembolism. Further results from ongoing clinical trials from these antagonistic anti-CD40 mAbs will surely shed more light on the relative role of target cell depletion, survival blockade and costimulation blockade in cancer versus autoimmune indications.

The partial agonist SGN-40 is unique in that it induces apoptosis in neoplastic B-cells but does not, by itself, deliver a strong proliferative signal to normal B-cells. Weekly doses of SGN-40 at 8 mg/kg appear to induce less inflammatory side effects than either rhuCD40L or the agonistic anti-CD40 mAb CP-870,893.[240,252,254,278] It would be important to develop diagnostic tools for identifying the lymphoma and leukemia subsets that are most susceptible to CD40-mediated signaling in the clinical development of SGN-40. The apoptosis-inducing activity of SGN-40 also provides the opportunities in clinical trials to evaluate the ability of SGN-40 to sensitize neoplastic B-cells to currently available standard therapeutic regimens.

Conclusions

The CD40-CD40L pathway is definitely one of the most crucial pathways in the pathogenesis and effector phase of many autoimmune diseases. CD40 signaling modulates proliferation, survival and the immunogenicity of neoplastic cells. Compelling evidence has been generated from preclinical animal models and early phase clinical trials to make both CD40 and CD40L promising drug targets. However, an approved therapeutics targeting this pathway is yet to be developed. Because of the diverse biological effects and functions mediated by the CD40-CD40L interaction, future research to explore the therapeutic potential of interfering with this costimulation pathway should include better elucidation of how distinct functions of this pathway contribute to the pathogenesis of specific diseases. Likewise, pharmacogenomic investigations will enable the identification of biomarkers associated with and/or predicative of responses to targeting the CD40-CD40L pathway. With this knowledge it would be more likely that custom designed molecules with precise targeting capability will be generated to achieve the therapeutic activities sought.

References

1. Aggarwal BB. Signalling pathways of the TNF superfamily: a double-edged sword. Nat Rev Immunol 2003; 3:745-56.
2. Bishop GA, Hostager BS, Brown KD. Mechanisms of TNF receptor-associated factor (TRAF) regulation in B-lymphocytes. J Leukoc Biol 2002; 72:19-23.
3. Bradley JR, Pober JS. Tumor necrosis factor receptor-associated factors (TRAFs). Oncogene 2001; 20:6482-91.
4. Biancone L, Cantaluppi V, Camussi G. CD40-CD154 interaction in experimental and human disease. Int J Mol Med 1999; 3:343-53.
5. van Kooten C, Banchereau J. CD40-CD40 ligand. J Leukoc Biol 2000; 67:2-17.
6. Freedman JE. CD40-CD40L and platelet function: beyond hemostasis. Circ Res 2003; 92:944-6.
7. Banchereau J, Bazan F, Blanchard D et al. The CD40 antigen and its ligand. Annu Rev Immunol 1994; 12:881-922.
8. van Kooten C, Banchereau J. Functions of CD40 on B-cells, dendritic cells and other cells. Curr Opin Immunol 1997; 9:330-7.
9. Young LS, Eliopoulos AG, Gallagher NJ et al. CD40 and epithelial cells: across the great divide. Immunol Today 1998; 19:502-6.
10. Grewal IS, Flavell RA. CD40 and CD154 in cell-mediated immunity. Annu Rev Immunol 1998; 16:111-35.
11. Gauchat JF, Aubry JP, Mazzei G et al. Human CD40-ligand: molecular cloning, cellular distribution and regulation of expression by factors controlling IgE production. FEBS Lett 1993; 315:259-66.
12. Henn V, Slupsky JR, Grafe M et al. CD40 ligand on activated platelets triggers an inflammatory reaction of endothelial cells. Nature 1998; 391:591-4.
13. Mach F, Schonbeck U, Sukhova GK et al. Reduction of atherosclerosis in mice by inhibition of CD40 signalling. Nature 1998; 394:200-3.
14. Clark EA, Ledbetter JA. How B and T-cells talk to each other. Nature 1994; 367:425-8.
15. Aruffo A, Farrington M, Hollenbaugh D et al. The CD40 ligand, gp39, is defective in activated T-cells from patients with X-linked hyper-IgM syndrome. Cell 1993; 72:291-300.
16. Hayward AR, Levy J, Facchetti F et al. Cholangiopathy and tumors of the pancreas, liver and biliary tree in boys with X-linked immunodeficiency with hyper-IgM. J Immunol 1997; 158:977-83.
17. Kinlen LJ, Webster AD, Bird AG et al. Prospective study of cancer in patients with hypogammaglobulinaemia. Lancet 1985; 1:263-6.
18. Laman JD, Claassen E, Noelle RJ. Immunodeficiency due to a faulty interaction between T-cells and B-cells. Curr Opin Immunol 1994; 6:636-41.
19. Ramesh N, Morio T, Fuleihan R et al. CD40-CD40 ligand (CD40L) interactions and X-linked hyperIgM syndrome (HIGMX-1). Clin Immunol Immunopathol 1995; 76:S208-S13.
20. Castigli E, Fuleihan R, Ramesh N et al. CD40 ligand/CD40 deficiency. Int Arch Allergy Immunol 1995; 107:37-39.
21. Kawabe T, Naka T, Yoshida K et al. The immune responses in CD40-deficient mice: impaired immunoglobulin class switching and germinal center formation. Immunity 1994; 1:167-78.
22. Castigli E, Alt FW, Davidson L et al. CD40-deficient mice generated by recombination-activating gene-2-deficient blastocyst complementation. Proc Natl Acad Sci USA 1994; 91:12135-9.
23. Xu J, Foy TM, Laman JD et al. Mice deficient for the CD40 ligand. Immunity 1994; 1:423-31.
24. Foy TM, Laman JD, Ledbetter JA et al gp39-CD40 interactions are essential for germinal center formation and the development of B-cell memory. J Exp Med 1994; 180:157-63.
25. Van den Eertwegh AJ, Noelle RJ, Roy M et al. In vivo CD40-gp39 interactions are essential for thymus-dependent humoral immunity. I. In vivo expression of CD40 ligand, cytokines and antibody production delineates sites of cognate T-B-cell interactions. J Exp Med 1993; 178:1555-65.
26. Renshaw BR, Fanslow WC, III, Armitage RJ et al. Humoral immune responses in CD40 ligand-deficient mice. J Exp Med 1994; 180:1889-900.
27. Borrow P, Tishon A, Lee S et al. CD40L-deficient mice show deficits in antiviral immunity and have an impaired memory CD8+ CTL response. J Exp Med 1996; 183:2129-42.
28. Grewal IS, Xu J, Flavell RA. Impairment of antigen-specific T-cell priming in mice lacking CD40 ligand. Nature 1995; 378:617-20.
29. Oxenius A, Campbell KA, Maliszewski CR et al. CD40-CD40 ligand interactions are critical in T-B cooperation but not for other anti-viral CD4+ T-cell functions. J Exp Med 1996; 183:2209-18.
30. Whitmire JK, Slifka MK, Grewal IS et al. CD40 ligand-deficient mice generate a normal primary cytotoxic T-lymphocyte response but a defective humoral response to a viral infection. J Virol 1996; 70:8375-81.

31. Whitmire JK, Flavell RA, Grewal IS et al. CD40-CD40 ligand costimulation is required for generating antiviral CD4 T-cell responses but is dispensable for CD8 T-cell responses. J Immunol 1999; 163:3194-201.

32. Borrow P, Tough DF, Eto D et al. CD40 ligand-mediated interactions are involved in the generation of memory CD8$^{(+)}$ cytotoxic T-lymphocytes (CTL) but are not required for the maintenance of CTL memory following virus infection. J Virol 1998; 72:7440-9.

33. Soong L, Xu JC, Grewal IS et al. Disruption of CD40-CD40 ligand interactions results in an enhanced susceptibility to Leishmania amazonensis infection. Immunity 1996; 4:263-73.

34. Roy M, Aruffo A, Ledbetter J et al. Studies on the interdependence of gp39 and B7 expression and function during antigen-specific immune responses. Eur J Immunol 1995; 25:596-603.

35. Sin JI, Kim JJ, Zhang D et al. Modulation of cellular responses by plasmid CD40L: CD40L plasmid vectors enhance antigen-specific helper T-cell type 1 CD4$^+$ T-cell-mediated protective immunity against herpes simplex virus type 2 in vivo. Hum Gene Ther 2001; 12:1091-102.

36. Kiener PA, Moran-Davis P, Rankin BM et al. Stimulation of CD40 with purified soluble gp39 induces proinflammatory responses in human monocytes. J Immunol 1995; 155:4917-25.

37. Cella M, Scheidegger D, Palmer-Lehmann K et al. Ligation of CD40 on dendritic cells triggers production of high levels of interleukin-12 and enhances T-cell stimulatory capacity: T-T help via APC activation. J Exp Med 1996; 184:747-52.

38. Bleharski JR, Niazi KR, Sieling PA et al. Signaling lymphocytic activation molecule is expressed on CD40 ligand-activated dendritic cells and directly augments production of inflammatory cytokines. J Immunol 2001; 167:3174-81.

39. Heath WR, Carbone FR. Cytotoxic T-lymphocyte activation by cross-priming. Curr Opin Immunol 1999; 11:314-8.

40. Toes RE, Schoenberger SP, van der Voort EI et al. CD40-CD40Ligand interactions and their role in cytotoxic T-lymphocyte priming and anti-tumor immunity. Semin Immunol 1998; 10:443-8.

41. French RR, Chan HT, Tutt AL et al. CD40 antibody evokes a cytotoxic T-cell response that eradicates lymphoma and bypasses T-cell help. Nat Med 1999; 5:548-53.

42. Singh SR, Casper K, Summers S et al. CD40 expression and function on human dermal microvascular endothelial cells: role in cutaneous inflammation. Clin Exp Dermatol 2001; 26:434-40.

43. Ciferska H, Horak P, Hermanova Z et al. The levels of sCD30 and of sCD40L in a group of patients with systemic lupus erythematodes and their diagnostic value. Clin Rheumatol 2007; 26:723-8.

44. Goules A, Tzioufas AG, Manousakis MN et al. Elevated levels of soluble CD40 ligand (sCD40L) in serum of patients with systemic autoimmune diseases. J Autoimmun 2006; 26:165-71.

45. Vakkalanka RK, Woo C, Kirou KA et al. Elevated levels and functional capacity of soluble CD40 ligand in systemic lupus erythematosus sera. Arthritis Rheum 1999; 42:871-81.

46. Ludwiczek O, Kaser A, Tilg H. Plasma levels of soluble CD40 ligand are elevated in inflammatory bowel diseases. Int J Colorectal Dis 2003; 18:142-7.

47. Heeschen C, Dimmeler S, Hamm CW et al. Soluble CD40 ligand in acute coronary syndromes. N Engl J Med 2003; 348:1104-11.

48. Desideri G, Cipollone F, Valeri L et al. Enhanced plasma soluble CD40 ligand levels in essential hypertensive patients with blunted nocturnal blood pressure decrease. Am J Hypertens 2007; 20:70-6; discussion 77.

49. Kato K, Santana-Sahagun E, Rassenti LZ et al. The soluble CD40 ligand sCD154 in systemic lupus erythematosus. J Clin Invest 1999; 104:947-55.

50. Desai-Mehta A, Lu L, Ramsey-Goldman R et al. Hyperexpression of CD40 ligand by B and T-cells in human lupus and its role in pathogenic autoantibody production. J Clin Invest 1996; 97:2063-73.

51. Koshy M, Berger D, Crow MK. Increased expression of CD40 ligand on systemic lupus erythematosus lymphocytes. J Clin Invest 1996; 98:826-37.

52. Liu MF, Chao SC, Wang CR et al. Expression of CD40 and CD40 ligand among cell populations within rheumatoid synovial compartment. Autoimmunity 2001; 34:107-13.

53. MacDonald KP, Nishioka Y, Lipsky PE et al. Functional CD40 ligand is expressed by T-cells in rheumatoid arthritis. J Clin Invest 1997; 100:2404-14.

54. Harigai M, Hara M, Nakazawa S et al. Ligation of CD40 induced tumor necrosis factor-alpha in rheumatoid arthritis: a novel mechanism of activation of synoviocytes. J Rheumatol 1999; 26:1035-43.

55. Wagner UG, Kurtin PJ, Wahner A et al. The role of CD8$^+$ CD40L$^+$ T-cells in the formation of germinal centers in rheumatoid synovitis. J Immunol 1998; 161:6390-7.

56. Huang WX, Huang P, Hillert J. Systemic upregulation of CD40 and CD40 ligand mRNA expression in multiple sclerosis. Mult Scler 2000; 6:61-5.

57. Gerritse K, Laman JD, Noelle RJ et al. CD40-CD40 ligand interactions in experimental allergic encephalomyelitis and multiple sclerosis. Proc Natl Acad Sci USA 1996; 93:2499-504.

58. Daoussis D, Antonopoulos I, Andonopoulos AP et al. Increased expression of CD154 (CD40L) on stimulated T-cells from patients with psoriatic arthritis. Rheumatology (Oxford) 2007; 46:227-31.
59. Liu Z, Geboes K, Colpaert S et al. IL-15 is highly expressed in inflammatory bowel disease and regulates local T-cell-dependent cytokine production. J Immunol 2000; 164:3608-15.
60. Ohlsson M, Szodoray P, Loro LL et al. CD40, CD154, Bax and Bcl-2 expression in Sjogren's syndrome salivary glands: a putative anti-apoptotic role during its effector phases. Scand J Immunol 2002; 56:561-71.
61. Devi BS, Van Noordin S, Krausz T et al. Peripheral blood lymphocytes in SLE—hyperexpression of CD154 on T- and B-lymphocytes and increased number of double negative T-cells. J Autoimmun 1998; 11:471-5.
62. Katsiari CG, Liossis SN, Dimopoulos AM et al. CD40L overexpression on T-cells and monocytes from patients with systemic lupus erythematosus is resistant to calcineurin inhibition. Lupus 2002; 11:370-8.
63. Katsiari CG, Liossis SN, Souliotis VL et al. Aberrant expression of the costimulatory molecule CD40 ligand on monocytes from patients with systemic lupus erythematosus. Clin Immunol 2002; 103:54-62.
64. Battaglia E, Biancone L, Resegotti A et al. Expression of CD40 and its ligand, CD40L, in intestinal lesions of Crohn's disease. Am J Gastroenterol 1999; 94:3279-84.
65. Sawada-Hase N, Kiyohara T, Miyagawa J et al. An increased number of CD40-high monocytes in patients with Crohn's disease. Am J Gastroenterol 2000; 95:1516-23.
66. Kitagawa M, Mitsui H, Nakamura H et al. Differential regulation of rheumatoid synovial cell interleukin-12 production by tumor necrosis factor alpha and CD40 signals. Arthritis Rheum 1999; 42:1917-26.
67. Mach F, Schonbeck U, Libby P. CD40 signaling in vascular cells: a key role in atherosclerosis? Atherosclerosis 1998; 137(Suppl):S89-95.
68. Lutgens E, Gorelik L, Daemen MJ et al. Requirement for CD154 in the progression of atherosclerosis. Nat Med 1999; 5:1313-6.
69. Monaco C, Andreakos E, Young S et al. T-cell-mediated signaling to vascular endothelium: induction of cytokines, chemokines and tissue factor. J Leukoc Biol 2002; 71:659-68.
70. Becher B, Blain M, Antel JP. CD40 engagement stimulates IL-12 p70 production by human microglial cells: basis for Th1 polarization in the CNS. J Neuroimmunol 2000; 102:44-50.
71. Cho CS, Cho ML, Min SY et al. CD40 engagement on synovial fibroblast up-regulates production of vascular endothelial growth factor. J Immunol 2000; 164:5055-61.
72. Danese S, Scaldaferri F, Vetrano S et al. Critical role of the CD40-CD40 ligand pathway in governing mucosal inflammation-driven angiogenesis in inflammatory bowel disease. Gut, 2007;56:1248-56.
73. Flaxenburg JA, Melter M, Lapchak PH et al. The CD40-induced signaling pathway in endothelial cells resulting in the overexpression of vascular endothelial growth factor involves Ras and phosphatidylinositol 3-kinase. J Immunol 2004; 172:7503-9.
74. Blazar BR, Taylor PA, Panoskaltsis-Mortari A et al. Blockade of CD40 ligand-CD40 interaction impairs CD4+ T-cell-mediated alloreactivity by inhibiting mature donor T-cell expansion and function after bone marrow transplantation. J Immunol 1997; 158:29-39.
75. De Jong YP, Comiskey M, Kalled SL et al. Chronic murine colitis is dependent on the CD154/CD40 pathway and can be attenuated by anti-CD154 administration. Gastroenterology 2000; 119:715-23.
76. Pollard KM, Arnush M, Hultman P et al. Costimulation requirements of induced murine systemic autoimmune disease. J Immunol 2004; 173:5880-7.
77. Grewal IS, Foellmer HG, Grewal KD et al. Requirement for CD40 ligand in costimulation induction, T-cell activation and experimental allergic encephalomyelitis. Science 1996; 273:1864-7.
78. Breslow JL. Mouse models of atherosclerosis. Science 1996; 272:685-8.
79. Ma J, Xu J, Madaio MP et al. Autoimmune lpr/lpr mice deficient in CD40 ligand: spontaneous Ig class switching with dichotomy of autoantibody responses. J Immunol 1996; 157:417-26.
80. Kawamura T, Kanai T, Dohi T et al. Ectopic CD40 ligand expression on B-cells triggers intestinal inflammation. J Immunol 2004; 172:6388-97.
81. Higuchi T, Aiba Y, Nomura T et al. Cutting Edge: Ectopic expression of CD40 ligand on B-cells induces lupus-like autoimmune disease. J Immunol 2002; 168:9-12.
82. Mehling A, Loser K, Varga G et al. Overexpression of CD40 ligand in murine epidermis results in chronic skin inflammation and systemic autoimmunity. J Exp Med 2001; 194:615-28.
83. Saito K, Sakurai J, Ohata J et al. Involvement of CD40 ligand-CD40 and CTLA4-B7 pathways in murine acute graft-versus-host disease induced by allogeneic T-cells lacking CD28. J Immunol 1998; 160:4225-31.
84. Durie FH, Aruffo A, Ledbetter J et al. Antibody to the ligand of CD40, gp39, blocks the occurrence of the acute and chronic forms of graft-vs-host disease. J Clin Invest 1994; 94:1333-8.

85. Stuber E, Strober W, Neurath M. Blocking the CD40L-CD40 interaction in vivo specifically prevents the priming of T helper 1 cells through the inhibition of interleukin 12 secretion. J Exp Med 1996; 183:693-8.
86. Banu N, Zhang Y, Meyers CM. Immune reactivity following CD40L blockade: role in autoimmune glomerulonephritis in susceptible recipients. Autoimmunity 1999; 30:21-33.
87. Larsen CP, Alexander DZ, Hollenbaugh D et al. CD40-gp39 interactions play a critical role during allograft rejection. Suppression of allograft rejection by blockade of the CD40-gp39 pathway. Transplantation 1996; 61:4-9.
88. Bumgardner GL, Li J, Heininger M et al. Costimulation pathways in host immune responses to allogeneic hepatocytes. Transplantation 1998; 66:1841-5.
89. Molano RD, Berney T, Li H et al. Prolonged islet graft survival in NOD mice by blockade of the CD40-CD154 pathway of T-cell costimulation. Diabetes 2001; 50:270-6.
90. Tung TH, Mackinnon SE, Mohanakumar T. Long-term limb allograft survival using anti-CD40L antibody in a murine model. Transplantation 2003; 75:644-50.
91. Larsen CP, Elwood ET, Alexander DZ et al. Long-term acceptance of skin and cardiac allografts after blocking CD40 and CD28 pathways. Nature 1996; 381:434-8.
92. Li Y, Li XC, Zheng XX et al. Blocking both signal 1 and signal 2 of T-cell activation prevents apoptosis of alloreactive T-cells and induction of peripheral allograft tolerance. Nat Med 1999; 5:1298-302.
93. Elwood ET, Larsen CP, Cho HR et al. Prolonged acceptance of concordant and discordant xenografts with combined CD40 and CD28 pathway blockade. Transplantation 1998; 65:1422-8.
94. Parker DC, Greiner DL, Phillips NE et al. Survival of mouse pancreatic islet allografts in recipients treated with allogeneic small lymphocytes and antibody to CD40 ligand. Proc Natl Acad Sci USA 1995; 92:9560-4.
95. Markees TG, Phillips NE, Noelle RJ et al. Prolonged survival of mouse skin allografts in recipients treated with donor splenocytes and antibody to CD40 ligand. Transplantation 1997; 64:329-35.
96. Durie FH, Fava RA, Foy TM et al. Prevention of collagen-induced arthritis with an antibody to gp39, the ligand for CD40. Science 1993; 261:1328-30.
97. Kyburz D, Carson DA, Corr M. The role of CD40 ligand and tumor necrosis factor alpha signaling in the transgenic K/BxN mouse model of rheumatoid arthritis. Arthritis Rheum 2000; 43:2571-7.
98. Tighe H, Heaphy P, Baird S et al. Human immunoglobulin (IgG) induced deletion of IgM rheumatoid factor B-cells in transgenic mice. J Exp Med 1995; 181:599-606.
99. Tighe H, Warnatz K, Brinson D et al. Peripheral deletion of rheumatoid factor B-cells after abortive activation by IgG. Proc Natl Acad Sci USA 1997; 94:646-51.
100. Kyburz D, Corr M, Brinson DC et al. Human rheumatoid factor production is dependent on CD40 signaling and autoantigen. J Immunol 1999; 163:3116-22.
101. Mohan C, Shi Y, Laman JD et al. Interaction between CD40 and its ligand gp39 in the development of murine lupus nephritis. J Immunol 1995; 154:1470-80.
102. Early GS, Zhao W, Burns CM. Anti-CD40 ligand antibody treatment prevents the development of lupus-like nephritis in a subset of New Zealand black x New Zealand white mice. Response correlates with the absence of an anti-antibody response. J Immunol 1996; 157:3159-64.
103. Wang X, Huang W, Schiffer LE et al. Effects of anti-CD154 treatment on B-cells in murine systemic lupus erythematosus. Arthritis Rheum 2003; 48:495-506.
104. Kalled SL, Cutler AH, Datta SK et al. Anti-CD40 ligand antibody treatment of SNF1 mice with established nephritis: preservation of kidney function. J Immunol 1998; 160:2158-65.
105. Kalled SL, Cutler AH, Ferrant JL. Long-term anti-CD154 dosing in nephritic mice is required to maintain survival and inhibit mediators of renal fibrosis. Lupus 2001; 10:9-22.
106. Daikh DI, Finck BK, Linsley PS et al. Long-term inhibition of murine lupus by brief simultaneous blockade of the B7/CD28 and CD40/gp39 costimulation pathways. J Immunol 1997; 159:3104-8.
107. Wang X, Huang W, Mihara M et al. Mechanism of action of combined short-term CTLA4Ig and anti-CD40 ligand in murine systemic lupus erythematosus. J Immunol 2002; 168:2046-53.
108. Laman JD, Maassen CB, Schellekens MM et al. Therapy with antibodies against CD40L (CD154) and CD44-variant isoforms reduces experimental autoimmune encephalomyelitis induced by a proteolipid protein peptide. Mult Scler 1998; 4:147-53.
109. Howard LM, Miga AJ, Vanderlugt CL et al. Mechanisms of immunotherapeutic intervention by anti-CD40L (CD154) antibody in an animal model of multiple sclerosis. J Clin Invest 1999; 103:281-90.
110. Schaub M, Issazadeh S, Stadlbauer TH et al. Costimulatory signal blockade in murine relapsing experimental autoimmune encephalomyelitis. J Neuroimmunol 1999; 96:158-66.
111. Liu Z, Geboes K, Colpaert S et al. Prevention of experimental colitis in SCID mice reconstituted with CD45RB^high CD4^+ T-cells by blocking the CD40-CD154 interactions. J Immunol 2000; 164:6005-14.

112. Cong Y, Brandwein SL, McCabe RP et al. CD4⁺ T-cells reactive to enteric bacterial antigens in spontane-
     ously colitic C3H/HeJBir mice: increased T helper cell type 1 response and ability to transfer disease.
     J Exp Med 1998; 187:855-64.
113. Cong Y, Weaver CT, Lazenby A et al. Colitis induced by enteric bacterial antigen-specific CD4⁺ T-cells
     requires CD40-CD40 ligand interactions for a sustained increase in mucosal IL-12. J Immunol 2000;
     165:2173-82.
114. Schonbeck U, Sukhova GK, Shimizu K et al. Inhibition of CD40 signaling limits evolution of established
     atherosclerosis in mice. Proc Natl Acad Sci USA 2000; 97:7458-63.
115. Lederman S, Yellin MJ, Krichevsky A et al. Identification of a novel surface protein on activated CD4⁺
     T-cells that induces contact-dependent B-cell differentiation (help). J Exp Med 1992; 175:1091-101.
116. Wagner DH Jr, Stout RD, Suttles J. Role of the CD40-CD40 ligand interaction in CD4⁺ T-cell
     contact-dependent activation of monocyte interleukin-1 synthesis. Eur J Immunol 1994; 24:3148-54.
117. Yellin MJ, Sinning J, Covey LR et al. T-lymphocyte T-cell-B-cell-activating molecule/CD40-L molecules
     induce normal B-cells or chronic lymphocytic leukemia B-cells to express CD80 (B7/BB-1) and enhance
     their costimulatory activity. J Immunol 1994; 153:666-74.
118. Nishioka Y, Lipsky PE. The role of CD40-CD40 ligand interaction in human T-cell-B-cell collaboration.
     J Immunol 1994; 153:1027-36.
119. Lederman S, Yellin MJ, Cleary AM et al. T-BAM/CD40-L on helper T-lymphocytes augments lympho-
     kine-induced B-cell Ig isotype switch recombination and rescues B-cells from programmed cell death. J
     Immunol 1994; 152:2163-71.
120. Kirk AD, Harlan DM, Armstrong NN et al. CTLA4-Ig and anti-CD40 ligand prevent renal allograft
     rejection in primates. Proc Natl Acad Sci USA 1997; 94:8789-94.
121. Gobburu JV, Tenhoor C, Rogge MC et al. Pharmacokinetics/dynamics of 5c8, a monoclonal antibody
     to CD154 (CD40 ligand) suppression of an immune response in monkeys. J Pharmacol Exp Ther 1998;
     286:925-30.
122. Kirk AD, Burkly LC, Batty DS et al. Treatment with humanized monoclonal antibody against CD154
     prevents acute renal allograft rejection in nonhuman primates. Nat Med 1999; 5:686-93.
123. Cho CS, Burkly LC, Fechner JH Jr, et al. Successful conversion from conventional immunosuppression
     to anti-CD154 monoclonal antibody costimulatory molecule blockade in rhesus renal allograft recipients.
     Transplantation 2001; 72:587-97.
124. Xu H, Tadaki DK, Elster EA et al. Humanized anti-CD154 antibody therapy for the treatment of
     allograft rejection in nonhuman primates. Transplantation 2002; 74:940-3.
125. Kenyon NS, Chatzipetrou M, Masetti M et al. Long-term survival and function of intrahepatic
     islet allografts in rhesus monkeys treated with humanized anti-CD154. Proc Natl Acad Sci USA 1999;
     96:8132-7.
126. Kenyon NS, Fernandez LA, Lehmann R et al. Long-term survival and function of intrahepatic islet al-
     lografts in baboons treated with humanized anti-CD154. Diabetes 1999; 48:1473-81.
127. Pierson RN 3rd, Chang AC, Blum MG et al. Prolongation of primate cardiac allograft survival by treat-
     ment with ANTI-CD40 ligand (CD154) antibody. Transplantation 1999; 68:1800-5.
128. Elster EA, Xu H, Tadaki DK et al. Treatment with the humanized CD154-specific monoclonal antibody,
     hu5C8, prevents acute rejection of primary skin allografts in nonhuman primates. Transplantation 2001;
     72:1473-8.
129. Jochum C, Beste M, Zellmer E et al. CD154 blockade and donor-specific transfusions in DLA-identical
     marrow transplantation in dogs conditioned with 1-Gy total body irradiation. Biol Blood Marrow
     Transplant 2007; 13:164-71.
130. Huang W, Sinha J, Newman J et al. The effect of anti-CD40 ligand antibody on B-cells in human
     systemic lupus erythematosus. Arthritis Rheum 2002; 46:1554-62.
131. Boumpas DT, Furie R, Manzi S et al. A short course of BG9588 (anti-CD40 ligand antibody) improves
     serologic activity and decreases hematuria in patients with proliferative lupus glomerulonephritis. Arthritis
     Rheum 2003; 48:719-27.
132. Grammer AC, Slota R, Fischer R et al. Abnormal germinal center reactions in systemic lupus erythe-
     matosus demonstrated by blockade of CD154-CD40 interactions. J Clin Invest 2003; 112:1506-20.
133. Brams P, Black A, Padlan EA et al. A humanized anti-human CD154 monoclonal antibody blocks
     CD154-CD40 mediated human B-cell activation. Int Immunopharmacol 2001; 1:277-94.
134. Crowe JE Jr, Sannella EC, Pfeiffer S et al. CD154 regulates primate humoral immunity to influenza.
     Am J Transplant 2003; 3:680-8.
135. Xu H, Montgomery SP, Preston EH et al. Studies investigating pretransplant donor-specific blood
     transfusion, rapamycin and the CD154-specific antibody IDEC-131 in a nonhuman primate model of
     skin allotransplantation. J Immunol 2003; 170:2776-82.
136. Azimzadeh AM, Pfeiffer S, Wu G et al. Alloimmunity in primate heart recipients with CD154 blockade:
     evidence for alternative costimulation mechanisms. Transplantation 2006; 81:255-64.

137. Preston EH, Xu H, Dhanireddy KK et al. IDEC-131 (anti-CD154), sirolimus and donor-specific transfusion facilitate operational tolerance in non-human primates. Am J Transplant 2005; 5:1032-41.

138. Kuwana M, Nomura S, Fujimura K et al. Effect of a single injection of humanized anti-CD154 monoclonal antibody on the platelet-specific autoimmune response in patients with immune thrombocytopenic purpura. Blood 2004; 103:1229-36.

139. Nomura S, Uehata S, Saito S et al. Enzyme immunoassay detection of platelet-derived microparticles and RANTES in acute coronary syndrome. Thromb Haemost 2003; 89:506-12.

140. Davis JC Jr, Totoritis MC, Rosenberg J et al. Phase I clinical trial of a monoclonal antibody against CD40-ligand (IDEC-131) in patients with systemic lupus erythematosus. J Rheumatol 2001; 28:95-101.

141. Kalunian KC, Davis JC Jr, Merrill JT et al. Treatment of systemic lupus erythematosus by inhibition of T-cell costimulation with anti-CD154: a randomized, double-blind, placebo-controlled trial. Arthritis Rheum 2002; 46:3251-8.

142. Schuler W, Bigaud M, Brinkmann V et al. Efficacy and safety of ABI793, a novel human anti-human CD154 monoclonal antibody, in cynomolgus monkey renal allotransplantation. Transplantation 2004; 77:717-26.

143. Kanmaz T, Fechner JJ Jr, Torrealba J et al. Monotherapy with the novel human anti-CD154 monoclonal antibody ABI793 in rhesus monkey renal transplantation model. Transplantation 2004; 77:914-20.

144. Knosalla C, Ryan DJ, Moran K et al. Initial experience with the human anti-human CD154 monoclonal antibody, ABI793, in pig-to-baboon xenotransplantation. Xenotransplantation 2004; 11:353-60.

145. Kawai T, Andrews D, Colvin RB et al. Thromboembolic complications after treatment with monoclonal antibody against CD40 ligand. Nat Med 2000; 6:114.

146. Buhler L, Alwayn IP, Appel JZ 3rd et al. Anti-CD154 monoclonal antibody and thromboembolism. Transplantation 2001; 71:491.

147. Roth GA, Zuckermann A, Klepetko W et al. Thrombophilia associated with anti-CD154 monoclonal antibody treatment and its prophylaxis in nonhuman primates. Transplantation 2004; 78:1238-9; author reply 39.

148. Knosalla C, Gollackner B, Cooper DK. Anti-CD154 monoclonal antibody and thromboembolism revisted. Transplantation 2002; 74:416-7.

149. Koyama I, Kawai T, Andrews D et al. Thrombophilia associated with anti-CD154 monoclonal antibody treatment and its prophylaxis in nonhuman primates. Transplantation 2004; 77:460-2.

150. Sanchez-Fueyo A, Domenig C, Strom TB et al. The complement dependent cytotoxicity (CDC) immune effector mechanism contributes to anti-CD154 induced immunosuppression. Transplantation 2002; 74:898-900.

151. Monk NJ, Hargreaves RE, Marsh JE et al. Fc-dependent depletion of activated T-cells occurs through CD40L-specific antibody rather than costimulation blockade. Nat Med 2003; 9:1275-80.

152. Ferrant JL, Benjamin CD, Cutler AH et al. The contribution of Fc effector mechanisms in the efficacy of anti-CD154 immunotherapy depends on the nature of the immune challenge. Int Immunol 2004; 16:1583-94.

153. Waldmann H. The new immunosuppression: just kill the T-cell. Nat Med 2003; 9:1259-60.

154. Nagelkerken L, Haspels I, van Rijs W et al. FcR interactions do not play a major role in inhibition of experimental autoimmune encephalomyelitis by anti-CD154 monoclonal antibodies. J Immunol 2004; 173:993-9.

155. Schuler W, Bigaud M, Di Padova F et al. ABI793, a novel, fully human anti-CD154 monoclonal antibody: efficacy in cynomolgus monkey kidney allo-transplantation Am J Transpl 2003; 3:290.

156. Armour KL, van de Winkel JG, Williamson LM et al. Differential binding to human FcgammaRIIa and FcgammaRIIb receptors by human IgG wildtype and mutant antibodies. Mol Immunol 2003; 40:585-93.

157. Schuler W, Bigaud M, Gram H et al. Efficacy of human anti-human CD154 monoclonal antibodies in allotransplantation is dependent on Fc-mediated effector functions. 12th International Congress of Immunology 2004:Abstract # 3117.

158. Shields RL, Namenuk AK, Hong K et al. High resolution mapping of the binding site on human IgG1 for Fc gamma RI, Fc gamma RII, Fc gamma RIII and FcRn and design of IgG1 variants with improved binding to the Fc gamma R. J Biol Chem 2001; 276:6591-604.

159. Presta LG. Engineering of therapeutic antibodies to minimize immunogenicity and optimize function. Adv Drug Deliv Rev 2006; 58:640-56.

160. Blick SK, Curran MP. Certolizumab pegol: in Crohn's disease. BioDrugs 2007; 21:195-201; discussion 02-3.

161. Molineux G. The design and development of pegfilgrastim (PEG-rmetHuG-CSF, Neulasta). Curr Pharm Des 2004; 10:1235-44.

162. Wang YS, Youngster S, Grace M et al. Structural and biological characterization of pegylated recombinant interferon alpha-2b and its therapeutic implications. Adv Drug Deliv Rev 2002; 54:547-70.

163. Allen SD, Rawale SV, Whitacre CC et al. Therapeutic peptidomimetic strategies for autoimmune diseases: costimulation blockade. J Pept Res 2005; 65:591-604.
164. Fournel S, Wieckowski S, Sun W et al. C3-symmetric peptide scaffolds are functional mimetics of trimeric CD40L. Nat Chem Biol 2005; 1:377-82.
165. Kitagawa M, Goto D, Mamura M et al. Identification of three novel peptides that inhibit CD40-CD154 interaction. Mod Rheumatol 2005; 15:423-6.
166. Hargreaves RE, Monk NJ, Jurcevic S. Selective depletion of activated T-cells: the CD40L-specific antibody experience. Trends Mol Med 2004; 10:130-5.
167. McEarchern JA, Oflazoglu E, Francisco L et al. Engineered anti-CD70 antibody with multiple effector functions exhibits in vitro and in vivo antitumor activities. Blood 2007; 109:1185-92.
168. Wu AM, Senter PD. Arming antibodies: prospects and challenges for immunoconjugates. Nat Biotechnol 2005; 23:1137-46.
169. Pagano L, Fianchi L, Caira M et al. The role of gemtuzumab ozogamicin in the treatment of acute myeloid leukemia patients. Oncogene 2007; 26:3679-90.
170. Wong BY, Gregory SA, Dang NH. Denileukin diftitox as novel targeted therapy for lymphoid malignancies. Cancer Invest 2007; 25:495-501.
171. Francisco JA, Cerveny CG, Meyer DL et al cAC10-vcMMAE, an anti-CD30-monomethyl auristatin E conjugate with potent and selective antitumor activity. Blood 2003; 102:1458-65.
172. Law CL, Gordon KA, Toki BE et al. Lymphocyte activation antigen CD70 expressed by renal cell carcinoma is a potential therapeutic target for anti-CD70 antibody-drug conjugates. Cancer Res 2006; 66:2328-37.
173. Ziebold JL, Hixon J, Boyd A et al. Differential effects of CD40 stimulation on normal and neoplastic cell growth. Arch Immunol Ther Exp (Warsz) 2000; 48:225-33.
174. Costello RT, Gastaut JA, Olive D. What is the real role of CD40 in cancer immunotherapy? Immunol Today 1999; 20:488-93.
175. Clark EA, Ledbetter JA. Activation of human B-cells mediated through two distinct cell surface differentiation antigens, Bp35 and Bp50. Proc Natl Acad Sci USA 1986; 83:4494-8.
176. Inui S, Kaisho T, Kikutani H et al. Identification of the intracytoplasmic region essential for signal transduction through a B-cell activation molecule, CD40. Eur J Immunol 1990; 20:1747-53.
177. Heath AW, Chang R, Harada N et al. Antibodies to murine CD40 stimulate normal B-lymphocytes but inhibit proliferation of B-lymphoma cells. Cell Immunol 1993; 152:468-80.
178. Funakoshi S, Longo DL, Beckwith M et al. Inhibition of human B-cell lymphoma growth by CD40 stimulation. Blood 1994; 83:2787-94.
179. Funakoshi S, Longo DL, Murphy WJ. Differential in vitro and in vivo antitumor effects mediated by anti-CD40 and anti-CD20 monoclonal antibodies against human B-cell lymphomas. J Immunother Emphasis Tumor Immunol 1996; 19:93.
180. Francisco JA, Donaldson KL, Chace D et al. Agonistic properties and in vivo antitumor activity of the anti-CD40 antibody SGN-14. Cancer Res 2000; 60:3225-31.
181. Szocinski JL, Khaled AR, Hixon J et al. Activation-induced cell death of aggressive histology lymphomas by CD40 stimulation: induction of bax. Blood 2002; 100:217-23.
182. Garrone P, Neidhardt EM, Garcia E et al. Fas ligation induces apoptosis of CD40-activated human B-lymphocytes. J Exp Med 1995; 182:1265-73.
183. Rothstein TL, Wang JK, Panka DJ et al. Protection against Fas-dependent Th1-mediated apoptosis by antigen receptor engagement in B-cells. Nature 1995; 374:163-5.
184. Schattner EJ, Elkon KB, Yoo DH et al. CD40 ligation induces Apo-1/Fas expression on human B-lymphocytes and facilitates apoptosis through the Apo-1/Fas pathway. J Exp Med 1995; 182:1557-65.
185. Schattner EJ, Mascarenhas J, Bishop J et al. CD4+ T-cell induction of Fas-mediated apoptosis in Burkitt's lymphoma B-cells. Blood 1996; 88:1375-82.
186. Wang D, Freeman GJ, Levine H et al. Role of the CD40 and CD95 (APO-1/Fas) antigens in the apoptosis of human B-cell malignancies. Br J Haematol 1997; 97:409-17.
187. luczynski W, Kowalczuk O, Ilendo E et al. CD40L and IL-4 stimulation of acute lymphoblastic leukemia cells results in upregulation of mRNA level of FLICE—an important component of apoptosis. Folia Histochem Cytobiol 2007; 45:15-20.
188. Segui B, Andrieu-Abadie N, Adam-Klages S et al. CD40 signals apoptosis through FAN-regulated activation of the sphingomyelin-ceramide pathway. J Biol Chem 1999; 274:37251-8.
189. Hollmann CA, Owens T, Nalbantoglu J et al. Constitutive activation of extracellular signal-regulated kinase predisposes diffuse large B-cell lymphoma cell lines to CD40-mediated cell death. Cancer Res 2006; 66:3550-7.
190. Hollmann AC, Gong Q, Owens T. CD40-mediated apoptosis in murine B-lymphoma lines containing mutated p53. Exp Cell Res 2002; 280:201-11.

191. Dicker F, Kater AP, Prada CE et al. CD154 induces p73 to overcome the resistance to apoptosis of chronic lymphocytic leukemia cells lacking functional p53. Blood 2006; 108:3450-7.

192. Lotz M, Ranheim E, Kipps TJ. Transforming growth factor beta as endogenous growth inhibitor of chronic lymphocytic leukemia B-cells. J Exp Med 1994; 179:999-1004.

193. Planken EV, Dijkstra NH, Willemze R et al. Proliferation of B-cell malignancies in all stages of differentiation upon stimulation in the 'CD40 system'. Leukemia 1996; 10:488-93.

194. Younes A, Snell V, Consoli U et al. Elevated levels of biologically active soluble CD40 ligand in the serum of patients with chronic lymphocytic leukaemia. Br J Haematol 1998; 100:135-41.

195. Kitada S, Zapata JM, Andreeff M et al. Bryostatin and CD40-ligand enhance apoptosis resistance and induce expression of cell survival genes in B-cell chronic lymphocytic leukaemia. Br J Haematol 1999; 106:995-1004.

196. Schattner EJ. CD40 ligand in CLL pathogenesis and therapy. Leuk Lymphoma 2000; 37:461-72.

197. Romano MF, Lamberti A, Tassone P et al. Triggering of CD40 antigen inhibits fludarabine-induced apoptosis in B chronic lymphocytic leukemia cells. Blood 1998; 92:990-5.

198. Ranheim EA, Kipps TJ. Activated T-cells induce expression of B7/BB1 on normal or leukemic B-cells through a CD40-dependent signal. J Exp Med 1993; 177:925-35.

199. Van den Hove LE, Van Gool SW, Vandenberghe P et al. CD40 triggering of chronic lymphocytic leukemia B-cells results in efficient alloantigen presentation and cytotoxic T-lymphocyte induction by up-regulation of CD80 and CD86 costimulatory molecules. Leukemia 1997; 11:572-80.

200. Wierda WG, Kipps TJ. Gene therapy and active immune therapy of hematologic malignancies. Best Pract Res Clin Haematol 2007; 20:557-68.

201. Takahashi S, Yotnda P, Rousseau RF et al. Transgenic expression of CD40L and interleukin-2 induces an autologous antitumor immune response in patients with non-Hodgkin's lymphoma. Cancer Gene Ther 2001; 8:378-87.

202. Willimott S, Baou M, Naresh K et al. CD154 induces a switch in pro-survival Bcl-2 family members in chronic lymphocytic leukaemia. Br J Haematol 2007; 138:721-32.

203. de Totero D, Tazzari PL, Capaia M et al. CD40 triggering enhances fludarabine-induced apoptosis of chronic lymphocytic leukemia B-cells through autocrine release of tumor necrosis factor-alpha and interferon-gama and tumor necrosis factor receptor-I-II upregulation. Haematologica 2003; 88:148-58.

204. Dicker F, Kater AP, Fukuda T et al. Fas-ligand (CD178) and TRAIL synergistically induce apoptosis of CD40-activated chronic lymphocytic leukemia B-cells. Blood 2005; 105:3193-8.

205. Kater AP, Dicker F, Mangiola M et al. Inhibitors of XIAP sensitize CD40-activated chronic lymphocytic leukemia cells to CD95-mediated apoptosis. Blood 2005; 106:1742-8.

206. de Totero D, Meazza R, Zupo S et al. Interleukin-21 receptor (IL-21R) is up-regulated by CD40 triggering and mediates proapoptotic signals in chronic lymphocytic leukemia B-cells. Blood 2006; 107:3708-15.

207. Tong AW, Zhang BQ, Mues G et al. Anti-CD40 antibody binding modulates human multiple myeloma clonogenicity in vitro. Blood 1994; 84:3026-33.

208. Westendorf JJ, Ahmann GJ, Armitage RJ et al. CD40 expression in malignant plasma cells. Role in stimulation of autocrine IL-6 secretion by a human myeloma cell line. J Immunol 1994; 152:117-28.

209. Zhou ZH, Wang JF, Wang YD et al. An agonist anti-human CD40 monoclonal antibody that induces dendritic cell formation and maturation and inhibits proliferation of a myeloma cell line. Hybridoma 1999; 18:471-8.

210. Pellat-Deceunynck C, Amiot M, Robillard N et al. CD11a-CD18 and CD102 interactions mediate human myeloma cell growth arrest induced by CD40 stimulation. Cancer Res 1996; 56:1909-16.

211. Bergamo A, Bataille R, Pellat-Deceunynck C. CD40 and CD95 induce programmed cell death in the human myeloma cell line XG2. Br J Haematol 1997; 97:652-55.

212. Tai YT, Catley LP, Mitsiades CS et al. Mechanisms by which SGN-40, a humanized anti-CD40 antibody, induces cytotoxicity in human multiple myeloma cells: clinical implications. Cancer Res 2004; 64:2846-52.

213. Tai YT, Li XF, Catley L et al. Immunomodulatory drug lenalidomide (CC-5013, IMiD3) augments anti-CD40 SGN-40-induced cytotoxicity in human multiple myeloma: clinical implications. Cancer Res 2005; 65:11712-20.

214. Hess S, Engelmann H. A novel function of CD40: induction of cell death in transformed cells. J Exp Med 1996; 183:159-67.

215. Hirano A, Longo DL, Taub DD et al. Inhibition of human breast carcinoma growth by a soluble recombinant human CD40 ligand. Blood 1999; 93:2999-3007.

216. Alexandroff AB, Jackson AM, Paterson T et al. Role for CD40-CD40 ligand interactions in the immune response to solid tumours. Mol Immunol 2000; 37:515-26.

217. Tong AW, Stone MJ. Prospects for CD40-directed experimental therapy of human cancer. Cancer Gene Ther 2003; 10:1-13.
218. Ghamande S, Hylander BL, Oflazoglu E et al. Recombinant CD40 ligand therapy has significant antitumor effects on CD40-positive ovarian tumor xenografts grown in SCID mice and demonstrates an augmented effect with cisplatin. Cancer Res 2001; 61:7556-62.
219. Gallagher NJ, Eliopoulos AG, Agathangelo A et al. CD40 activation in epithelial ovarian carcinoma cells modulates growth, apoptosis and cytokine secretion. Mol Pathol 2002; 55:110-20.
220. Eliopoulos AG, Davies C, Knox PG et al. CD40 induces apoptosis in carcinoma cells through activation of cytotoxic ligands of the tumor necrosis factor superfamily. Mol Cell Biol 2000; 20:5503-15.
221. Eliopoulos AG, Dawson CW, Mosialos G et al. CD40-induced growth inhibition in epithelial cells is mimicked by Epstein-Barr Virus-encoded LMP1: involvement of TRAF3 as a common mediator. Oncogene 1996; 13:2243-54.
222. Eliopoulos AG, Stack M, Dawson CW et al. Epstein-Barr virus-encoded LMP1 and CD40 mediate IL-6 production in epithelial cells via an NF-kappaB pathway involving TNF receptor-associated factors. Oncogene 1997; 14:2899-916.
223. Mackey MF, Gunn JR, Ting PP et al. Protective immunity induced by tumor vaccines requires interaction between CD40 and its ligand, CD154. Cancer Res 1997; 57:2569-74.
224. van Mierlo GJ, den Boer AT, Medema JP et al. CD40 stimulation leads to effective therapy of CD40(−) tumors through induction of strong systemic cytotoxic T-lymphocyte immunity. Proc Natl Acad Sci USA 2002; 99:5561-6.
225. Antonia SJ, Extermann M, Flavell RA. Immunologic nonresponsiveness to tumors. Crit Rev Oncog 1998; 9:35-41.
226. Yamada M, Shiroko T, Kawaguchi Y et al. CD40-CD40 ligand (CD154) engagement is required but not sufficient for modulating MHC class I, ICAM-1 and Fas expression and proliferation of human non-small cell lung tumors. Int J Cancer 2001; 92:589-99.
227. Gruss HJ, Hirschstein D, Wright B et al. Expression and function of CD40 on Hodgkin and Reed-Sternberg cells and the possible relevance for Hodgkin's disease. Blood 1994; 84:2305-14.
228. Gruss HJ, Ulrich D, Braddy S et al. Recombinant CD30 ligand and CD40 ligand share common biological activities on Hodgkin and Reed-Sternberg cells. Eur J Immunol 1995; 25:2083-9.
229. Barr TA, Heath AW. Functional activity of CD40 antibodies correlates to the position of binding relative to CD154. Immunology 2001; 102:39-43.
230. Malmborg Hager AC, Ellmark P, Borrebaeck CA et al. Affinity and epitope profiling of mouse anti-CD40 monoclonal antibodies. Scand J Immunol 2003; 57:517-24.
231. Bjorck P, Braesch-Andersen S, Paulie S. Antibodies to distinct epitopes on the CD40 molecule co-operate in stimulation and can be used for the detection of soluble CD40. Immunology 1994; 83:430-37.
232. Pound JD, Challa A, Holder MJ et al. Minimal cross-linking and epitope requirements for CD40-dependent suppression of apoptosis contrast with those for promotion of the cell cycle and homotypic adhesions in human B-cells. Int Immunol 1999; 11:11-20.
233. Schwabe RF, Hess S, Johnson JP et al. Modulation of soluble CD40 ligand bioactivity with anti-CD40 antibodies. Hybridoma 1997; 16:217-26.
234. Kwekkeboom J, De Boer M, Tager JM et al. CD40 plays an essential role in the activation of human B-cells by murine EL4B5 cells. Immunology 1993; 79:439-44.
235. Bjorck P, Paulie S. CD40 antibodies defining distinct epitopes display qualitative differences in their induction of B-cell differentiation. Immunology 1996; 87:291-5.
236. Challa A, Pound JD, Armitage RJ et al. Epitope-dependent synergism and antagonism between CD40 antibodies and soluble CD40 ligand for the regulation of CD23 expression and IgE synthesis in human B-cells. Allergy 1999; 54:576-83.
237. Hasbold J, Johnson-Leger C, Atkins CJ et al. Properties of mouse CD40: cellular distribution of CD40 and B-cell activation by monoclonal anti-mouse CD40 antibodies. Eur J Immunol 1994; 24:1835-42.
238. Heath AW, Wu WW, Howard MC. Monoclonal antibodies to murine CD40 define two distinct functional epitopes. Eur J Immunol 1994; 24:1828-34.
239. Morris AE, Remmele RL Jr, Klinke R et al. Incorporation of an isoleucine zipper motif enhances the biological activity of soluble CD40L (CD154). J Biol Chem 1999; 274:418-23.
240. Vonderheide RH, Dutcher JP, Anderson JE et al. Phase I study of recombinant human CD40 ligand in cancer patients. J Clin Oncol 2001; 19:3280-7.
241. Schultze JL, Anderson KC, Gilleece MH et al. A pilot study of combined immunotherapy with autologous adoptive tumour-specific T-cell transfer, vaccination with CD40-activated malignant B-cells and interleukin 2. Br J Haematol 2001; 113:455-60.
242. Wierda WG, Cantwell MJ, Woods SJ et al. CD40-ligand (CD154) gene therapy for chronic lymphocytic leukemia. Blood 2000; 96:2917-24.
243. Younes A. CD40 ligand therapy of lymphoma patients. J Clin Oncol 2001; 19:4351-3.

244. Koho H, Paulie S, Ben Aissa H et al. Monoclonal antibodies to antigens associated with transitional cell carcinoma of the human urinary bladder. I. Determination of the selectivity of six antibodies by cell ELISA and immunofluorescence. Cancer Immunol Immunother 1984; 17:165-72.

245. Paulie S, Koho H, Ben Aissa H et al. Monoclonal antibodies to antigens associated with transitional cell carcinoma of the human urinary bladder. II. Identification of the cellular target structures by immunoprecipitation and SDS-PAGE analysis. Cancer Immunol Immunother 1984; 17:173-9.

246. Paulie S, Ehlin-Henriksson B, Mellstedt H et al. A p50 surface antigen restricted to human urinary bladder carcinomas and B-lymphocytes. Cancer Immunol Immunother 1985; 20:23-8.

247. Shorts L, Weiss JM, Lee JK et al. Stimulation through CD40 on mouse and human renal cell carcinomas triggers cytokine production, leukocyte recruitment and antitumor responses that can be independent of host CD40 expression. J Immunol 2006; 176:6543-52.

248. Hayashi T, Treon SP, Hideshima T et al. Recombinant humanized anti-CD40 monoclonal antibody triggers autologous antibody-dependent cell-mediated cytotoxicity against multiple myeloma cells. Br J Haematol 2003; 121:592-6.

249. Law CL, Gordon KA, Collier J et al. Preclinical antilymphoma activity of a humanized anti-CD40 monoclonal antibody, SGN-40. Cancer Res 2005; 65:8331-8.

250. Law C-L, McEarchern JA, Cerveny CG et al. The humanized anti-CD40 monoclonal antibody SGN-40 targets hodgkin's disease cells through multiple mechanisms. Blood 2005; 106:Abstract # 1476.

251. Lewis TS, Sutherland MSK, Jonas M et al. The humanized anti-CD40 antibody, SGN-40, promotes apoptosis signaling and is effective in combination with standard therapies in lymphoma xenograft models. Blood 2006; 108:Abstract # 2499.

252. Hussein MA, Berenson JR, Niesvizky R et al. Results of a phase I trial of SGN-40 (Anti-huCD40 mAb) in patients with relapsed multiple myeloma. Blood 2006; 108:Abstract # 3576.

253. Kelley SK, Gelzleichter T, Xie D et al. Preclinical pharmacokinetics, pharmacodynamics and activity of a humanized anti-CD40 antibody (SGN-40) in rodents and non-human primates. Br J Pharmacol 2006; 148:1116-23.

254. Advani R, Forero-Torres A, Furman RR et al. SGN-40 (Anti-huCD40 mAb) monotherapy induces durable objective responses in patients with relapsed aggressive non-Hodgkins lymphoma: evidence of antitumor activity from a phase I study. Blood 2006; 108:Abstract # 695.

255. Long L, Patawaran M, Tong X et al. Efficacy of an antagonistic anti-CD40 monoclonal antibody, HCD122 (CHIR-12.12), in preclinical models of human non-Hodgkins lymphoma and Hodgkins disease. Blood 2006; 108:Abstract # 230.

256. Tai YT, Li X, Tong X et al. Human anti-CD40 antagonist antibody triggers significant antitumor activity against human multiple myeloma. Cancer Res 2005; 65:5898-906.

257. Hsu SJ, Esposito LA, Aukerman SL et al. HCD122, an antagonist human anti-CD40 monoclonal antibody, inhibits tumor growth in xenograft models of human diffuse large B-cell lymphoma, a subset of non-Hodgkins lymphoma. Blood 2006; 108:Abstract # 2519.

258. Tong X, Georgakis GV, Long L et al. In vitro activity of a novel fully human anti-CD40 antibody CHIR-12.12 in chronic lymphocytic leukemia: blockade of CD40 activation and induction of ADCC. Blood 2004; 104:Abstract # 2504.

259. Weng W-K, Tong X, Luqman M et al. A fully human anti-CD40 antagonistic antibody, CHIR-12.12, inhibit the proliferation of human B-cell non-Hodgkin's lymphoma. Blood 2004; 104:Abstract # 3279.

260. Jeffry UB, Huh K, Tong X et al. Safety evaluation of an fully human antagonist anti-CD40 antibody, CHIR-12.12, in a dose range-finding study in cynomolgus monkeys. Blood 2004; 104:Abstract # 3282.

261. Jeffry UB, Luqman M, Huh K et al. Immunological profile and safety evaluation in a 23-week single dose study in cynomolgus monkey with CHIR-12.12, a fully human antagonist anti-CD40 antibody. Blood 2004; 104:Abstract # 4638.

262. Byrd JC, Flinn IW, Khan KD et al. Pharmacokinetics and Pharmacodynamics from a first-in-human phase 1 dose escalation study with antagonist anti-CD40 antibody, HCD122 (Formerly CHIR-12.12), in patients with relapsed and refractory chronic lymphocytic leukemia. Blood 2006; 108:Abstract # 2837.

263. Bensinger W, Jagannath S, Becker PS et al. A phase 1 dose escalation study of a fully human, antagonist anti-CD40 antibody, HCD122 (Formerly CHIR-12.12) in patients with relapsed and refractory multiple myeloma. Blood 2006; 108:Abstract # 3575.

264. de Boer M, Conroy L, Min HY et al. Generation of monoclonal antibodies to human lymphocyte cell surface antigens using insect cells expressing recombinant proteins. J Immunol Methods 1992; 152:15-23.

265. Kwekkeboom J, de Rijk D, Kasran A et al. Helper effector function of human T-cells stimulated by anti-CD3 mAb can be enhanced by costimulatory signals and is partially dependent on CD40-CD40 ligand interaction. Eur J Immunol 1994; 24:508-17.

266. Laman JD, t Hart BA, Brok H et al. Protection of marmoset monkeys against EAE by treatment with a murine antibody blocking CD40 (mu5D12). Eur J Immunol 2002; 32:2218-28.
267. Boon L, Laman JD, Ortiz-Buijsse A et al. Preclinical assessment of anti-CD40 Mab 5D12 in cynomolgus monkeys. Toxicology 2002; 174:53-65.
268. Boon L, Brok HP, Bauer J et al. Prevention of experimental autoimmune encephalomyelitis in the common marmoset (Callithrix jacchus) using a chimeric antagonist monoclonal antibody against human CD40 is associated with altered B-cell responses. J Immunol 2001; 167:2942-9.
269. t Hart BA, Blezer EL, Brok HP et al. Treatment with chimeric anti-human CD40 antibody suppresses MRI-detectable inflammation and enlargement of pre-existing brain lesions in common marmosets affected by MOG-induced EAE. J Neuroimmunol 2005; 163:31-9.
270. de Vos AF, Melief MJ, van Riel D et al. Antagonist anti-human CD40 antibody inhibits germinal center formation in cynomolgus monkeys. Eur J Immunol 2004; 34:3446-55.
271. Kasran A, Boon L, Wortel CH et al. Safety and tolerability of antagonist anti-human CD40 Mab ch5D12 in patients with moderate to severe Crohn's disease. Aliment Pharmacol Ther 2005; 22:111-22.
272. Hunter TB, Alsarraj M, Gladue RP et al. An agonist antibody specific for CD40 induces dendritic cell maturation and promotes autologous anti-tumour T-cell responses in an in vitro mixed autologous tumour cell/lymph node cell model. Scand J Immunol 2007; 65:479-86.
273. Kimura K, Moriwaki H, Nagaki M et al. Pathogenic role of B-cells in anti-CD40-induced necroinflammatory liver disease. Am J Pathol 2006; 168:786-95.
274. Kimura K, Nagaki M, Takai S et al. Pivotal role of nuclear factor kappaB signaling in anti-CD40-induced liver injury in mice. Hepatology 2004; 40:1180-9.
275. Adams AB, Shirasugi N, Jones TR et al. Development of a chimeric anti-CD40 monoclonal antibody that synergizes with LEA29Y to prolong islet allograft survival. J Immunol 2005; 174:542-50.
276. Pearson TC, Trambley J, Odom K et al. Anti-CD40 therapy extends renal allograft survival in rhesus macaques. Transplantation 2002; 74:933-40.
277. Geldart TR, Harvey M, Carr N et al. Cancer immunotherapy with a chimeric anti-CD40 monoclonal antibody: Evidence of preclinical efficacy. J Clin Oncol 2004; 22:Abstract # 2577.
278. Vonderheide RH, Flaherty KT, Khalil M et al. Clinical activity and immune modulation in cancer patients treated with CP-870,893, a novel CD40 agonist monoclonal antibody. J Clin Oncol 2007; 25:876-83.

CHAPTER 3

Targeting TNF for Treatment of Cancer and Autoimmunity

Gautam Sethi, Bokyung Sung, Ajaikumar B. Kunnumakkara
and Bharat B. Aggarwal*

Abstract

Tumor necrosis factor-α (TNF-α) was first isolated two decades ago as a macrophage-produced protein that can effectively kill tumor cells. TNF-α is also an essential component of the immune system and is required for hematopoiesis, for protection from bacterial infection and for immune cell-mediated cytotoxicity. Extensive research, however, has revealed that TNF-α is one of the major players in tumor initiation, proliferation, invasion, angiogenesis and metastasis. The proinflammatory activities link TNF-α with a wide variety of autoimmune diseases, including psoriasis, inflammatory bowel disease, rheumatoid arthritis, systemic sclerosis, systemic lupus erythematosus, multiple sclerosis, diabetes and ankylosing spondylitis. Systemic inhibitors of TNF such as etanercept (Enbrel) (a soluble TNF receptor) and infliximab (Remicade) and adalimumab (Humira) (anti-TNF antibodies) have been approved for the treatment inflammatory bowel disease, psoriasis and rheumatoid arthritis. These drugs, however, exhibit severe side effects and are expensive. Hence orally active blockers of TNF-α that are safe, efficacious and inexpensive are urgently needed. Numerous products from fruits, vegetable and traditional medicinal plants have been described which can suppress TNF expression and TNF signaling but their clinical potential is yet uncertain.

Discovery of TNF

Tumor necrosis factor (TNF), an activity in the serum of endotoxin-injected animals, was first identified in 1944, rediscovered in the mid-1970s and chemically isolated from macrophage-conditioned medium as a cytokine that kills tumor cells in culture in 1984.[1,2] Two distinct factors were identified in macrophages and lymphocytes: TNF-α and TNF-β, respectively. The identification of their primary amino acid sequences led to the cloning of their genes and the availability of large amounts of pure cytokines for preclinical and clinical evaluation. Intravenous administration of TNF to cancer patients produced numerous toxic reactions including fever.[3] In animal studies, TNF-α has been shown to mediate endotoxin-mediated septic shock.[4] Several reports over the past years have indicated that dysregulation of TNF-α synthesis mediates a wide variety of autoimmune diseases and cancer.[2]

Signaling Mechanism(s) by TNF-α

TNF-α mediates its effects through two different receptors: TNF receptor I (also known as p55 or p60) and TNF receptor II (also known as p75 or p80). Whereas TNF receptor I is expressed

*Corresponding Author: Bharat B. Aggarwal—Cytokine Research Laboratory, Department of Experimental Therapeutics, The University of Texas MD Anderson Cancer Center, Unit 143, 1515 Holcombe Boulevard, Houston, Texas 77030, USA. Email: aggarwal@mdanderson.org

Therapeutic Targets of the TNF Superfamily, edited by Iqbal S. Grewal.
©2009 Landes Bioscience and Springer Science+Business Media.

on all cell types in the body, TNF receptor II is expressed selectively on endothelial cells and on cells of the immune system.[2,5] The cytoplasmic domain of the TNF receptor I has a death domain, which has been shown to sequentially recruit TNF receptor-associated death domain (TRADD), Fas-associated death domain (FADD) and FADD-like ICE (FLICE) (also called caspase-8) lead to caspase-3 activation, which in turn induces apoptosis by inducing degradation of multiple proteins.[6] TRADD also recruits TNF receptor-associated factor (TRAF2), which through receptor-interacting protein (RIP) activates IκBα kinase (IKK) leading to IκBα phosphorylation, ubiquitination and degradation, which finally leads to NF-κB activation. Through recruitment of TRAF2, TNF also activates various mitogen-activated protein kinases (MAPK), including the c-jun N-terminal kinases (JNK) p38 MAPK and p42/p44 MAPK. TRAF2 is also essential for the TNF-induced activation of AKT, another cell-survival signaling pathway. Thus TNFRI activates both apoptosis and cell survival signaling pathways simultaneously.[7-9]

Gene-deletion studies have shown that TNFR2 can also activate NF-κB, JNK, p38 MAPK and p42/p44 MAPK.[10] TNFR2 can also mediate TNF-induced apoptosis.[11] Because TNFR2 cannot recruit TRADD-FADD-FLICE, how TNFR2 mediates apoptosis is not understood. However, the true physiological role of TNF, its receptors and associated proteins has been explored through gene-deletion experiments. It was found that animals with homologous gene deletion are fully viable but are more susceptible to infection[12-24] (Table 1). Overall the deletion of TNF, its receptors and associated proteins indicates the critical role of this cytokine in protection from microorganisms, the formation of lymph nodes and the development of the immune system.

Role of TNF-α in Cancer

TNF-α, initially discovered as a result of its antitumor activity, has now been shown to mediate all steps involved in tumorigenesis, including cellular transformation, promotion, survival, proliferation, invasion, angiogenesis and metastasis[25] (Fig. 1). These are discussed in detail as follows.

TNF-α Can Induce Tumor Initiation and Promotion

A number of reports indicate that TNF-α induces tumor initiation and tumor promotion[5,26,27] Komori's group reported that human TNF-α is 1000 times more effective than the chemical tumor promoters okadaic acid and 12-O-tetradecanoylphorbol-13-acetate in inducing cancer. Once initiated with these chemical carcinogens and exposed for 2 weeks to TNF-α, BALB/3T3 cells underwent transformation and yielded tumors in nude mice.[28] The essential role of TNF-α in tumor promotion has also been demonstrated using TNF-α-deficient mice. Specifically, okadaic acid did not show any tumor-promoting activity in TNF[-/-] mice after up to 19 weeks of tumor promotion, whereas okadaic acid induced strong tumor-promoting activity in TNF[+/+] mice. Tumor development in TPA-treated TNF[-/-] mice was delayed and both the average number of tumors per mouse and the tumor size were dramatically reduced compared with results for TNF[+/+] CD-1 mice.[29] Similarly, in a model of chemically induced liver cancer, TNF-α production by hepatocytes was implicated in tumor development.[30] All these reports establish that TNF-α plays a critical role in tumor promotion.

Tumor Cells Produce TNF-α and Mediate Proliferation

TNF-α is also produced by a wide variety of tumor cells, including B-cell lymphoma,[31,32] cutaneous T-cell lymphoma,[33] megakaryoblastic leukemia,[34] adult T-cell leukemia,[35] CLL,[36] ALL,[37] breast carcinoma,[38] lung carcinoma,[39] pancreatic cancer,[40] ovarian carcinoma,[41] cervical epithelial cancer,[42] glioblastoma[43] and neuroblastoma.[44] In most of these cells, TNF-α acts as an autocrine growth factor; however; in some cell types TNF-α induces the expression of other growth factors that mediate proliferation of tumors. For instance, in cervical cells TNF-α induces amphiregulin, which induces the proliferation of cells,[42] whereas in pancreatic cells TNF-α induces the expression of epidermal growth factor receptor (EGFR) and transforming growth factor (TGF-α), which mediate proliferation.[40]

Table 1. Phenotype of mice with gene deletion for TNF, TNF receptor and receptor-associated proteins

Gene	Phenotype	Ref.
TNF	• Homozygous mutants viable • Readily succumb to *Listeria monocytogenes* infection • Show reduced contact hypersensitivity responses • Resistant to lipopolysaccharide toxicity • Lack splenic primary B-cell follicle follicular dendritic cell network • Exhibit resistance to skin carcinogenesis	12-14
TNFR1	• Resistant to low levels of lipopolysaccharide • Increased susceptibility to *Listeria monocytogenes* infection	15
TNFR2	• Resistant to low levels of lipopolysaccharide • Impaired T-cell development • Reduced cytotoxic T-lymphocyte proliferation • Increased resistance to TNF-induced necrotic cell death	16
TRAF1	• Exhibit stronger proliferation than wild-type T-cell to anti-CD3 • Respond to TNF-induced NF-κB and AP-1 signaling pathways • Skin hypersensitive to TNF-induced necrosis	17
TRAF2	• Defective Th-dependent antibody response • CD40-mediated proliferation and NF-κB activation • Thymus and spleen atrophied and B-cell precursors depleted • Thymocytes and hematopoietic progenitors sensitive to TNF-induced apoptosis • Serum TNF levels elevated • Reduced TNF-mediated JNK/SAPK activation Mild effect on NF-κB activation	18, 19
RIP1	• Appear normal at birth but fail to thrive • Die at 1-3 days of age • Extensive apoptosis in lymphoid and adipose tissue • RIP$^{-/-}$ cells highly sensitive to TNFα-induced cell death • No NF-κB activation	20
FADD	• Do not survive beyond day 11.5 of embryogenesis • Cardiac failure and abdominal hemorrhage • Chimeric embryos showing a high contribution of FADD null mutantcells to the heart reproduce the phenotype of FADD$^{-/-}$ mutants • Activates rearrangement of the immunoglobulin and TCR genes • Fas-induced apoptosis completely blocked • Fas-mediated activation-induced proliferation impaired	21, 22
Caspase-8	• Embryos exhibit impaired heart muscle development • Congested accumulation of erythrocytes in embryos • TNF receptors, Fas/Apo1 and DR3 fail to induce cell death	23
IKKβ	• Die at mid-gestation from uncontrolled liver apoptosis • IKKβ-deficientcells lack activation of IKK and NF-κB in response to TNF-α or IL-1β	24

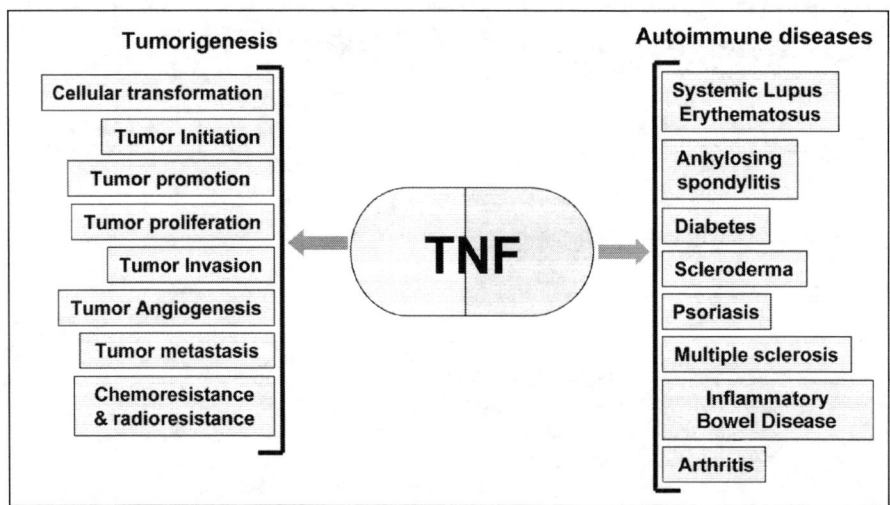

Figure 1. Pro-inflammatory effects of TNF are involved in tumorigenesis and in autoimmune diseases.

TNF-α Can Induce Invasion and Angiogenesis of Tumor Cells

That TNF-α can induce invasion and angiogenesis of tumor cells is well documented. TNF-α has been shown to confer an invasive, transformed phenotype on mammary epithelial cells.[38] TNF-α has been reported to induce angiogenic factor upregulation in malignant glioma cells.[45] This upregulation in turn promotes angiogenesis and tumor progression. TNF-α also stimulates epithelial tumor cell motility, which is a critical function in embryonic development, tissue repair and tumor invasion.[46] TNF-α has been even reported to mediate macrophage-induced angiogenesis.[47]

Role of TNF-α in Tumor Metastasis

TNF-α also plays a role in the metastasis of cancer cells. In a model of experimental lung metastasis of colon adenocarcinoma, injection of LPS into mice enhanced the development of metastatic lesions. The increased metastasis was dependent on TNF-α production by host hematopoietic cells. This TNF-α activated NF-κB in the tumor cells, increasing their proliferation and survival.[48] Moreover, endogenous and exogenous TNF-α administration enhanced metastasis in an experimental fibrosarcoma metastasis model.[49] Mice injected with fibrosarcoma cells showed enhanced metastasis to the lungs in the presence of exogenous TNF. Neutralization of endogenous tumor-induced TNF led to a significant decrease of the number of pulmonary metastases. An essential role of TNFR p55 has been found in liver metastases following intrasplenic administration of colon 26 cells.[50] Malik et al described found that overexpression of TNF-α conferred invasive properties on xenograft tumors.[51] Neutralization of endogenous TNF-α reversed the hepatic metastases and prolonged survival in mouse models.[52]

Role of TNF-α in the Immune System

TNF-α is a critical component of effective immune surveillance and is required for proper proliferation and function of natural killer cells (NK-cells), T-cells, B-cells, macrophages and dendritic cells.[5] TNF-α can influence inflammation and innate immunity, lymphoid organization and activation of APCs and can provide direct signals to T-cells.[2,53-55] TNFR2 can augment T-cell proliferation and thus may also provide a costimulatory signal for T-cells.[56] Mice strains in which the TNF-α gene or its p55 receptor has been deleted (TNF-KO or TNFR1-KO mice) have severe defects in lymph node follicle and germinal center formation.[57-59] TNF-α acting through TNF receptor p55 is involved in the development/maturation of dendritic cells (DCs) in bone marrow progenitor cultures.[60] Moreover, the microenvironment in peripheral lymphoid organs is associated with TNF-α signaling and chemokine production is critical for recruitment efficiency of DCs.[60] Follicular DCs are specialized mesenchymal cells that collect antigens in draining lymph nodes, interact with clonally expanding B-cells and form networks in the follicle under the influence of TNF-α and TNF-β.[53]

TNFR1 is a costimulator of T-cell activation and is expressed by activated T-cells. The initiation of an immune response by dendritic cells originating in epithelial barriers and stimulating naive T-cells in draining lymph nodes involves active involvement of TNF/TNFR1. Moreover, TNF-α regulates the expansion and survival of CD4+ and CD8+ T-cells.[53,54] T-cell-derived TNF-α is important for protection against high bacterial load, whereas mastcell-derived TNF-α is a critical and early component of the allergic response.[61]

TNF-α also plays a central role in initiating the inflammatory reactions of the innate immune system. Bacterial pathogens and several other proinflammatory and environmental stimuli induce TNF-α and NF-κB signaling cascade via Toll-like receptors and also enhance its translational efficiency.[62] Early production of TNF-α is prominent in the subsequent initiation of a highly complex biological cascade involving chemokines, cytokines and endothelial adhesions that recruits and activates neutrophils, macrophages and lymphocytes at the sites of infections. Release of preformed TNF-α acts as a positive autocrine feedback signal to activate NF-κB and to induce further TNF-α and other cytokines such as granulocte-monocyte colony-stimulating factor (GM-CSF) and IL-8.[61] Thus TNF-α exerts a global regulatory effect on the immune system.

Role of TNF-α in Autoimmune Diseases

Dysregulation of TNF-α has been implicated in a wide variety of autoimmune diseases, including rheumatoid arthritis, Crohn's disease, multiple sclerosis, psoriasis, scleroderma, systemic lupus erythromatosus, ankylosing spondylitis and diabetes (Fig. 1). How TNF-α mediates disease-causing effects is incompletely understood. The induction of proinflammatory genes by TNF-α has been linked to most diseases. The proinflammatory effects of TNF-α are primarily due to its ability to activate NF-κB.[63] Almost all cell types, when exposed to TNF-α, activate NF-κB, leading to the expression of inflammatory genes. The role of TNF-α in some of the autoimmune diseases is discussed in detail below.

Psoriasis

Psoriasis is a chronic inflammatory disease of the skin, affecting 2-3% of the world's population. Histopathologically, psoriasis is characterized by hyperproliferation of epidermal keratinocytes and hyperkeratosis, as well as infiltration of immunocytes along with angiogenesis.[64] T-cells play a major role in the initiation of psoriatic lesions. Activated T-cells in the region of the dermal epidermal junction promote the hyperplastic proliferative response through increased production of Th1 cytokines, among which TNF-α is the major player.[65] In psoriatic lesions, levels of TNF-α-induced genes, such as IL-1β, IL-8 and IL-6, are greatly increased.[66-68] Furthermore, in psoriatic plaques, there is a significant upregulation of activated phosphorylated NF-κB compared with normal epidermis and uninvolved epidermis from psoriasis patients.[69] TNF blockers have been shown to reverse the epidermal hyperplasia and cutaneous inflammation characteristic of psoriatic plaques.[70] All these findings together suggest a major role for TNF-α in both initiation and progression of psoriasis.

Inflammatory Bowel Disease

Inflammatory bowel disease (IBD) is characterized by a chronic relapsing inflammation of the gastrointestinal tract and is divided into two primary forms: Crohn's disease and ulcerative colitis.[71] IBD is associated with the activation of local intestinal and systemic immune responses and is caused by the loss of tolerance against intestinal antigens.[72] TNF-α levels are elevated in the serum, mucosa and stool of IBD patients and *TNF*-/- mice show a marked reduction in chemically induced intestinal inflammation.[73-76] Increased nuclear translocation of NF-κB has also been shown in lamina propria mononuclear cells derived from IBD patients.[77] Hence TNF-α is considered to be an attractive target for the treatment of IBD and several antiTNF reagents have been developed, but most of them have not proven safe and efficacious in the treatment of IBD.

Arthritis

As a proinflammatory cytokine, TNF-α has perhaps the most dominant role in the etiology of rheumatoid arthritis.[78] Patients with rheumatoid arthritis have high concentrations of TNF-α in the synovial fluid and at the cartilage-pannus junction, which leads to the erosion of bone.[79,80] In cultures of synovial cells from patients with rheumatoid arthritis, blocking TNF-α with antibodies significantly reduced the production of IL-1β, IL-6, IL-8 and GM-CSF.[81] Hence, the inhibition of TNF-α has a more global effect on inflammation than the suppression of other cytokines present in high concentrations in synovial fluids, such as IL-1β. The results of studies in animals provide further evidence of the importance of TNF-α in rheumatoid arthritis. In transgenic mice that expressed a deregulated human TNF-α gene, an inflammatory and destructive polyarthritis similar to rheumatoid arthritis spontaneously developed.[82] AntiTNF-α therapies are being used for the treatment of rheumatoid arthritis, but these agents are associated with side effects, some of them quite serious.[83] Hence novel agents are needed for the management of rheumatoid arthritis.

Systemic Sclerosis (Scleroderma)

Systemic sclerosis (scleroderma) is a generalized connective tissue disorder, characterized by a wide spectrum of microvascular and immunological abnormalities, leading to progressive thickening and fibrosis of the skin and other visceral organs, such as the lungs, gastrointestinal tract, heart and kidneys.[84,85] Compelling evidence indicates that the increased production of TNF-α is involved in the pathogenesis of scleroderma.[86] Patients with systemic sclerosis exhibit a systemic and local rise in TNF-α levels that leads to pulmonary fibrosis.[87] The serum levels of TNFR1 are directly correlated to the severity of the disease.[88] TNF-α gene polymorphism is also associated with scleroderma.[89] Thus dysregulation of TNF-α plays a critical role in the development of systemic sclerosis in normal human subjects.

Systemic Lupus Erythematosus

Systemic lupus erythematosus (SLE) is a multifactorial autoimmune disease characterized by the breakdown of self-tolerance, B-cell hyperactivity, autoantibody production, aberrant formation of immune complexes and inflammation of multiple organs.[90] The TNF-α level is increased and seems to be bioactive in the serum of patients with active SLE. The levels of TNF-α have been shown to correlate with SLE disease activity.[91,92] Various antiTNF-α agents are currently being used for the treatment of SLE.

Ankylosing Spondylitis

Ankylosing spondylitis (AS) is an autoimmune disease characterized by prominent inflammation of the spinal joints and adjacent structures leading to progressive bony fusion of the spine.[93] Pathophysiologically, TNF-α appears to play a role in promoting the inflammatory pattern associated with AS. Increased TNF-α protein is found in the sacroiliac joints[94] and peripheral synovium[95,96] as well as the serum[97,98] of patients with active AS. While disease activity cannot be predicted from levels of TNF-α, blockade of this protein has been shown to have benefits in animal models and human studies of AS. Considering the critical role of TNF-α in the pathogenesis of AS, the molecules targeted at blocking the effects of TNF-α are likely to play a crucial role in the management of this disease.

Diabetes Mellitus

Autoimmune diabetes, or insulin-dependent diabetes mellitus (IDDM), is characterized by selective destruction of insulin-producing cells.[99] The role of TNF-α in the pathogenesis of autoimmune diabetes has received increasing attention recently.[100] It was shown that TNF-α in combination with IFN-γ could induce the aberrant expression of class II major histocompatibility complex

(MHC) molecules on pancreatic beta cells, suggesting a role for these cytokines in the induction of the autoimmune process in diabetes.[101] A different group of investigators has suggested that IL-1β is toxic to pancreatic beta cells and that TNF-α significantly enhances this toxicity.[102] Transgenic mice, expressing constitutively active IKK-β, a kinase required for activation of NF-κB, exhibited type 2 diabetes phenotype and increased hepatic production of TNF-α. Hepatic expression of the IκBα super repressor reversed this diabetic phenotype in transgenic mice as well as wild-type mice fed a high-fat diet.[103] These findings indicate that lipid accumulation in the liver leads to subacute hepatic 'inflammation' through NF-κB activation and downstream cytokine production. This causes insulin resistance both locally in liver and systemically. Thus novel blockers of TNF-α have significant implications for future new therapeutic strategies for insulin-dependent diabetes mellitus.

Multiple Sclerosis

Multiple sclerosis (MS) is an inflammatory disease of the central nervous system characterized by localized areas of demyelination.[104] TNF-α plays an important role in the pathogenesis of MS and its animal model, experimental autoimmune encephalomyelitis.[105,106] TNF-α has been detected in MS plaques[107,108] and circulating levels of TNF-α and its receptor have been found in cerebro-spinal fluid of MS patients.[109,110] All these findings support an enormous role for TNF-α inhibitors in the treatment of multiple sclerosis.

TNF Inhibitors

On the basis of the above descriptions, TNF blockers have tremendous potential for the treatment of various cancers and autoimmune diseases. Several classes of TNF-α inhibitors are available and these are discussed below.

TNF Antibodies

The best studied of the monoclonal TNF-α antibodies is infliximab (Remicade), originally referred to as cA2. Infliximab binds with high specificity and affinity to free and membrane-bound TNF-α, which is expressed at the cell surface by activated T-cells and macrophages.[111] Adalimumab (Humira) is a human monoclonal IgG$_1$ antibody containing only human peptide sequences. It binds with high specificity and affinity to soluble and membrane-bound TNF-α and blocks its interaction with the p55 and p75 cell surface TNF receptors, thereby neutralizing the biological activities of this cytokine.[112] However, these antibodies have demonstrated several potentially serious adverse effects that include greater predisposition towards infection, congestive heart failure, neurologic changes (e.g., demyelination), lymphomas, re-exacerbation of latent tuberculosis and problems related to autoimmunity, for example lupus-like syndrome.[113]

Soluble TNF Receptors

In the second approach to TNF-α inhibition, soluble TNF receptors have been engineered as fusion proteins in which the extracellular ligand-binding portion of TNFRI or TNFR2 is coupled to a human immunoglobulin-like molecule. Etanercept (Enbrel) is a recombinant human fusion protein that consists of two soluble p75 TNF receptors and the F$_c$ portion of human IgG$_1$.[114] Etanercept possesses a dimeric structure with high affinity to TNF-α and the linkage to the F$_c$ portion of human IgG produces a longer half-life. Etanercept is better at neutralizing TNF-α than is the monomeric soluble p75 receptor. The various side effects observed include lymphomas, re-exacerbation of latent tuberculosis and problems related to autoimmunity.[113] Recent studies indicate that administration of TNF-α inhibitors can even lead to psoriasis[115] and contribute to the severity of the disease in paracoccidioidomycosis.[116]

Besides p75, TNF has been shown to bind to p55 receptor with an affinity either equal or even greater than p75.[117] Although soluble p75 receptors clearly can sequester TNF, very little is known about the ability of the soluble form of the p55 receptor to sequester TNF in vivo.

Inhibitors of TNF Expression

Several compounds that can inhibit both TNF-α expression and synthesis are also available. These include thalidomide ([+]-alpha-phthalimidoglutarimide), which is currently being used for treatment of multiple myeloma[118,119] and pentoxifylline, used to treat leg pain caused by poor blood circulation.[120] Thus these agents may be useful for the treatment of various cancers and autoimmune diseases mediated by TNF.

Inhibitors of TNF Oligomerization

Some inhibitors that can suppress oligomerization of TNF are also known. Steed and coworkers[121] designed a novel dominant-negative variant TNF protein that rapidly forms heterotrimers with native TNF to give complexes that neither bind to nor stimulate signaling through TNF receptors and thus inactivate TNF by sequestration. He et al[122] identified another small-molecule inhibitor that promotes subunit disassembly of trimeric TNF. This compound inhibited TNF activity in biochemical and cell-based assays, with median inhibitory concentrations of 22 and 4.6 micromolar, respectively. Formation of an intermediate complex between the compound and the intact trimer resulted in a 600-fold accelerated subunit dissociation rate that led to trimer dissociation.

Inhibitors of TNF-α-Induced Signaling Pathways

TNF-α activates cell survival signaling pathways, i.e., NF-κB, Akt and MAPK pathways, as well as apoptotic pathways such as JNK, p38 and AP-1. Hence, inhibitors that target these pathways also have potential against various proinflammatory conditions mediated by TNF-α. For example, TNF-α activates NF-κB, which in turn regulates TNF-α production. Hence various NF-κB blockers (both synthetic and natural) are currently available on the market and effective against a wide variety of inflammatory conditions.

Natural Products as Inhibitors of TNF

Numerous plant-derived products have been identified that can suppress TNF-α expression from macrophages activated by numerous inflammatory stimuli (129-165, see Table 2). These include curcumin, resveratrol, emodin, silymarin and others. Thus these products are likely to be useful for the treatment of cancer and autoimmune diseases mediated by TNF.

Table 2. A list of natural products that inhibit the expression of TNF

• 1'-acetoxychavicol acetate[123]	• *Lonicera japonica*[143]
• 1'-acetoxyeugenol acetate[124]	• Neolignans and lignans[144]
• *Allium sativum*[125]	• Patridoids I, II and IIA[145]
• *Aloe vera*[126]	• Phthalide lactone[146]
• *Aloe barbadensis*[127]	• Phloroglucinol derivatives[147]
• *Asparagus cochinchinensis*[128]	• Platycodin D and D3[148]
• Bisdemethoxycurcumin[129]	• *Phlebodium decumanum*[149]
• Butein[130]	• *Phyllanthus amarus*[150]
• Cardamomin[131]	• Resveratrol[151]
• Curcumin[132, 133]	• 14,15-Secopregnanederivatives argelosides[152]
• Diphenyl dimethyl bicarboxylate[134]	• Silymarin[153]
• Emodin inhibits IL-1β and IL-6[135]	• *Tanacetum microphyllum*[154]
• Epigallocatechin gallate[136]	• *Taraxacum officinale*[155]
• F022[137]	• Δ9-Tetrahydrocannabinoid[156]
• Ginkgolide B[138, 139]	• *Theobroma cacao*[157]
• 2'-Hydroxychalcone[140, 141]	• *Uncaria guianensis*[158]
• Hypoestoxide[142]	• *Zostera japonica*[159]

Conclusion

TNF clearly plays a major role in cancer and in autoimmune diseases. Because TNF is also needed for the proper functioning of the immune system, complete suppression of TNF over a long period is likely to prove harmful. The potential of TNF inhibitors in the treatment of autoimmune diseases as employed currently is just "the tip of the iceberg." Any chronic inflammatory condition, linked to majority of the inflammatory diseases, could be a potential target for antiTNF therapy. Thus the development of inhibitors that are orally active, safe and inexpensive would have major potential. Because of long-term safety and cost, nutraceuticals derived from fruits and vegetables, that can suppress TNF expression and TNF signaling, should be explored clinically for efficacy.

References

1. Pennica D, Nedwin GE, Hayflick JS et al. Human tumour necrosis factor: precursor structure, expression and homology to lymphotoxin. Nature 1984; 312:724-729.
2. Aggarwal BB. Signalling pathways of the TNF superfamily: a double-edged sword. Nat Rev Immunol 2003; 3:745-756.
3. Kurzrock R, Rosenblum MG, Sherwin SA et al. Pharmacokinetics, single-dose tolerance and biological activity of recombinant gamma-interferon in cancer patients. Cancer Res 1985; 45:2866-2872.
4. Beutler B, Milsark IW, Cerami AC. Passive immunization against cachectin/tumor necrosis factor protects mice from lethal effect of endotoxin. Science 1985; 229:869-871.
5. Aggarwal BB, Shishodia S, Ashikawa K et al. The role of TNF and its family members in inflammation and cancer: lessons from gene deletion. Curr Drug Targets Inflamm Allergy 2002; 1:327-341.
6. Nagata S and Golstein P. The Fas death factor. Science 1995; 267:1449-1456.
7. Darnay BG Aggarwal BB. Early events in TNF signaling: a story of associations and dissociations. J Leukoc Biol 1997; 61:559-566.
8. Bhardwaj A and Aggarwal BB. Receptor-mediated choreography of life and death. J Clin Immunol 2003; 23:317-332.
9. Aggarwal BB and Takada Y. Pro-apoptotic and anti-apoptotic effects of tumor necrosis factor in tumor cells. Role of nuclear transcription factor NF-kappaB. Cancer Treat Res 2005; 126:103-127.
10. Mukhopadhyay A, Suttles J, Stout RD et al. Genetic deletion of the tumor necrosis factor receptor p60 or p80 abrogates ligand-mediated activation of nuclear factor-kappa B and of mitogen-activated protein kinases in macrophages. J Biol Chem 2001; 276:31906-31912.
11. Haridas V, Darnay BG, Natarajan K et al. Overexpression of the p80 TNF receptor leads to TNF-dependent apoptosis, nuclear factor-kappa B activation and c-Jun kinase activation. J Immunol 1998; 160:3152-3162.
12. Pasparakis M, Alexopoulou L, Episkopou V et al. Immune and inflammatory responses in TNF-alpha-deficient mice: a critical requirement for TNF-alpha in the formation of primary B-cell follicles, follicular dendritic cell networks and germinal centers and in the maturation of the humoral immune response. J Exp Med 1996; 184:1397-1411.
13. Marino MW, Dunn A, Grail D et al. Characterization of tumor necrosis factor-deficient mice. Proc Natl Acad Sci USA 1997; 94:8093-8098.
14. Moore RJ, Owens DM, Stamp G et al. Mice deficient in tumor necrosis factor-alpha are resistant to skin carcinogenesis. Nat Med 1999; 5:828-831.
15. Rothe J, Lesslauer W, Lotscher H et al. Mice lacking the tumour necrosis factor receptor 1 are resistant to TNF-mediated toxicity but highly susceptible to infection by Listeria monocytogenes. Nature 1993; 364:798-802.
16. Erickson SL, de Sauvage FJ, Kikly K et al. Decreased sensitivity to tumour-necrosis factor but normal T-cell development in TNF receptor-2-deficient mice. Nature 1994; 372:560-563.
17. Tsitsikov EN, Laouini D, Dunn IF et al. TRAF1 is a negative regulator of TNF signaling. enhanced TNF signaling in TRAF1-deficient mice. Immunity 2001; 15:647-657.
18. Yeh WC, Shahinian A, Speiser D et al. Early lethality, functional NF-kappaB activation and increased sensitivity to TNF-induced cell death in TRAF2-deficient mice. Immunity 1997; 7:715-725.
19. Nguyen LT, Duncan GS, Mirtsos C et al. TRAF2 deficiency results in hyperactivity of certain TNFR1 signals and impairment of CD40-mediated responses. Immunity 1999; 11:379-389.
20. Kelliher MA, Grimm S, Ishida Y et al. The death domain kinase RIP mediates the TNF-induced NF-kappaB signal. Immunity 1998; 8:297-303.
21. Yeh JH, Hsu SC, Han SH et al. Mitogen-activated protein kinase kinase antagonized fas-associated death domain protein-mediated apoptosis by induced FLICE-inhibitory protein expression. J Exp Med 1998; 188:1795-1802.

22. Zhang J, Cado D, Chen A et al. Fas-mediated apoptosis and activation-induced T-cell proliferation are defective in mice lacking FADD/Mort.1 Nature 1998; 392:296-300.
23. Varfolomeev EE, Schuchmann M, Luria V et al. Targeted disruption of the mouse Caspase 8 gene ablates cell death induction by the TNF receptors, Fas/Apo,1 and DR3 and is lethal prenatally. Immunity 1998; 9:267-276.
24. Li ZW, Chu W, Hu Y et al. The IKKbeta subunit of IkappaB kinase (IKK) is essential for nuclear factor kappaB activation and prevention of apoptosis. J Exp Med 1999; 189:1839-1845.
25. Balkwill F. Tumor necrosis factor or tumor promoting factor? Cytokine Growth Factor Rev 2002; 13:135-141.
26. Aggarwal BB, Shishodia S, Takada Y et al. TNF blockade: an inflammatory issue. Ernst Schering Res Found Workshop, 2006:161-186.
27. Aggarwal BB, Shishodia S, Sandur SK et al. Inflammation and cancer: how hot is the link? Biochem Pharmacol 2006; 72:1605-1621.
28. Komori A, Yatsunami J, Suganuma M et al. Tumor necrosis factor acts as a tumor promoter in BALB/3T3 cell transformation. Cancer Res 1993; 53:1982-1985.
29. Suganuma M, Okabe S, Marino MW et al. Essential role of tumor necrosis factor alpha (TNF-alpha) in tumor promotion as revealed by TNF-alpha-deficient mice. Cancer Res 1999; 59:4516-4518.
30. Knight B, Yeoh GC, Husk KL et al. Impaired preneoplastic changes and liver tumor formation in tumor necrosis factor receptor type 1 knockout mice. J Exp Med 2000; 192:1809-1818.
31. Digel W, Stefanic M, Schoniger W et al. Tumor necrosis factor induces proliferation of neoplastic B-cells from chronic lymphocytic leukemia. Blood 1989; 73:1242-1246.
32. Digel W, Schoniger W, Stefanic M et al. Receptors for tumor necrosis factor on neoplastic B-cells from chronic lymphocytic leukemia are expressed in vitro but not in vivo. Blood 1990; 76:1607-1613.
33. Giri DK and Aggarwal BB. Constitutive activation of NF-kappaB causes resistance to apoptosis in human cutaneous T-cell lymphoma HuT-78 cells. Autocrine role of tumor necrosis factor and reactive oxygen intermediates. J Biol Chem 1998; 273:14008-14014.
34. Liu RY, Fan C, Mitchell S et al. The role of type I and type II tumor necrosis factor (TNF) receptors in the ability of TNF-alpha to transduce a proliferative signal in the human megakaryoblastic leukemic cell line Mo7e. Cancer Res 1998; 58:2217-2223.
35. Tsukasaki K, Miller CW, Kubota T et al. Tumor necrosis factor alpha polymorphism associated with increased susceptibility to development of adult T-cell leukemia/lymphoma in human T-lymphotropic virus type 1 carriers. Cancer Res 2001; 61:3770-3774.
36. Duncombe AS, Heslop HE, Turner M et al. Tumor necrosis factor mediates autocrine growth inhibition in a chronic leukemia. J Immunol 1989; 143:3828-3834.
37. Elbaz O and Mahmoud LA. Tumor necrosis factor and human acute leukemia. Leuk Lymphoma 1994; 12:191-195.
38. Montesano R, Soulie P, Eble JA et al. Tumour necrosis factor lpha confers an invasive, transformed phenotype on mammary epithelial cells. J Cell Sci 2005; 118:3487-3500.
39. Kalthoff H, Roeder C, Gieseking J et al. Inverse regulation of human ERBB2 and epidermal growth factor receptors by tumor necrosis factor alpha. Proc Natl Acad Sci USA 1993; 90:8972-8976.
40. Schmiegel W, Roeder C, Schmielau J et al. Tumor necrosis factor alpha induces the expression of transforming growth factor alpha and the epidermal growth factor receptor in human pancreatic cancer cells. Proc Natl Acad Sci USA 1993; 90:863-867.
41. Wu S, Boyer CM, Whitaker RS et al. Tumor necrosis factor alpha as an autocrine and paracrine growth factor for ovarian cancer: monokine induction of tumor cell proliferation and tumor necrosis factor alpha expression. Cancer Res 1993; 53:1939-1944.
42. Woodworth CD, McMullin E, Iglesias M et al. Interleukin 1 alpha and tumor necrosis factor alpha stimulate autocrine amphiregulin expression and proliferation of human papillomavirus-immortalized and carcinoma-derived cervical epithelial cells. Proc Natl Acad Sci USA 1995; 92:2840-2844.
43. Aggarwal BB, Schwarz L, Hogan ME et al. Triple helix-forming oligodeoxyribonucleotides targeted to the human tumor necrosis factor (TNF) gene inhibit TNF production and block the TNF-dependent growth of human glioblastoma tumor cells. Cancer Res 1996; 56:5156-5164.
44. Goillot E, Combaret V, Ladenstein R et al. Tumor necrosis factor as an autocrine growth factor for neuroblastoma. Cancer Res 1992; 52:3194-3200.
45. Nabors LB, Suswam E, Huang Y et al. Tumor necrosis factor alpha induces angiogenic factor up-regulation in malignant glioma cells: a role for RNA stabilization and HuR. Cancer Res 2003; 63:4181-4187.
46. Rosen EM, Goldberg ID, Liu D et al. Tumor necrosis factor stimulates epithelial tumor cell motility. Cancer Res 1991; 51:5315-5321.
47. Leibovich SJ, Polverini PJ, Shepard HM et al. Macrophage-induced angiogenesis is mediated by tumour necrosis factor-alpha. Nature 1987; 329:630-632.

48. Luo JL, Maeda S, Hsu LC et al. Inhibition of NF-kappaB in cancer cells converts inflammation-induced tumor growth mediated by TNF-alpha to TRAIL-mediated tumor regression. Cancer Cell 2004; 6:297-305.
49. Orosz P, Echtenacher B, Falk W et al. Enhancement of experimental metastasis by tumor necrosis factor. J Exp Med 1993; 177:1391-1398.
50. Kitakata H, Nemoto-Sasaki Y, Takahashi Y et al. Essential roles of tumor necrosis factor receptor p55 in liver metastasis of intrasplenic administration of colon 26 cells. Cancer Res 2002; 62:6682-6687.
51. Malik ST, Naylor MS, East N et al. Cells secreting tumour necrosis factor show enhanced metastasis in nude mice. Eur J Cancer 1990; 26:1031-1034.
52. Orosz P, Kruger A, Hubbe M et al. Promotion of experimental liver metastasis by tumor necrosis factor. Int J Cancer 1995; 60:867-871.
53. Locksley RM, Killeen N, Lenardo MJ. The TNF and TNF receptor superfamilies: integrating mammalian biology. Cell 2001; 104:487-501.
54. Pfeffer K. Biological functions of tumor necrosis factor cytokines and their receptors. Cytokine Growth Factor Rev 2003; 14:185-191.
55. Croft M. Costimulatory members of the TNFR family: keys to effective T-cell immunity? Nat Rev Immunol 2003; 3:609-620.
56. Kim EY and Te HS. TNF type 2 receptor (p75) lowers the threshold of T-cell activation. J Immunol 2001; 167:6812-6820.
57. Fu YX and Chaplin DD. Development and maturation of secondary lymphoid tissues. Annu Rev Immunol 1999; 17:399-433.
58. Pasparakis M, Alexopoulou L, Grell M et al. Peyer's patch organogenesis is intact yet formation of B lymphocyte follicles is defective in peripheral lymphoid organs of mice deficient for tumor necrosis factor and its 55-kDa receptor. Proc Natl Acad Sci USA 1997; 94:6319-6323.
59. Kuprash DV, Tumanov AV, Liepinsh DJ et al. Novel tumor necrosis factor-knockout mice that lack Peyer's patches. Eur J Immunol 2005; 35:1592-1600.
60. Abe K, Yarovinsky FO, Murakami T et al. Distinct contributions of TNF and LT cytokines to the development of dendritic cells in vitro and their recruitment in vivo. Blood 2003; 101:1477-1483.
61. Grivennikov SI, Tumanov AV, Liepinsh DJ et al. Distinct and nonredundant in vivo functions of TNF produced by T-cells and macrophages/neutrophils: protective and deleterious effects. Immunity 2005; 22:93-104.
62. Akira S, Takeda K. Toll-like receptor signalling. Nat Rev Immunol 2004; 4:499-511.
63. Aggarwal BB. Nuclear factor-kappaB: the enemy within. Cancer Cell 2004; 6:203-208.
64. Schon MP and Boehncke WH. Psoriasis. N Engl J Med 2005; 352:1899-1912.
65. Okubo Y and Koga M. Peripheral blood monocytes in psoriatic patients overproduce cytokines. J Dermatol Sci 1998; 17:223-232.
66. Nickoloff BJ, Karabin GD, Barker JN et al. Cellular localization of interleukin-8 and its inducer, tumor necrosis factor-alpha in psoriasis. Am J Pathol 1991; 138:129-140.
67. Gomi T, Shiohara T, Munakata T et al. Interleukin 1 alpha, tumor necrosis factor alpha and interferon gamma in psoriasis. Arch Dermatol 1991; 127:827-830.
68. Ettehadi P, Greaves MW, Wallach D et al. Elevated tumour necrosis factor-alpha (TNF-alpha) biological activity in psoriatic skin lesions. Clin Exp Immunol 1994; 96:146-151.
69. Lizzul PF, Aphale A, Malaviya R et al. Differential expression of phosphorylated NF-kappaB/RelA in normal and psoriatic epidermis and downregulation of NF-kappaB in response to treatment with etanercept. J Invest Dermatol 2005; 124:1275-1283.
70. Gottlieb AB, Chamian F, Masud S et al. TNF inhibition rapidly down-regulates multiple proinflammatory pathways in psoriasis plaques. J Immunol 2005; 175:2721-2729.
71. Bouma G, Strober W. The immunological and genetic basis of inflammatory bowel disease. Nat Rev Immunol 2003; 3:521-533.
72. Podolsky DK. Inflammatory bowel disease. N Engl J Med 2002; 347:417-429.
73. Komatsu M, Kobayashi D, Saito K et al. Tumor necrosis factor-alpha in serum of patients with inflammatory bowel disease as measured by a highly sensitive immuno-PCR. Clin Chem 2001; 47:1297-1301.
74. Braegger CP, Nicholls S, Murch SH et al. Tumour necrosis factor alpha in stool as a marker of intestinal inflammation. Lancet 1992; 339:89-91.
75. Breese EJ, Michie CA, Nicholls SW et al. Tumor necrosis factor alpha-producing cells in the intestinal mucosa of children with inflammatory bowel disease. Gastroenterology 1994; 106:1455-1466.
76. Neurath MF, Fuss I, Pasparakis M et al. Predominant pathogenic role of tumor necrosis factor in experimental colitis in mice. Eur J Immunol 1997; 27:1743-1750.
77. Schreiber S, Nikolaus S, Hampe J. Activation of nuclear factor kappa B inflammatory bowel disease. Gut 1998; 42:477-484.
78. Firestein GS. Evolving concepts of rheumatoid arthritis. Nature 2003; 423:356-361.

79. Saxne T, Palladino MA Jr, Heinegard D et al. Detection of tumor necrosis factor alpha but not tumor necrosis factor beta in rheumatoid arthritis synovial fluid and serum. Arthritis Rheum 1988; 31:1041-1045.

80. Chu CQ, Field M, Feldmann M et al. Localization of tumor necrosis factor alpha in synovial tissues and at the cartilage-pannus junction in patients with rheumatoid arthritis. Arthritis Rheum 1991; 34:1125-1132.

81. Butler DM, Maini RN, Feldmann M et al. Modulation of proinflammatory cytokine release in rheumatoid synovial membrane cell cultures. Comparison of monoclonal anti TNF-alpha antibody with the interleukin-1 receptor antagonist. Eur Cytokine Netw 1995; 6:225-230.

82. Keffer J, Probert L, Cazlaris H et al. Transgenic mice expressing human tumour necrosis factor: a predictive genetic model of arthritis. EMBO J 1991; 10:4025-4031.

83. Roos JC and Ostor AJ. Tumor necrosis factor inhibitors for rheumatoid arthritis. N Engl J Med 2006; 355:2046-2047; author reply 2048.

84. Johnson RW, Tew MB, Arnett FC. The genetics of systemic sclerosis. Curr Rheumatol Rep 2002; 4:99-107.

85. Medsger TA, Jr. Assessment of damage and activity in systemic sclerosis. Curr Opin Rheumatol 2000; 12:545-548.

86. Gruschwitz MS, Albrecht M, Vieth G et al. In situ expression and serum levels of tumor necrosis factor-alpha receptors in patients with early stages of systemic sclerosis. J Rheumatol 1997; 24:1936-1943.

87. Hasegawa M, Fujimoto M, Kikuchi K et al. Elevated serum tumor necrosis factor-alpha levels in patients with systemic sclerosis: association with pulmonary fibrosis. J Rheumatol 1997; 24:663-665.

88. Majewski S, Wojas-Pelc A, Malejczyk M et al. Serum levels of soluble TNF-alpha receptor type I and the severity of systemic sclerosis. Acta Derm Venereol 1999; 79:207-210.

89. Pandey JP and Takeuchi F. TNF-alpha and TNF-beta gene polymorphisms in systemic sclerosis. Hum Immunol 1999; 60:1128-1130.

90. Manson JJ and Isenberg DA. The pathogenesis of systemic lupus erythematosus. Neth J Med 2003; 61:343-346.

91. Aringer M, Feierl E, Steiner G et al. Increased bioactive TNF in human systemic lupus erythematosus: associations with cell death. Lupus 2002; 11:102-108.

92. Gabay C, Cakir N, Moral F et al. Circulating levels of tumor necrosis factor soluble receptors in systemic lupus erythematosus are significantly higher than in other rheumatic diseases and correlate with disease activity. J Rheumatol 1997; 24:303-308.

93. Sieper J, Braun J, Rudwaleit M et al. Ankylosing spondylitis: an overview. Ann Rheum Dis 2002; 61 Suppl 3:iii8-18.

94. Braun J, Bollow M, Neure L et al. Use of immunohistologic and in situ hybridization techniques in the examination of sacroiliac joint biopsy specimens from patients with ankylosing spondylitis. Arthritis Rheum 1995; 38:499-505.

95. Grom AA, Murray KJ, Luyrink L et al. Patterns of expression of tumor necrosis factor alpha, tumor necrosis factor beta and their receptors in synovia of patients with juvenile rheumatoid arthritis and juvenile spondylarthropathy. Arthritis Rheum 1996; 39:1703-1710.

96. Canete JD, Llena J, Collado A et al. Comparative cytokine gene expression in synovial tissue of early rheumatoid arthritis and seronegative spondyloarthropathies. Br J Rheumatol 1997; 36:38-42.

97. Gratacos J, Collado A, Filella X et al. Serum cytokines (IL-6, TNF-alpha, IL-1 beta and IFN-gamma) in ankylosing spondylitis: a close correlation between serum IL-6 and disease activity and severity. Br J Rheumatol 1994; 33:927-931.

98. Toussirot E, Lafforgue P, Boucraut J et al. Serum levels of interleukin 1-beta, tumor necrosis factor-alpha, soluble interleukin 2 receptor and soluble CD8 in seronegative spondylarthropathies. Rheumatol Int 1994; 13:175-180.

99. Moller DE. Potential role of TNF-alpha in the pathogenesis of insulin resistance and type 2 diabetes. Trends Endocrinol Metab 2000; 11:212-217.

100. Zoppini G, Faccini G, Muggeo M et al. Elevated plasma levels of soluble receptors of TNF-alpha and their association with smoking and microvascular complications in young adults with type 1 diabetes. J Clin Endocrinol Metab 2001; 86:3805-3808.

101. Pujol-Borrell R, Todd I, Doshi M et al. HLA class II induction in human isletcells by interferon-gamma plus tumour necrosis factor or lymphotoxin. Nature 1987; 326:304-306.

102. Mandrup-Poulsen T, Bendtzen K, Dinarello CA et al. Human tumor necrosis factor potentiates human interleukin 1-mediated rat pancreatic beta-cell cytotoxicity. J Immunol 1987; 139:4077-4082.

103. Cai D, Yuan M, Frantz DF et al. Local and systemic insulin resistance resulting from hepatic activation of IKK-beta and NF-kappaB. Nat Med 2005; 11:183-190.

104. Bernard CC, Kerlero de Rosbo N. Multiple sclerosis: an autoimmune disease of multifactorial etiology. Curr Opin Immunol 1992; 4:760-765.

105. Navikas V, Link H. Review: cytokines and the pathogenesis of multiple sclerosis. J Neurosci Res 1996; 45:322-333.
106. Selmaj K, Papierz W, Glabinski A et al. Prevention of chronic relapsing experimental autoimmune encephalomyelitis by soluble tumor necrosis factor receptor I. J Neuroimmunol 1995; 56:135-141.
107. Hofman FM, Hinton DR, Johnson K et al. Tumor necrosis factor identified in multiple sclerosis brain. J Exp Med 1989; 170:607-612.
108. Selmaj K, Raine CS, Cannella B et al. Identification of lymphotoxin and tumor necrosis factor in multiple sclerosis lesions. J Clin Invest 1991; 87:949-954.
109. Sharief MK, Hentges R. Association between tumor necrosis factor-alpha and disease progression in patients with multiple sclerosis. N Engl J Med 1991; 325:467-472.
110. Tsukada N, Matsuda M, Miyagi K et al. Increased levels of intercellular adhesion molecule-1 (ICAM-1) and tumor necrosis factor receptor in the cerebrospinal fluid of patients with multiple sclerosis. Neurology 1993; 43:2679-2682.
111. Maini R, St Clair EW, Breedveld F et al. Infliximab (chimeric antitumour necrosis factor alpha monoclonal antibody) versus placebo in rheumatoid arthritis patients receiving concomitant methotrexate: a randomised phase III trial. ATTRACT Study Group. Lancet 1999; 354:1932-1939.
112. Keystone EC, Kavanaugh AF, Sharp JT et al. Radiographic, clinical and functional outcomes of treatment with adalimumab (a human antitumor necrosis factor monoclonal antibody) in patients with active rheumatoid arthritis receiving concomitant methotrexate therapy: a randomized, placebo-controlled, 52-week trial. Arthritis Rheum 2004; 50:1400-1411.
113. Hasan U. Tumour necrosis factor inhibitors—what we need to know. N Z Med J 2006; 119:U2336.
114. Bathon JM, Martin RW, Fleischmann RM et al. A comparison of etanercept and methotrexate in patients with early rheumatoid arthritis. N Engl J Med 2000; 343:1586-1593.
115. Ubriani R, Van Voorhees AS. Onset of psoriasis during treatment with TNF-{alpha} antagonists: a report of 3 cases. Arch Dermatol 2007; 143:270-272.
116. Corvino CL, Mamoni RL, Fagundes GZ et al. Serum interleukin-18 and soluble tumour necrosis factor receptor 2 are associated with disease severity in patients with paracoccidioidomycosis. Clin Exp Immunol 2007; 147:483-490.
117. Higuchi M, Aggarwal BB. Modulation of two forms of tumor necrosis factor receptors and their cellular response by soluble receptors and their monoclonal antibodies. J Biol Chem 1992; 267:20892-20899.
118. Majumdar S, Lamothe B, Aggarwal BB. Thalidomide suppresses NF-kappa B activation induced by TNF and H_2O_2, but not that activated by ceramide, lipopolysaccharides, or phorbol ester. J Immunol 2002; 168:2644-2651.
119. Harousseau JL. Thalidomide in multiple myeloma: past, present and future. Future Oncol 2006; 2:577-589.
120. Zabel P, Schade FU, Schlaak M. Inhibition of endogenous TNF formation by pentoxifylline. Immunobiology 1993; 187:447-463.
121. Steed PM, Tansey MG, Zalevsky J et al. Inactivation of TNF signaling by rationally designed dominant-negative TNF variants. Science 2003; 301:1895-1898.
122. He MM, Smith AS, Oslob JD et al. Small-molecule inhibition of TNF-alpha. Science 2005; 310:1022-1025.
123. Grzanna R, Phan P, Polotsky A et al. Ginger extract inhibits beta-amyloid peptide-induced cytokine and chemokine expression in cultured THP-1 monocytes. J Altern Complement Med 2004; 10:1009-1013.
124. Matsuda H, Morikawa T, Managi H et al. Antiallergic principles from Alpinia galanga: structural requirements of phenylpropanoids for inhibition of degranulation and release of TNF-alpha and IL-4 in RBL-2H3 cells. Bioorg Med Chem Lett 2003; 13:3197-3202.
125. Makris A, Thornton CE, Xu B et al. Garlic increases IL-10 and inhibits TNF-alpha and IL-6 production in endotoxin-stimulated human placental explants. Placenta 2005; 26:828-834.
126. Duansak D, Somboonwong J, Patumraj S. Effects of Aloe vera on leukocyte adhesion and TNF-alpha and IL-6 levels in burn wounded rats. Clin Hemorheol Microcirc 2003; 29:239-246.
127. Qiu Z, Jones K, Wylie M et al. Modified Aloe barbadensis polysaccharide with immunoregulatory activity. Planta Med 2000; 66:152-156.
128. Kim H, Lee E, Lim T et al. Inhibitory effect of Asparagus cochinchinensis on tumor necrosis factor-alpha secretion from astrocytes. Int J Immunopharmacol 1998; 20:153-162.
129. Matsuda H, Tewtrakul S, Morikawa T et al. Anti-allergic principles from Thai zedoary: structural requirements of curcuminoids for inhibition of degranulation and effect on the release of TNF-alpha and IL-4 in RBL-2H3 cells. Bioorg Med Chem 2004; 12:5891-5898.
130. Lee SH, Seo GS, Sohn DH. Inhibition of lipopolysaccharide-induced expression of inducible nitric oxide synthase by butein in RAW 264.7 cells. Biochem Biophys Res Commun 2004; 323:125-132.

131. Lee JH, Jung HS, Giang PM et al. Blockade of nuclear factor-kappaB signaling pathway and anti-inflammatory activity of cardamomin, a chalcone analog from Alpinia conchigera. J Pharmacol Exp Ther 2006; 316:271-278.
132. Chan MM. Inhibition of tumor necrosis factor by curcumin, a phytochemical. Biochem Pharmacol 1995; 49:1551-1556.
133. Shishodia S, Amin HM, Lai R et al. Curcumin (diferuloylmethane) inhibits constitutive NF-kappaB activation, induces G1/S arrest, suppresses proliferation and induces apoptosis in mantle cell lymphoma. Biochem Pharmacol 2005; 70:700-713.
134. Gao M, Zhang J, Liu G. Effect of diphenyl dimethyl bicarboxylate on concanavalin A-induced liver injury in mice. Liver Int 2005; 25:904-912.
135. Kuo YC, Tsai WJ, Meng HC et al. Immune reponses in human mesangial cells regulated by emodin from Polygonum hypoleucum Ohwi. Life Sci 2001; 68:1271-1286.
136. Matsunaga K, Klein TW, Friedman H et al. Epigallocatechin gallate, a potential immunomodulatory agent of tea components, diminishes cigarette smoke condensate-induced suppression of antiLegionella pneumophila activity and cytokine responses of alveolar macrophages. Clin Diagn Lab Immunol 2002; 9:864-871.
137. Lin AH, Fang SX, Fang JG et al. [Studies on anti-endotoxin activity of F022 from Radix Isatidis]. Zhongguo Zhong Yao Za Zhi 2002; 27:439-442.
138. Nie ZG, Peng SY, Wang WJ. [Effects of ginkgolide B on lipopolysaccharide-induced TNF-alpha production in mouse peritoneal macrophages and NF-kappaB activation in rat pleural polymorphonuclear leukocytes]. Yao Xue Xue Bao 2004; 39:415-418.
139. Wadsworth TL, McDonald TL, Koop DR. Effects of Ginkgo biloba extract (EGb 761) and quercetin on lipopolysaccharide-induced signaling pathways involved in the release of tumor necrosis factor-alpha. Biochem Pharmacol 2001; 62:963-974.
140. Abuarqoub H, Foresti R, Green CJ et al. Heme oxygenase-1 mediates the anti-inflammatory actions of 2'-hydroxychalcone in RAW 264.7 murine macrophages. Am J Physiol Cell Physiol 2006; 290: C1092-1099.
141. Ban HS, Suzuki K, Lim SS et al. Inhibition of lipopolysaccharide-induced expression of inducible nitric oxide synthase and tumor necrosis factor-alpha by 2'-hydroxychalcone derivatives in RAW 264.7 cells. Biochem Pharmacol 2004; 67:1549-1557.
142. Ojo-Amaize EA, Kapahi P, Kakkanaiah VN et al. Hypoestoxide, a novel anti-inflammatory natural diterpene, inhibits the activity of IkappaB kinase. Cell Immunol 2001; 209:149-157.
143. Kang OH, Choi YA, Park HJ et al. Inhibition of trypsin-induced mastcell activation by water fraction of Lonicera japonica. Arch Pharm Res 2004; 27:1141-1146.
144. Cho JY, Park J, Yoo ES et al. Inhibitory effect of lignans from the rhizomes of Coptis japonica var. dissecta on tumor necrosis factor-alpha production in lipopolysaccharide-stimulated RAW264.7 cells. Arch Pharm Res 1998; 21:12-16.
145. Ju HK, Moon TC, Lee E et al. Inhibitory effects of a new iridoid, patridoid II and its isomers, on nitric oxide and TNF-alpha production in cultured murine macrophages. Planta Med 2003; 69:950-953.
146. Liu L, Ning ZQ, Shan S et al. Phthalide Lactones from Ligusticum chuanxiong inhibit lipopolysaccharide-induced TNF-alpha production and TNF-alpha-mediated NF-kappaB Activation. Planta Med 2005; 71:808-813.
147. Ishii R, Horie M, Saito K et al. Inhibition of lipopolysaccharide-induced pro-inflammatory cytokine expression via suppression of nuclear factor-kappaB activation by Mallotus japonicus phloroglucinol derivatives. Biochim Biophys Acta 2003; 1620:108-118.
148. Wang C, Schuller Levis GB, Lee EB et al. Platycodin D and D3 isolated from the root of Platycodon grandiflorum modulate the production of nitric oxide and secretion of TNF-alpha in activated RAW 264.7 cells. Int Immunopharmacol 2004; 4:1039-1049.
149. Punzon C, Alcaide A, Fresno M. In vitro anti-inflammatory activity of Phlebodium decumanum. Modulation of tumor necrosis factor and soluble TNF receptors. Int Immunopharmacol 2003; 3:1293-1299.
150. Kiemer AK, Hartung T, Huber C et al. Phyllanthus amarus has anti-inflammatory potential by inhibition of iNOS, COX-2 and cytokines via the NF-kappaB pathway. J Hepatol 2003; 38:289-297.
151. Bi XL, Yang JY, Dong YX et al. Resveratrol inhibits nitric oxide and TNF-alpha production by lipopolysaccharide-activated microglia. Int Immunopharmacol 2005; 5:185-193.
152. Perrone A, Plaza A, Ercolino SF et al. 14,15-secopregnane derivatives from the leaves of Solenostemma argel. J Nat Prod 2006; 69:50-54.
153. Zi X, Mukhtar H, Agarwal R. Novel cancer chemopreventive effects of a flavonoid antioxidant silymarin: inhibition of mRNA expression of an endogenous tumor promoter TNF-alpha. Biochem Biophys Res Commun 1997; 239:334-339.

154. Abad MJ, Bermejo P, Alvarez M et al. Flavonoids and a sesquiterpene lactone from Tanacetum micro-phyllum inhibit anti-inflammatory mediators in LPS-stimulated mouse peritoneal macrophages. Planta Med 2004; 70:34-38.
155. Kim HM, Shin HY, Lim KH et al. Taraxacum officinale inhibits tumor necrosis factor-alpha production from rat astrocytes. Immunopharmacol Immunotoxicol 2000; 22:519-530.
156. Verhoeckx KC, Korthout HA, van Meeteren-Kreikamp AP et al. Unheated Cannabis sativa extracts and its major compound THC-acid have potential immuno-modulating properties not mediated by CB1 and CB2 receptor coupled pathways. Int Immunopharmacol 2006; 6:656-665.
157. Ramiro E, Franch A, Castellote C et al. Effect of Theobroma cacao flavonoids on immune activation of a lymphoid cell line. Br J Nutr 2005; 93:859-866.
158. Piscoya J, Rodriguez Z, Bustamante SA et al. Efficacy and safety of freeze-dried cat's claw in osteoarthritis of the knee: mechanisms of action of the species Uncaria guianensis. Inflamm Res 2001; 50:442-448.
159. Hua KF, Hsu HY, Su YC et al. Study on the antiinflammatory activity of methanol extract from seagrass Zostera japonica. J Agric Food Chem 2006; 54:306-311.

CHAPTER 4

Targeting of BAFF and APRIL for Autoimmunity and Oncology

Maureen C. Ryan* and Iqbal S. Grewal

Abstract

BLyS and APRIL are tumor necrosis factor superfamily members shown to be important for B-cell development, maturation and survival. Recent data also indicate that these cytokines regulate the survival and maintenance of malignant B-cells in cancer patients. The key role of BLyS/APRIL in the immune system and their potential role in cancers have attracted the attention of basic scientists and biotechnology companies alike. As a result, the pathways regulated by BLyS and APRIL have been quickly elevated as attractive targets for antibody-based and non-antibody based therapeutics. Exploitation of these pathways has not only given us enormous insights into the basic biology of the APRIL/BLyS system but it has also identified potential clinical candidates for cancer and autoimmunity. As such, multiple biotechnology companies are currently testing various therapeutic candidates in the clinic. This chapter will review BLyS and APRIL functions and discuss alternative therapeutic approaches to target BLyS and APRIL pathways for human malignancies and autoimmunity.

Introduction

B-cell activating factor (BAFF)[1-4] and a proliferation inducing ligand (APRIL)[5] are TNF ligands that regulate immune function, tolerance and malignancy. BAFF, also called BLyS,[1] TALL-1[4] and THANK,[2] is a costimulatory factor for normal B-cells and plays a vital role in B-cell homeostasis. BAFF's closest relative amongst the TNF superfamily is APRIL. APRIL was originally noted for its ability to stimulate proliferation of tumor cells.[5,6] A functional relationship between BAFF and APRIL became apparent when it was shown that APRIL regulates tumor cell proliferation[6] and humoral immunity[28] by binding to some of the same TNF receptors as BAFF. Thus, while BAFF and APRIL act as essential regulators of normal T- and B-cell function, they also have the potential to be permissive in autoimmunity and cancer. This chapter will review the biology behind an emerging class of therapeutics aimed at targeting BAFF and APRIL for immunology and oncology.

The BAFF and APRIL Receptor/Ligand System

BAFF and APRIL are type II transmembrane proteins produced by monocytes,[1,8] macrophages,[4] neutrophils,[9] dendritic cells[10] and T-cells.[3,7] Elevated expression and release of these factors is often stimulated by pro-inflammatory cytokines.[1,8-11] BAFF and APRIL can also be expressed by nonhematopoietic cells in normal tissue[12] and disease states.[13,14] Remarkably, it is the constitutive expression of BAFF by a radiation-resistant population of nonhematopoietic cells in bone marrow that is essential for the maintenance of peripheral B-cells in mice.[12]

*Corresponding Author: Maureen C. Ryan—Seattle Genetics, Inc. 21823—30th Drive SE Bothell, WA 98021. Email: mryan@seagen.com

Therapeutic Targets of the TNF Superfamily, edited by Iqbal S. Grewal.
©2009Landes Bioscience and Springer Science+Business Media.

BAFF and APRIL both contain a multibasic consensus motif that is proteolytically cleaved to generate a soluble, active form of the ligand. Although APRIL and BAFF are typically expressed as homotrimers, biologically active heterotrimers have been reported in the serum samples of patients with systemic immune-based rheumatic diseases.[15] APRIL is processed intracellularly by a furin convertase and is solely active in a soluble form.[16] A possible exception occurs when APRIL is expressed as TWE-PRIL.[17,18] TWE-PRIL is a hybrid transcript that combines a TWEAK intracellular, transmembrane and stalk region with an APRIL receptor-binding domain. The function of this unique hybrid transcript is unknown but it potentially enables the receptor-binding domain of APRIL to be presented in a membrane-associated form. BAFF can exist as a membrane bound or secreted form and is reported to have activity in either form.[8] BAFF activity can be modulated by the production of ΔBAFF.[19] ΔBAFF is an alternative splice variant that is uncleavable and leads to the formation of multimeric BAFF complexes with diminished biologic activity in vitro an in vivo.[19,20]

BAFF binds three distinct TNF receptors (see Fig. 1): B-cell maturation antigen (BCMA),[21,22] transmembrane activator and calcium-modulator and cyclophilin ligand interactor (TACI)[22] and BAFF receptor (BAFF-R),[23-26] also known as BR3.[36] APRIL, in contrast, binds to TACI and BCMA[6,21,27,28] but not BAFF-R.[23] BAFF-R, TACI and BCMA each contain a limited number of cysteine-rich domains (CRDs) when compared to other TNF receptors. The extracellular domain of TNF receptors typically contains 4 CRDs for ligand binding.[29] In contrast, BAFF-R, BCMA and TACI contain 1/2, 1 and 2 CRDs, respectively. BAFF-R, BCMA and TACI also lack the death domain that is prevalent in many TNF receptors and instead transduce signals through the TRAF family of adaptor proteins.[30] Pro-survival signals proceed through NFκB using either the canonical or alternative pathways.[59]

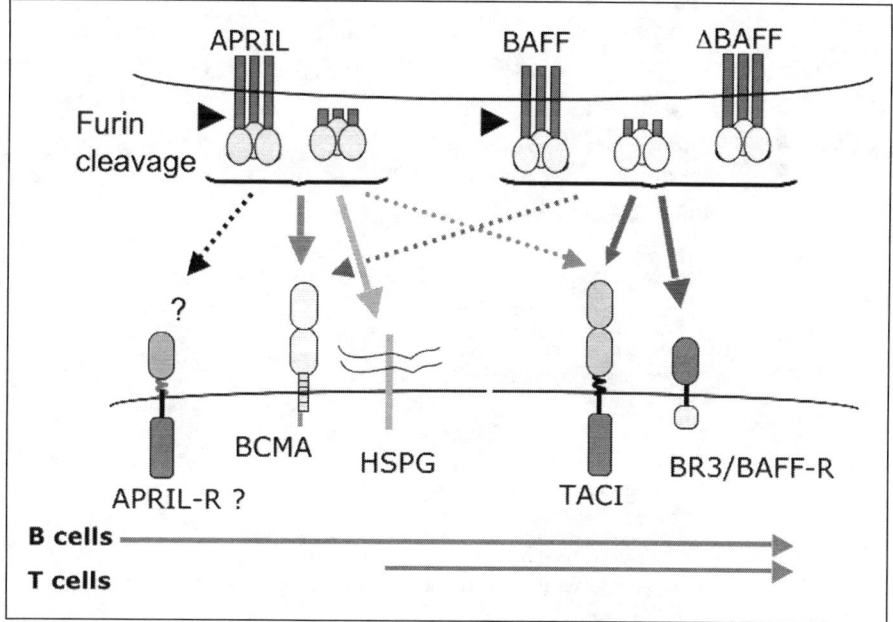

Figure 1. APRIL and BAFF bind to multiple receptors. Solid lines depict primary receptors for APRIL and BAFF and doted lines indicate low affinity alternative receptors. Both APRIL and BAFF exist in soluble and membrane expressed forms. ΔBAFF is a membrane expressed without Furin Cleavage site. APRIL is also suspected to have a yet unknown receptor, which is depicted as APRIL-R. All receptors are predominantly expressed on B- and T-cells as indicated in the figure.

Interestingly, APRIL was noted to support proliferation of tumor cells that lack expression of either TACI or BCMA. This observation lead to the prediction that there is a third APRIL receptor.[6] Recently, heparin sulphate proteoglycans (HSPGs) were identified as a nonTNF binding moiety for APRIL.[31,32] The HSPG binding domain in APRIL occurs within a stretch of basic amino acid residues that are not present in BAFF, conferring a unique binding interaction between APRIL and HSPGs.[31] Although HSPGs are prevalent on a wide variety of normal and malignant cells, the biological significance of APRIL interaction with HSPGs remains unknown. It is speculated, however, that HSPGs may augment APRIL function through oligomerization of the ligand or by retaining the ligand in the bone marrow microenvironment.[31]

BAFF and APRIL Regulate Immune Functions

Early studies on BAFF and APRIL showed that these ligands are key regulators of immune function.[7,21,26,28] The precise roles and dominant contributions of each ligand were discovered through in vivo models that examined over-expression or deficiency of BAFF, APRIL and their receptors (Table 1). Additionally, the contribution of individual receptor/ligand interactions has been resolved through the use of targeting molecules that neutralize or antagonize ligand function (Table 2). These

Table 1. Mouse models to examine BlyS, APRIL, BAFF-R, TACI and BCMA function

Deficiency or Over-Expression of BAFF, APRIL and Their Receptors

Gene Symbol/ Protein	Phenotype	Ref.
BAFF(-/-)	Severe ↓ mature follicular and marginal zone B-lymphocytes Blockade at T1 to T2 cell transition	24
A/WySnJ	↓ Mature follicular and marginal zone B cells	24,36
APRIL(-/-)	Impaired IgA class switching Normal immune system development	51,52
TACI(-/-)	B-cell accumulation and splenomegaly	38
BCMA(-/-)	Normal B-cell development and homeostasis No defects in humoral immunity Impaired long-term survival of plasma cells	24,106 40
BAFF Transgenic	B-cell hyperplasia Enlarged spleen, lymph nodes and Peyers patches ↑ B220+ cells ↓ T-cells (Thy-1.2 positive, CD4 and CD8) Hypergammaglobulinemia Autoantibodies to nuclear antigens Immune complexes in kidney	22,55
APRIL Transgenic	Enhanced survival of transgenic T-cells in vitro Enhanced survival of staphylococcal enterotoxin B-reactive CD4t T cells in vivo Increased IgM but not IgG response to T-cell dependent antigens	7
BAFF-Tg in TNF(-/-) back-ground	Autoimmunity with predisposition of B-cell lymphoma Expansion of T2 and marginal zone B-cells Enhanced T-independent immune responses ↑ B-cell lymphomas	64

studies clearly establish that BAFF regulates development and homeostasis of B-cells following their exit from the bone marrow.[23,24] In particular, BAFF supports the survival of splenic immature transitional B-cells and mature B-cells. Consistently, targeted disruption of BAFF in mice results in impaired differentiation at the transitional type 1 stage and a substantial loss of follicular and marginal zone B-cells.[24] Blockade at the T1 to T2 transition may be a direct effect on B-cell differentiation or an indirect effect related to the survival function of BAFF. Over-expression of Bcl-2 can partially compensate for loss of BAFF signaling but does not rescue all B-cell defects, suggesting that B-cell defects in BAFF-deficient mice are not exclusively due to loss of survival signals.[33] BAFF deficient mice also have decreased serum immunoglobulin levels and an impaired antibody response to T-cell dependent antigens.[24] Concordantly, neutralization of BAFF through the use of soluble receptor decoys blocks the T1 to T2 transition of B-cells,[34] inhibits antigen-specific antibody production,[26] abolishes splenic germinal center (GC) formation[26] and decreases the number of peripheral B-cells.[35] BAFF-R is the major receptor mediating BAFF-dependent survival of B-cells because A/WySnJ mice, which have a natural mutation in the BAFF-R locus, display a phenotype that is qualitatively similar to BAFF-deficient mice.[23,36] Interestingly, APRIL does not substitute for BAFF despite historic data showing that APRIL can stimulate in vivo expansion of B-cells.[28] Likewise, the presence of TACI or BCMA does not compensate for loss of BAFF-R during peripheral B-cell development. On the contrary, TACI acts as a negative regulator of B-cell expansion[37,38] while BCMA appears to have a unique role in regulating the survival of terminally differentiated plasma cells.[39,40] The BCMA-dependent survival of plasmablasts and plasma cells can be supported by either BAFF or APRIL. The varied expression of BAFF-R, TACI and BCMA throughout B-cell ontogeny is consistent with the unique functional roles of these receptors on B-cells.[41,42]

BAFF and its receptors are routinely highlighted for their dominant role in B-cell homeostasis. However, BAFF-R[43] and TACI[44] are also expressed by activated T-cells and they can modulate T-cell function. BAFF costimulation of activated CD4+ T-cells mediates allo-proliferation in vivo through BAFF-R.[43,45] Mice that are deficient for BAFF or BAFF-R show prolonged cardiac allograft survival when compared to controls.[43] Moreover, BAFF transgenic mice show enhanced Th1-mediated response,[46] suggesting that BAFF can directly or indirectly regulate T-cell function. TACI may also modulate T-cell dependent function. In a mouse model for rheumatoid arthritis (RA), an autoimmune disease that involves both B- and T-cell components, TACI-Fc treatment substantially inhibited inflammation, and bone and cartilage destruction.[47]

Table 2. *Potential contribution of individual receptors to B-cell biology and candidate targeting molecules*

Receptor	Key Function	Potential Targeting Molecule
BAFF-R/BR3	B-cell survival; Plasma cell survival; T-cell costimulation; T-dependent Ab production; Germinal center formation; Ig class switching (IgG, IgE)	TACI-Ig BR3-Ig Anti-BAFF Ab Anti-BR3 Ab
TACI	T-dependent Ab production Germinal center formation Ig class switching (IgG, IgE, IgA) T-independent responses B1 B-cell survival	TACI-Ig BR3-Ig BCMA-Ig Anti-BAFF Ab Anti-TACI Ab
BCMA	Plasma cell survival	TACI-Ig BR3-Ig BCMA-Ig Anti-BLyS Ab Anti-BCMA Ab
HGPS	Unknown	Anti-APRIL Ab

Mice transgenic for APRIL under control of a T-cell-specific promoter display altered T- and B-cell mediated functions[7] (Table 1). The heightened humoral response to T-cell dependent antigens observed in APRIL transgenic mice agrees with recent in vitro data showing that APRIL can promote antigen presentation in B-cells through BCMA.[48] APRIL transgenic mice also showed enhanced T-cell survival in vitro and a significant increase in a rare population of T-cells that are distinct from classically activated T-cells.[7] APRIL transgenic mice also develop lymphoid tumors that originate from expansion of the peritoneal B-1 B-cell population.[49] Overall, however, the in vivo function of APRIL in normal tissues has remained a bit more elusive when compared to BAFF. The ambiguity is due in part to disparate results from APRIL ($-/-$) mice.[50, 51] The disparity may be due to different background strains used to create APRIL deficient mice. One group reported that APRIL ($-/-$) mice have typical T- and B-cell development and normal humoral response to antigen challenge.[51] A second group observed concurrent normal T- and B-cell development in APRIL ($-/-$) mice but also detected increased numbers of CD44high/CD62low effector memory T-cells, increased IgG response to T-cell-dependent antibody responses and impaired IgA class switching.[50] In vitro studies on B-cells support a role for APRIL and BAFF in class switching.[52] Class switching via APRIL is mediated by TACI whereas BAFF can promote class switch in B-cells by either TACI or BAFF-R.[52] Mutations in TACI that impair interactions with APRIL have also been implicated in combined variable immunodeficiency (CVID) and selective IgA deficiency in humans.[53,54]

BAFF and APRIL in Autoimmunity

B-cell numbers and humoral immunity can be heightened or dampened by modulating the levels of available BAFF or APRIL. BAFF levels, in particular, must be carefully regulated to maintain B-cell homeostasis. Systemic administration of soluble BAFF in mice causes B-cell expansion and increased levels of serum IgM and IgA.[1] A similar but augmented B-cell response occurs in BAFF transgenic mice,[22,55,56] which is characterized by B-cell hyperplasia, hypergammaglobulinemia, the presence of circulating autoantibodies and formation of immune complexes. As BAFF transgenic mice age, the hyperimmune phenotype culminates into a condition that resembles human systemic lupus erythematosus (SLE)[22,55-57] and Sjögren's syndrome.[57] Similarly, NZB/W(F1) and MRL-lpr/lpr mouse strains that are predisposed to SLE or mice with chemically-induced autoimmunity show heightened levels of BAFF with the onset and progression of disease.[22,58] Treatment of lupus-prone NZB/W(F1) mice with soluble receptor decoys, such as BR3-Fc or TACI-Ig, blocks BAFF-dependent signaling,[59] attenuates disease[59] and prolongs survival of the animals.[22]

In the human population, BAFF and APRIL are frequently elevated in the serum and target organs of patients with a variety of autimmune disorders.[60-63] Increased BAFF levels are associated with pathogenic antibodies in patients with SLE, suggesting that BAFF may contribute to loss of B-cell tolerance in some autoimmune patients.[60,61,63] A role for BAFF in tolerance is supported by in vivo studies showing that BAFF allows survival of immature, transitional type 2 cells in spleen that would otherwise be removed by negative selection.[64] In agreement with this notion, escape of marginal zone B-cells is observed in BAFF-transgenic mice where they home to salivary glands and contribute to the autoimmune phenotype.[57]

Examination of APRIL levels in SLE patients has led to conflicting results.[65,66] One group examined 40 patients with SLE and found a positive correlation between anti-DNA antibodies and APRIL levels.[65] A second group examined 68 patients and found APRIL levels were inversely correlated with disease activity in SLE.[66] Additional studies will be required to elucidate the significance of APRIL in autoimmunity. However, a connection between APRIL and SLE has been identified at the genetic level[67] with three polymorphisms in the gene for APRIL showing association with autoimmunity.

BAFF and APRIL are elevated in rheumatoid arthritis (RA), with significantly higher levels in the synovial fluid than in the serum.[63,68] Lymphocytes that infiltrate into the joints of RA patients can remain diffuse or they can take on an architecture that is reminiscent of a lymphoid follicle.[69] Examination of APRIL and BAFF in the inflamed joints of RA patients showed expression of these ligands varied with distinct lymphoid architectures. APRIL was present at the highest levels in germinal-centre-positive synovitis whereas BAFF was present at similar levels independent of lymphoid architecture. Importantly, the authors found that inhibition of BAFF/APRIL by TACI-Ig was most effective in mice transplanted with human tissues with germinal-center-positive synovitis. It was noted that the differential effects they observed correlated with the presence of TACI+ T-cells in the other two forms of synovitis.[70] In previous studies that used a mouse model for rheumatoid arthritis (RA), treatment with TACI-Fc substantially inhibited inflammation, bone and cartilage destruction and disease development.[34,47] Taken together, these studies suggest that inhibition of BAFF and APRIL might have therapeutic benefits for autoimmune diseases, such as RA, that involve both B- and T-cells.

APRIL and BAFF in Cancer

APRIL and BAFF are potential survival factors for B-cell malignancies including chronic lymphocytic leukemia (B-CLL),[71,72] Hodgkin's lymphoma,[73] nonHodgkins lymphoma (NHL)[74-76] and multiple myeloma (MM).[77,78] This hypothesis is supported by the expression of one or more of the receptors for BAFF and APRIL on malignant B-cells, which generally correlates with the developmental origin of the tumor cell.[41] Malignancies derived from mature B-cells typically show prevalent expression of BAFF-R and TACI while plasma cell malignancies frequently express BCMA. The pro-survival ligands, BAFF and APRIL, can be expressed by the tumor cell itself[49,79] or by a neighboring cell in the tumor microenvironment.[13,80] Autocrine production of BAFF and APRIL have been detected in B-CLL cells where it is believed to protect these cells against spontaneous and drug-induced apoptosis.[49,79] Likewise, paracrine ligand production has been illustrated in a subset of NHL patients where the major source of APRIL concentrated at the tumor lesion is derived from neutrophils and correlates with decreased overall patient survival.[81] Hence, BAFF and APRIL can function as both autocrine and paracrine factors to promote tumor cell survival, thereby protecting tumor cells from death. Numerous studies confirm that BAFF and APRIL can also augment tumor cell growth by either stimulating proliferation,[73,78,82] inhibiting apoptosis,[72,73,76] or protecting malignant cells against drug-induced apoptosis.[79] The pro-survival role of BAFF and APRIL coupled with the prevalence of BAFF, APRIL and their receptors on malignant B-cells suggested that blockade of this pathway is a plausible therapeutic strategy for oncology. As predicted, in vitro studies consistently show that treatment of tumor cells with soluble receptor decoys attenuates tumor cell survival in a variety of malignant B-cells.[71,73,76,77,79,80] Alternatively, BAFF and APRIL receptors expressed on the surface of malignant B-cells can be targeted for antibody directed cytotoxicity[83] or delivery of potent cytotoxic drugs.[83-85]

Detection of APRIL in a variety of solid tumors[5,86] suggests that this ligand may regulate proliferation of solid tumors as well as B-cell malignancies. In agreement with this notion, transfection of APRIL into NIH3T3 cells stimulates their proliferation in vivo and in vitro,[5] showing that APRIL can regulate proliferation of transformed cells.[5] Likewise, APRIL-mediated stimulation of carcinoma cells in vivo is indicated by studies showing that blockade of APRIL binding by BCMA-Fc inhibits growth of HT29 cells in nude mice.[6]

Parallels between Autoimmunity and Cancer

Altered expression and function of BAFF and APRIL have identified connections between autoimmunity and cancer. Compelling data from in vivo animal models shows that transgenic expression of either BAFF or APRIL heightens immune response and predisposes mice to B-cell lymphomas. APRIL transgenic mice develop lymphoid tumors with significant frequency by 9- to 12-months of age. Tumors originate from expansion of the peritoneal B-1a B-cell population, reminiscent of human B-CLL, thereby solidifying a connection to human biology.[49] While aging BAFF transgenic mice show only a slight increase in the incidence of B-cell lymphomas, the frequency becomes elevated in the context of a TNF null background, escalating to an incidence of 33% by the first year.[64] Humans with autoimmunity are also at increased risk of developing lymphomas,[87] underscoring the need for effective therapeutic strategies that target the BAFF and APRIL subfamily.

New Therapeutics for Autoimmunity and Cancer

Several companies are developing therapeutics to target BAFF and APRIL (Table 3). GlaxoSmithKline (Brentford, London, UK) and Human Genome Sciences (Rockville, MD, USA) have developed LymphoStat-B®, also known as belimumab, which is a fully human IgG1 monoclonal antibody that targets BAFF.[88] Belimumab binds with high affinity to BAFF and blocks binding of BAFF to its receptors, BCMA, TACI and BAFF-R. Since belimumab binds specifically to the soluble, active form of BAFF rather than the membrane associated form, it should not induce ADCC. Belimumab inhibits BAFF mediated proliferation of B-cells in vitro and blocks the in vivo expansion of B-cells in mice following administration of recombinant human BAFF.[88] Phase II clinical trials on belimumab for efficacy in SLE[90-92] and RA[93,94] were completed in June of 2006. Belimumab showed statistically significant reduction in disease activity for RA patients and it reduced disease activity in patients with serologically active SLE (www.hgsi.com/products/LSB.html). In addition, Human Genome Science has a patent (US 7,189,820) claiming some antibodies against APRIL, representing yet another potential strategy to target this TNF subfamily.

Genentech, Inc. (South San Francisco, CA, USA) and Biogen Idec (Cambridge, MA, USA) are codeveloping BR3-Fc as a soluble BAFF antagonist[59,95] for the treatment of RA and SLE. The results of phase I clinical trials are yet to be reported. However, BR3-Fc was effective at significantly reducing B-cells from peripheral blood and lymphoid tissue in nonhuman primates, including the marginal zone B-cells.[96] The reduction of marginal zone B-cells has potential therapeutic significance because the marginal zone B-cells have been implicated in human autoimmunity.[64] BR3-Fc also has the potential to be synergistic with rituximab, Genentech's anti-CD20 B-cell depleting antibody. Rituximab is approved for treatment of rheumatoid arthritis. In preclinical studies with mice, blockade of BAFF signaling with BR3-Fc synergized with anti-CD20 antibodies resulting in more complete B-cell depletion.[97] Given that BAFF levels can be elevated in response to B-cell depletion, neutralization of BAFF may be critical to block the survival of nondepleted B-cells. In addition, Genentech and Biogen Idec are exploring the development of an antagonistic antibody against BAFF-R or BR3.[98] An antagonistic BR3 antibody would be dual functional, combining blockade of BAFF signaling with B- cell depletion in a single therapeutic reagent. Recently, B-cell depletion was compared in mice and nonhuman primates using the three prospective therapeutic agents: anti-BR3, BR3-Fc and anti-CD20.[98] While anti-BR3 achieved impressive B-cell depletion in mice, these findings did not translate into nonhuman primates.[98] Genentech has also created a BCMA-Ig that binds APRIL but not BAFF.[99] Although this potential therapeutic is not in

Table 3. Molecules in development to target BAFF/APRIL

Company	Target Ligand/Receptor	Candidate	Mechanism of Action	Status and Indication
Human Geneome Sciences	BAFF	Anti-BAFF	Blocking BAFF binding to its receptors	PhaseII/III SLE
Genentech	BAFF	BR3-Ig	Blocking BAFF binding to its receptors	Phase I
Amgen	BAFF	AMG 623	Blocking BAFF binding to its receptors	Phase II SLE
Genentech	BR3	Anti-BR3 Ab	Blocking BAFF binding to BR3/BAFF-R	Phase I CLL
Zymogenetics	BAFF/APRIL	TACI-Ig	Blocking both BAFF and APRIL binding to their receptors	Phase II SLE
Human Genome Sciences	BCMA/TACI/BR3	BAFF-radio-conjugate	Inducing cytotoxicity in cells positive for BAFF receptors	Phase I NHL

clinical trials, it represents a novel strategy to target APRIL without impacting BAFF-dependent signaling.

Zymogenetics, Inc. (Seattle, WA, USA) and Merck Serono International, S.A. (Geneva, Switzerland) are codeveloping TACI-Ig, also called Atacicept, for autoimmunity and B-cell malignancies. In contrast to BR3-Fc, which exclusively neutralizes BAFF, TACI-Ig can neutralize both BAFF and APRIL.[34] In addition, TACI-Ig neutralizes BAFF/APRIL heterotrimers, providing a potential advantage for systemic immune-based rheumatoid disease.[15] TACI-Ig is in Phase I clinical trials for SLE,[100] RA[101] and B-CLL[102] and thus far, appears to be well-tolerated (www.zymogenetics.com/clinical/TACI-Ig.html). RA patients treated with Atacicept showed a reduction in circulating Igs, decreased peripheral B-cells and positive trends in scores for disease activity, suggesting that Atacicept has the potential to improve disease in RA.

Finally, Amgen Inc. (Thousand Oaks, CA USA) has recently completed Phase I clinical studies for AMG 623 in SLE patients. AMG 623 is an Fc-peptide fusion protein or a "peptibody" that has the potential to inhibit B-cell maturation and survival by functioning as a BAFF antagonist.

Future Applications, New Research, Anticipated Developments

Rituximab, an anti-CD20 B-cell depleting monoclonal antibody, is efficacious for treatment of NHL and is now approved for RA based on successful clinical trials. However, the incomplete B-cell depletion observed with rituximab and an inability to modulate B-cell signaling intensifies the need to improve B-cell-based therapies for oncology and immunology. BAFF, APRIL and their receptors represent an alternative and potentially complementary path to target B-cells and modulate immune function. Neutralizing BAFF and APRIL in preclinical studies bodes well for the utility of targeting this TNF subfamily but efficacy in humans awaits the outcome of ongoing clinical trials. Key issues that remain unresolved are the possible immunosuppressive effects caused by prolonged depletion of vital B-cell subsets and safety concerns resulting from disruption of T-cell mediated functions. Also unknown is the required level of selectivity or the best therapeutic moiety to neutralize BAFF and APRIL function. TACI-Ig can neutralize BAFF and APRIL whereas BAFF-R-Ig or anti-BAFF will selectively target BAFF. All of these prospective therapeutic molecules can impact cells that express BAFF-R, TACI or BCMA but the biological effects of antagonizing BAFF, APRIL or a combination thereof, has yet to be studied within the context of the human immune system. A comparison of BAFF-R-Ig and TACI-Ig in a mouse model of lupus showed that both molecules can prolong the survival of SLE mice but only TACI-Ig resulted in depletion of IgM-secreting plasma cells in the spleen and bone marrow.[103] If this observation translates to humans then TACI-Ig may be the desirable therapeutic for autoimmune indications when IgM autoantibodies are present. Moreover, understanding which autoimmune patients will benefit from a neutralizing agent may depend on whether the ligand is a facilitator or contributor to the disease process[61] and whether the corresponding receptor is in the prebound state.[104] Recent data showing that BAFF-R on blood B-cells in SLE is consistently occupied suggests that therapeutic strategies for SLE may require overcoming the persistent binding of BAFF to BAFF-R.[104]

In summary, the pivotal role of BAFF and APRIL in cell survival and immune regulation has drawn considerable interest in these molecules as prospective therapeutic targets.[42,105] As strategies to modulate or deplete B-cells take center stage, BAFF- and APRIL-based targeting molecules will remain a fertile area of development to address unmet clinical needs in oncology and immunology.

References
1. Moore PA, Belvedere O, Orr A et al. BLyS: member of the tumor necrosis factor family and B-lymphocyte stimulator. Science 1999; 285:260-263.
2. Mukhopadhyay A, Ni J, Zhai Y et al. Identification and characterization of a novel cytokine, THANK, a TNF homologue that activates apoptosis, nuclear factor-kappaB and c-Jun NH2-terminal kinase. J Biol Chem 1999; 274:15978-15981.
3. Schneider P, MacKay F, Steiner V et al. BAFF, a novel ligand of the tumor necrosis factor family, stimulates B-cell growth. J Exp Med 1999; 189:1747-1756.

4. Shu HB, Hu WH, Johnson H. TALL-1 is a novel member of the TNF family that is down-regulated by mitogens. J Leukoc Biol 1999; 65:680-683.
5. Hahne M, Kataoka T, Schroter M et al. APRIL, a new ligand of the tumor necrosis factor family, stimulates tumor cell growth. J Exp Med 1998; 188:1185-1190.
6. Rennert P, Schneider P, Cachero TG et al. A soluble form of B-cell maturation antigen, a receptor for the tumor necrosis factor family member APRIL, inhibits tumor cell growth. J Exp Med 2000; 192:1677-1684.
7. Stein JV, Lopez-Fraga M, Elustondo FA et al. APRIL modulates B- and T-cell immunity. J Clin Invest 2002; 109:1587-1598.
8. Nardelli B, Belvedere O, Roschke V et al. Synthesis and release of B-lymphocyte stimulator from myeloid cells. Blood 2001; 97:198-204.
9. Scapini P, Nardelli B, Nadali G et al. G-CSF-stimulated neutrophils are a prominent source of functional BLyS. J Exp Med 2003; 197:297-302.
10. Litinskiy MB, Nardelli B, Hilbert DM et al. DCs induce CD40-independent immunoglobulin class switching through BLyS and APRIL. Nat Immunol 2002; 3:822-829.
11. Scapini P, Carletto A, Nardelli B et al. Proinflammatory mediators elicit secretion of the intracellular B-lymphocyte stimulator pool (BLyS) that is stored in activated neutrophils: implications for inflammatory diseases. Blood 2005; 105:830-837.
12. Gorelik L, Gilbride K, Dobles M et al. Normal B-cell homeostasis requires B-cell activation factor production by radiation-resistant cells. J Exp Med 2003; 198:937-945.
13. Moreaux J, Cremer FW, Reme T et al. The level of TACI gene expression in myeloma cells is associated with a signature of microenvironment dependence versus a plasmablastic signature. Blood 2005; 106:1021-1030.
14. Ohata J, Zvaifler NJ, Nishio M et al. Fibroblast-like synoviocytes of mesenchymal origin express functional B-cell-activating factor of the TNF family in response to proinflammatory cytokines. J Immunol 2005; 174:864-870.
15. Roschke V, Sosnovtseva S, Ward CD et al. BLyS and APRIL form biologically active heterotrimers that are expressed in patients with systemic immune-based rheumatic diseases. J Immunol 2002; 169:4314-4321.
16. Lopez-Fraga M, Fernandez R, Albar JP et al. Biologically active APRIL is secreted following intracellular processing in the Golgi apparatus by furin convertase. EMBO Rep 2001; 2:945-951.
17. Kolfschoten GM, Pradet-Balade B, Hahne M et al. TWE-PRIL; a fusion protein of TWEAK and APRIL. Biochem Pharmacol 2003; 66:1427-1432.
18. Pradet-Balade B, Medema JP, Lopez-Fraga M et al. An endogenous hybrid mRNA encodes TWE-PRIL, a functional cell surface TWEAK-APRIL fusion protein. EMBO J 2002; 21:5711-5720.
19. Gavin AL, Ait-Azzouzene D, Ware CF et al. DeltaBAFF, an alternate splice isoform that regulates receptor binding and biopresentation of the B-cell survival cytokine, BAFF. J Biol Chem 2003; 278:38220-38228.
20. Gavin AL, Duong B, Skog P et al. DeltaBAFF, a splice isoform of BAFF, opposes full-length BAFF activity in vivo in transgenic mouse models. J Immunol 2005; 175:319-328.
21. Marsters SA, Yan M, Pitti RM et al. Interaction of the TNF homologues BLyS and APRIL with the TNF receptor homologues BCMA and TACI. Curr Biol 2000; 10:785-788.
22. Gross JA, Johnston J, Mudri S et al. TACI and BCMA are receptors for a TNF homologue implicated in B-cell autoimmune disease. Nature 2000; 404:995-999.
23. Thompson JS, Bixler SA, Qian F et al. BAFF-R, a newly identified TNF receptor that specifically interacts with BAFF. Science 2001; 293:2108-2111.
24. Schiemann B, Gommerman JL, Vora K et al. An essential role for BAFF in the normal development of B-cells through a BCMA-independent pathway. Science 2001; 293:2111-2114.
25. Schneider P, Takatsuka H, Wilson A et al. Maturation of marginal zone and follicular B-cells requires B-cell activating factor of the tumor necrosis factor family and is independent of B-cell maturation antigen. J Exp Med 2001; 194:1691-1697.
26. Yan M, Marsters SA, Grewal IS et al. Identification of a receptor for BLyS demonstrates a crucial role in humoral immunity. Nat Immunol 2000; 1:37-41.
27. Wu Y, Bressette D, Carrell JA et al. Tumor necrosis factor (TNF) receptor superfamily member TACI is a high affinity receptor for TNF family members APRIL and BLyS. J Biol Chem 2000; 275:35478-35485.
28. Yu G, Boone T, Delaney J et al. APRIL and TALL-I and receptors BCMA and TACI: system for regulating humoral immunity. Nat Immunol 2000; 1:252-256.
29. Locksley RM, Killeen N, Lenardo MJ. The TNF and TNF receptor superfamilies: integrating mammalian biology. Cell 2001; 104:487-501.

30. Mackay F, Silveira PA, Brink R. B-cells and the BAFF/APRIL axis: fast-forward on autoimmunity and signaling. Curr Opin Immunol 2007; 19:327-336.
31. Ingold K, Zumsteg A, Tardivel A et al. Identification of proteoglycans as the APRIL-specific binding partners. J Exp Med 2005; 201:1375-1383.
32. Hendriks J, Planelles L, de Jong-Odding J et al. Heparan sulfate proteoglycan binding promotes APRIL-induced tumor cell proliferation. Cell Death Differ 2005; 12:637-648.
33. Tardivel A, Tinel A, Lens S et al. The anti-apoptotic factor Bcl-2 can functionally substitute for the B-cell survival but not for the marginal zone B-cell differentiation activity of BAFF. Eur J Immunol 2004; 34:509-518.
34. Gross JA, Dillon SR, Mudri S et al. TACI-Ig neutralizes molecules critical for B-cell development and autoimmune disease. Impaired B-cell maturation in mice lacking BLyS. Immunity 2001; 15:289-302.
35. Thompson JS, Schneider P, Kalled SL et al. BAFF binds to the tumor necrosis factor receptor-like molecule B-cell maturation antigen and is important for maintaining the peripheral B-cell population. J Exp Med 2000; 192:129-135.
36. Yan M, Brady JR, Chan B et al. Identification of a novel receptor for B-lymphocyte stimulator that is mutated in a mouse strain with severe B-cell deficiency. Curr Biol 2001; 11:1547-1552.
37. Seshasayee D, Valdez P, Yan M et al. Loss of TACI causes fatal lymphoproliferation and autoimmunity, establishing TACI as an inhibitory BLyS receptor. Immunity 2003; 18:279-288.
38. Yan M, Wang H, Chan B et al. Activation and accumulation of B-cells in TACI-deficient mice. Nat Immunol 2001; 2:638-643.
39. Avery DT, Kalled SL, Ellyard JI et al. BAFF selectively enhances the survival of plasmablasts generated from human memory B-cells. J Clin Invest 2003; 112:286-297.
40. O'Connor BP, Raman VS, Erickson LD et al. BCMA is essential for the survival of long-lived bone marrow plasma cells. J Exp Med 2004; 199:91-98.
41. Jelinek DF, Darce JR. Human B-lymphocyte malignancies: exploitation of BLyS and APRIL and their receptors. Curr Dir Autoimmun 2005; 8:266-288.
42. Sutherland AP, Mackay F, Mackay CR. Targeting BAFF: immunomodulation for autoimmune diseases and lymphomas. Pharmacol Ther 2006; 112:774-786.
43. Ye Q, Wang L, Wells AD et al. BAFF binding to T-cell-expressed BAFF-R costimulates T-cell proliferation and alloresponses. Eur J Immunol 2004; 34:2750-2759.
44. von Bulow GU, Bram RJ. NF-AT activation induced by a CAML-interacting member of the tumor necrosis factor receptor superfamily. Science 1997; 278:138-141.
45. Ng LG, Sutherland AP, Newton R et al. B-cell-activating factor belonging to the TNF family (BAFF)-R is the principal BAFF receptor facilitating BAFF costimulation of circulating T- and B-cells. J Immunol 2004; 173:807-817.
46. Sutherland AP, Ng LG, Fletcher CA et al. BAFF augments certain Th1-associated inflammatory responses. J Immunol 2005; 174:5537-5544.
47. Wang H, Marsters SA, Baker T et al. TACI-ligand interactions are required for T-cell activation and collagen-induced arthritis in mice. Nat Immunol 2001; 2:632-637.
48. Yang M, Hase H, Legarda-Addison D et al. B-cell maturation antigen, the receptor for a proliferation-inducing ligand and B-cell-activating factor of the TNF family, induces antigen presentation in B-cells. J Immunol 2005; 175:2814-2824.
49. Planelles L, Carvalho-Pinto CE, Hardenberg G et al. APRIL promotes B-1 cell-associated neoplasm. Cancer Cell 2004; 6:399-408.
50. Castigli E, Scott S, Dedeoglu F et al. Impaired IgA class switching in APRIL-deficient mice. Proc Natl Acad Sci USA 2004; 101:3903-3908.
51. Varfolomeev E, Kischkel F, Martin F et al. APRIL-deficient mice have normal immune system development. Mol Cell Biol 2004; 24:997-1006.
52. Castigli E, Wilson SA, Scott S et al. TACI and BAFF-R mediate isotype switching in B-cells. J Exp Med 2005; 201:35-39.
53. Castigli E, Wilson SA, Garibyan L et al. TACI is mutant in common variable immunodeficiency and IgA deficiency. Nat Genet 2005; 37:829-834.
54. Salzer U, Chapel HM, Webster AD et al. Mutations in TNFRSF13B encoding TACI are associated with common variable immunodeficiency in humans. Nat Genet 2005; 37:820-828.
55. Khare SD, Sarosi I, Xia XZ et al. Severe B-cell hyperplasia and autoimmune disease in TALL-1 transgenic mice. Proc Natl Acad Sci USA 2000; 97:3370-3375.
56. Mackay F, Woodcock SA, Lawton P et al. Mice transgenic for BAFF develop lymphocytic disorders along with autoimmune manifestations. J Exp Med. 1999; 190:1697-1710.
57. Groom J, Kalled SL, Cutler AH et al. Association of BAFF/BLyS overexpression and altered B-cell differentiation with Sjogren's syndrome 10.1172/JCI200214121. J Clin Invest 2002; 109:59-68.

58. Zheng Y, Gallucci S, Gaughan JP et al. A role for B-cell-activating factor of the TNF family in chemically induced autoimmunity. J Immunol 2005; 175:6163-6168.
59. Kayagaki N, Yan M, Seshasayee D et al. BAFF/BLyS receptor 3 binds the B-cell survival factor BAFF ligand through a discrete surface loop and promotes processing of NF-kappaB2. Immunity 2002; 17:515-524.
60. Zhang J, Roschke V, Baker KP et al. Cutting edge: a role for B-lymphocyte stimulator in systemic lupus erythematosus. J Immunol 2001; 166:6-10.
61. Stohl W, Metyas S, Tan SM et al. B-lymphocyte stimulator overexpression in patients with systemic lupus erythematosus: longitudinal observations. Arthritis Rheum 2003; 48:3475-3486.
62. Matsushita T, Hasegawa M, Yanaba K et al. Elevated serum BAFF levels in patients with systemic sclerosis: enhanced BAFF signaling in systemic sclerosis B-lymphocytes. Arthritis Rheum 2006; 54:192-201.
63. Cheema GS, Roschke V, Hilbert DM et al. Elevated serum B-lymphocyte stimulator levels in patients with systemic immune-based rheumatic diseases. Arthritis Rheum 2001; 44:1313-1319.
64. Batten M, Fletcher C, Ng LG et al. TNF deficiency fails to protect BAFF transgenic mice against autoimmunity and reveals a predisposition to B-cell lymphoma. J Immunol 2004; 172:812-822.
65. Koyama T, Tsukamoto H, Miyagi Y et al. Raised serum APRIL levels in patients with systemic lupus erythematosus. Ann Rheum Dis 2005; 64:1065-1067.
66. Stohl W, Metyas S, Tan SM et al. Inverse association between circulating APRIL levels and serological and clinical disease activity in patients with systemic lupus erythematosus. Ann Rheum Dis 2004; 63:1096-1103.
67. Koyama T, Tsukamoto H, Masumoto K et al. A novel polymorphism of the human APRIL gene is associated with systemic lupus erythematosus. Rheumatology (Oxford) 2003; 42:980-985.
68. Tan SM, Xu D, Roschke V et al. Local production of B-lymphocyte stimulator protein and APRIL in arthritic joints of patients with inflammatory arthritis. Arthritis Rheum 2003; 48:982-992.
69. Takemura S, Braun A, Crowson C et al. Lymphoid neogenesis in rheumatoid synovitis. J Immunol 2001; 167:1072-1080.
70. Seyler TM, Park YW, Takemura S et al. BLyS and APRIL in rheumatoid arthritis. J Clin Invest 2005; 115:3083-3092.
71. Novak AJ, Bram RJ, Kay NE et al. Aberrant expression of B-lymphocyte stimulator by B chronic lymphocytic leukemia cells: a mechanism for survival. Blood 2002; 100:2973-2979.
72. Endo T, Nishio M, Enzler T et al. BAFF and APRIL support chronic lymphocytic leukemia B-cell survival through activation of the canonical NF-{kappa}B pathway 10.1182/blood-2006-06-027755. Blood 2007; 109:703-710.
73. Chiu A, Xu W, He B et al. Hodgkin lymphoma cells express TACI and BCMA receptors and generate survival and proliferation signals in response to BAFF and APRIL. Blood 2007; 109:729-739.
74. Fu L, Lin-Lee YC, Pham LV et al. Constitutive NF-kappaB and NFAT activation leads to stimulation of the BLyS survival pathway in aggressive B-cell lymphomas. Blood 2006; 107:4540-4548.
75. Novak AJ, Grote DM, Stenson M et al. Expression of BLyS and its receptors in B-cell nonHodgkin lymphoma: correlation with disease activity and patient outcome. Blood 2004; 104:2247-2253.
76. He B, Chadburn A, Jou E et al. Lymphoma B-cells evade apoptosis through the TNF family members BAFF/BLyS and APRIL. J Immunol 2004; 172:3268-3279.
77. Moreaux J, Legouffe E, Jourdan E et al. BAFF and APRIL protect myeloma cells from apoptosis induced by interleukin 6 deprivation and dexamethasone. Blood 2004; 103:3148-3157.
78. Novak AJ, Darce JR, Arendt BK et al. Expression of BCMA, TACI and BAFF-R in multiple myeloma: a mechanism for growth and survival. Blood 2004; 103:689-694.
79. Kern C, Cornuel JF, Billard C et al. Involvement of BAFF and APRIL in the resistance to apoptosis of B-CLL through an autocrine pathway. Blood 2004; 103:679-688.
80. Nishio M, Endo T, Tsukada N et al. Nurselike cells express BAFF and APRIL, which can promote survival of chronic lymphocytic leukemia cells via a paracrine pathway distinct from that of SDF-1alpha. Blood 2005; 106:1012-1020.
81. Schwaller J, Schneider P, Mhawech-Fauceglia P et al. Neutrophil-derived APRIL concentrated in tumor lesions by proteoglycans correlates with human B-cell lymphoma aggressiveness. Blood 2007; 109:331-338.
82. Elsawa SF, Novak AJ, Grote DM et al. B-lymphocyte stimulator (BLyS) stimulates immunoglobulin production and malignant B-cell growth in Waldenstrom macroglobulinemia. Blood 2006; 107:2882-2888.
83. Ryan MC, Hering M, Peckham D et al. Antibody Targeting of BCMA on Malignant Plasma Cells. Mol Cancer Ther 2007; 6:3007-3018.
84. Nimmanapalli R, Lyu MA, Du M et al. The growth factor fusion construct containing B-lymphocyte stimulator (BLyS) and the toxin rGel induces apoptosis specifically in BAFF-R-positive CLL cells. Blood 2007; 109:2557-2564.

85. Lyu MA, Cheung LH, Hittelman WN et al. The rGel/BLyS fusion toxin specifically targets malignant B-cells expressing the BLyS receptors BAFF-R, TACI and BCMA. Mol Cancer Ther 2007; 6:460-470.

86. Kelly K, Manos E, Jensen G et al. APRIL/TRDL-1, a tumor necrosis factor-like ligand, stimulates cell death. Cancer Res 2000; 60:1021-1027.

87. Shaffer AL, Rosenwald A, Staudt LM. Lymphoid malignancies: the dark side of B-cell differentiation. Nat Rev Immunol 2002; 2:920-932.

88. Baker KP, Edwards BM, Main SH et al. Generation and characterization of LymphoStat-B, a human monoclonal antibody that antagonizes the bioactivities of B-lymphocyte stimulator. Arthritis Rheum 2003; 48:3253-3265.

89. Parry TJ, Riccobene TA, Strawn SJ et al. Pharmacokinetics and immunological effects of exogenously administered recombinant human B-lymphocyte stimulator (BLyS) in mice. J Pharmacol Exp Ther 2001; 296:396-404.

90. Wallace DJ LJ, Stohl W, McKay J et al. Belimumab (LymphoStat-B) shows bioactivity and reduces SLE disease activity. Belimumab (LymphoStat-B) shows bioactivity and reduces SLE disease activity. European Congress of Rheumatology; 2006.

91. Furie R LJ, Merrill JT, Petri M et al. Multiple SLE disease activity measures in a multi-center Phase 2 SLE trial demonstrate belimumab improves or stabilizes SLE activity in serologically active SLE patients. European Congress of Rheumatology; 2006.

92. Petri M WD, Stohl W, McKay J et al. SLE patients with active production of anti-nuclear autoantibodies (ANA positive) have distinct patterns of lupus activity and peripheral B-cell biomarkers compared to ANA negative patients. European Congress of Rheumatology; 2006.

93. Huizinga T, Boling E, Valente R et al. Genetic and environmental risk factors, disease outcome and responses to anti B-cell therapy belimumab indicate anti-CCP positive RA is a distinct disease entity. 70th Annual Scientific Meeting of the American College of Rheumatology/Association of Rheumatology Health Professionals; 2006.

94. McKay J C-SH, Boling E et al. Belimumab, a fully human monoclonal antibody to B-lymphocyte stimulator (BLyS), combined with standard of care therapy reduces the signs and symptoms of rheumatoid arthritis in a heterogeneous subject population. 69th Annual Scientific Meeting of the American College of Rheumatology/Association of Rheumatology Health Professionals; 2005.

95. Pelletier M, Thompson JS, Qian F et al. Comparison of soluble decoy IgG fusion proteins of BAFF-R and BCMA as antagonists for BAFF. J Biol Chem 2003; 278:33127-33133.

96. Vugmeyster Y, Seshasayee D, Chang W et al. A soluble BAFF antagonist, BR3-Fc, decreases peripheral blood B-cells and lymphoid tissue marginal zone and follicular B-cells in cynomolgus monkeys. Am J Pathol 2006; 168:476-489.

97. Gong Q, Ou Q, Ye S et al. Importance of cellular microenvironment and circulatory dynamics in B cell immunotherapy. J Immunol 2005; 174:817-826.

98. Lin WY, Gong Q, Seshasayee D et al. Anti-BR3 antibodies—a new class of B-cell immunotherapy combining cellular depletion and survival blockade. Blood 2007. In Press.

99. Patel DR, Wallweber HJ, Yin J et al. Engineering an APRIL-specific B-cell maturation antigen. J Biol Chem 2004; 279:16727-16735.

100. Dall'Era M, Chakravarty E, Genovese M et al. Trial of Atacicept in Patients with Systemic Lupus Erythematosus (SLE). American College of Rheumatology; 2006.

101. Tak PP, Thurlings RM, Dimic A et al. A Phase Ib Study to Investigate Atacicept (TACI-Ig) in Patients with Rhuematoid Arthritis. American College of Rheumatolgoy; 2007.

102. Kofler DM, Elter T, Gianella-Borradori A et al. A phase Ib trial of Atacicept (TACI-Ig) to neutralize APRIL and BlyS in patients with refractory or relapsed B-Cell Chronic Lymphocytic Leukemia (B-CLL). American Society of Clinical Oncology; 2007.

103. Ramanujam M, Wang X, Huang W et al. Similarities and differences between selective and nonselective BAFF blockade in murine SLE. J Clin Invest 2006; 116:724-734.

104. Carter RH, Zhao H, Liu X et al. Expression and occupancy of BAFF-R on B-cells in systemic lupus erythematosus. Arthritis Rheum 2005; 52:3943-3954.

105. Dillon SR, Gross JA, Ansell SM et al. An APRIL to remember: novel TNF ligands as therapeutic targets. Nat Rev Drug Discov 2006; 5:235-246.

106. Xu S, Lam KP. B-cell maturation protein, which binds the tumor necrosis factor family members BAFF and APRIL, is dispensable for humoral immune responses. Mol Cell Biol 2001; 21:4067-4074.

CHAPTER 5

The Role of FasL and Fas in Health and Disease

Martin Ehrenschwender* and Harald Wajant

Abstract

The FS7-associated cell surface antigen (Fas, also named CD95, APO-1 or TNFRSF6) attracted considerable interest in the field of apoptosis research since its discovery in 1989. The groups of Shin Yonehara and Peter Krammer were the first reporting extensive apoptotic cell death induction upon treating cells with Fas-specific monoclonal antibodies.[1,2] Cloning of Fas[3] and its ligand,[4,5] FasL (also known as CD178, CD95L or TNFSF6), laid the cornerstone in establishing this receptor-ligand system as a central regulator of apoptosis in mammals. Therapeutic exploitation of FasL-Fas-mediated cytotoxicity was soon an ambitous goal and during the last decade numerous strategies have been developed for its realization. In this chapter, we will briefly introduce essential general aspects of the FasL-Fas system before reviewing its physiological and pathophysiological relevance. Finally, FasL-Fas-related therapeutic tools and concepts will be addressed.

The FasL-Fas System

Structure of Fas

Fas is the prototypic representative of the death receptor subgroup of the tumor necrosis factor receptor family. In the human genome, the Fas gene is located on chromosome 10q24.1, containing 9 exons and spanning about 26 kb of DNA.[6] Consensus sequences for "TATA" and "CAAT" boxes are missing in the 5' upstream sequence resulting in multiple transcription initiation sites.[6] Due to alternative splicing seven variants of mRNA transcripts have to date been observed encoding several soluble forms of Fas with negative regulatory effects in vitro,[7] e.g., a Fas molecule lacking the transmembrane domain.[8] Mature Fas is a type I transmembrane protein of 319 aa, divided into a 157 aa extracellular and a 145 aa intracellular domain (Fig. 1).

The extracellular domain of Fas contains three cysteine rich domains (CRDs), the structural hallmark of the TNF receptor family.[9,10] Functionally all three CRDs of Fas are required for ligand binding,[11] but sites for direct contact are exclusively provided by CRD2 and CRD3.[12] Although CRD1 has no ligand specifity,[11] it is a prerequisite for efficient receptor-ligand interaction and Fas signaling.[13,14] As a major part of the so called preligand binding assembly domain (PLAD) it mediates formation of signaling incompetent Fas complexes which in contrast to Fas monomers have high affinity for FasL.

The C-terminal half of the intracellular domain of Fas comprises the death domain (DD) (Fig. 1), which is essential for apoptosis induction[15] and characteristic for the subgroup of death receptors.[16] The death domain is not limited to death receptors, but can also be found in cytoplasmic

*Corresponding Author: Martin Ehrenschwender—Department of Molecular Internal Medicine, Medical Clinic and Polyclinic II, University of Wuerzburg, Roentgenring 11 97070 Wuerzburg, Germany. Email: martin.ehrenschwender@uni-wuerzburg.de

Therapeutic Targets of the TNF Superfamily, edited by Iqbal S. Grewal.
©2009 Landes Bioscience and Springer Science+Business Media.

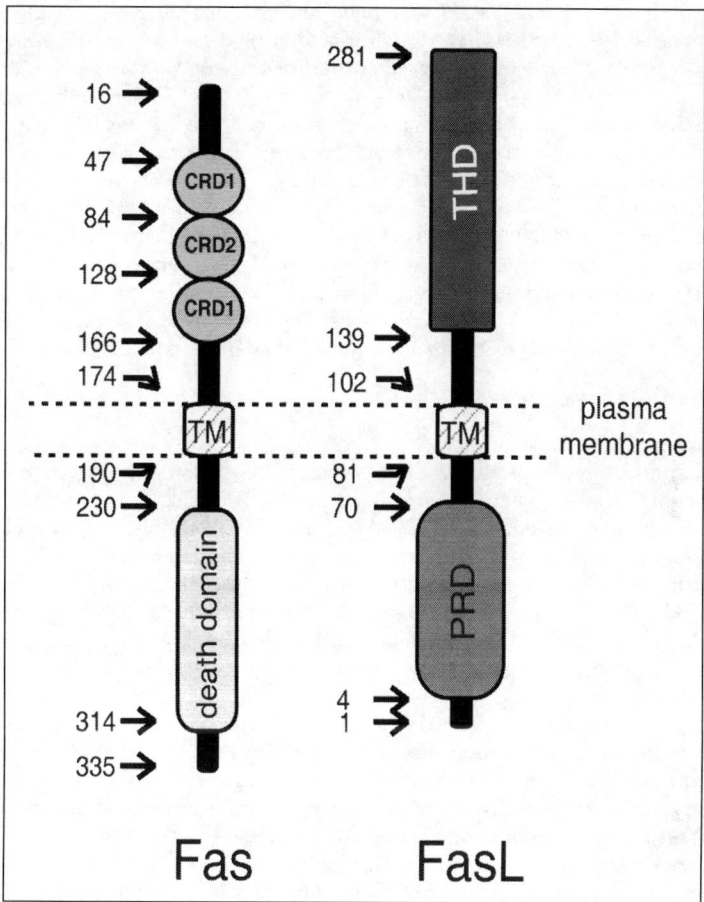

Figure 1. Domain architecture of FasL and Fas. Numbers indicate amino acid position. TM = transmembrane domain, PRD = proline rich domain, CRD = cysteine rich domain, THD = TNF homology domain.

adaptor proteins and kinases.[17] Serving as a homophilic interaction domain, the death domain mediates homo- or heteromerization of DD proteins, presumably facilitated through charged residues on the DD surface.[17] Expression of Fas has been reported for many types of cells, including fibroblasts, epithelial cells and cells of the hematopoetic system. In the latter, a correlation between Fas expression and maturation status has been observed.[18]

Structure of FasL

The gene of human FasL is located on chromosome 1q23, spanning about 8 kb of DNA and consisting of 4 exons.[5] Like the majority of ligands of the TNF family, mature FasL is a 40 kDa type II transmembrane glyco-protein.

The extracellular portion (179 aa) of FasL has three potential N-glycosylation sites[19] and contains two antiparallel ß-sheets forming a "jelly roll" known as the TNF homology domain (THD),[20] the characteristic structural feature of the TNF ligand family (Fig. 1).[21] Although sequence homology between THDs from different TNF family ligands does not exceed 35% the tertiary structure is essentially similar and mediates ligand homotrimerization and receptor binding.[21]

The intracellular portion of FasL (80 aa) contains an extended polyproline region (aa 45-65) enabling interaction with proteins having proline-binding motifs, such as Src homology 3 (SH3) and WW domains.[22,23] Furthermore, several tyrosine phosphorylation sites and a "double" casein kinase phosphorylation motif (aa 17-21) are present (Fig. 1).[24] Functionally these domains have been implicated in FasL sorting and reverse signaling.[23,24] FasL occurs in two forms, either membrane-bound or soluble. The soluble form is generated by alternative splicing or proteolytic processing of the membrane-bound form. Metalloproteinase-3 and metalloproteinase-7 are known to contribute to FasL shedding[25-27] through cleavage between K129 and Q130.[28] Although receptor binding was demonstrated for both forms of FasL only membrane-bound or immobilized FasL exerts robust Fas activation.[29,30] Soluble FasL may on the one hand compete with membrane-bound FasL for receptor binding and thus act antagonistically,[28,29] on the other hand it might convert to an agonist through binding to extracellular matrix components.[31] Furthermore, soluble FasL is a chemoattractant and increases migration of neutrophils and phagocytes in inflamed tissue.[32,33]

Pathways in Fas Signaling

Mechanisms of Fas Activation

Recently, a model of Fas activation has been proposed distinguishing five stages:[34] (1) ligand-induced conversion of preassociated, signaling-incompetent Fas complexes into stable Fas microaggregates and incipient death inducing signaling complex (DISC) assembly, (2) Fas association with lipid rafts forming signaling protein oligomeric transduction structures (SPOTS), (3) clustering and coalescence of Fas-containing lipid raft to large platforms, (4) receptor internalization and (5) high level DISC formation in the endosomal compartement. Inactive Fas complexes formed via the PLAD crucially depend on formation of high molecular weight ligand-receptor clusters, induced by membrane FasL, agonistic antibodies, immobilized soluble FasL,[31,35] synergistically acting mixtures of soluble FasL and non-agonistic Fas antibodies or oligomerized soluble FasL (see Fig. 2). Cluster formation is assisted by constitutive and induced association of Fas with lipid rafts[36-38] where further oligomerization of ligated Fas complexes arises (a conglomerate also referred to as SPOTS)[39] and facilitates recruitment of cytoplasmic signaling molecules. Although DISC formation starts at plasma membrane level, mounting of components predominantly occurs after receptor internalization in an endosomal compartment.[34] Beside FasL and Fas the DISC contains the Fas-associated death domain protein (FADD) and procaspase-8.[40] FADD binds directly to the DD of Fas by virtue of its own C-terminal DD and furthermore mediates procaspase-8 recruitment via its N-terminal death effector domain.[41,42] In context of supramolecular DISC pro-caspase-8 is initially activated by dimerization, but is readily converted into mature heterotetrameric caspase-8 by two-step autoproteolytic maturation.[43,44] Formation of procaspase-8 dimers and processing are impaired in the presence of the short isoform of cellular FLICE-inhibitory protein (FLIP).[7] Processing of procaspase-8 is blocked in addition by the long isoform of FLIP at an intermediate step. Active heterotetrameric caspase-8 is generated and released from the DISC. Subsequently, activation of downstream effector caspases (in particular caspase-3) by caspase-8 heralds the execution phase of apoptosis, whereby molecular mechanisms utilized in this phase depend on the cell type. In type I cells, direct activation of effector caspases by caspase-8 is sufficient for robustly triggering the cell death machinery and completing the apoptotic programm.[45,46] In sharp contrast, type II cells exhibit insufficient caspase activation due to low caspase-8 expression levels and/or presence of caspase inhibitory molecules. These cells require an amplification loop emanating from caspase-8 mediated cleavage of the BH3-only protein Bid. tBid, the caspase-8-processed from of Bid, translocates to the outer mitochondrial membrane (OMM) and activates Bak allosterically. Subsequently, Bak oligomerizes and forms pores in the OMM allowing proapoptotic proteins to leave the mitochondrial intermembrane space and enter the cytoplasm.[45,46] These proapoptotic proteins include cytochrome c, the second mitochondria-derived activator of caspase/direct IAP binding protein with low pI (SMAC/DIABLO) and HtrA2/Omi.[47,48] Once released, cytochrome c together with cytosolic ATP binds to the scaffold protein apoptosis promoting factor-1 (Apaf-1), forming the apoptosome which mediates caspase-9 activation. Caspase-9 is like

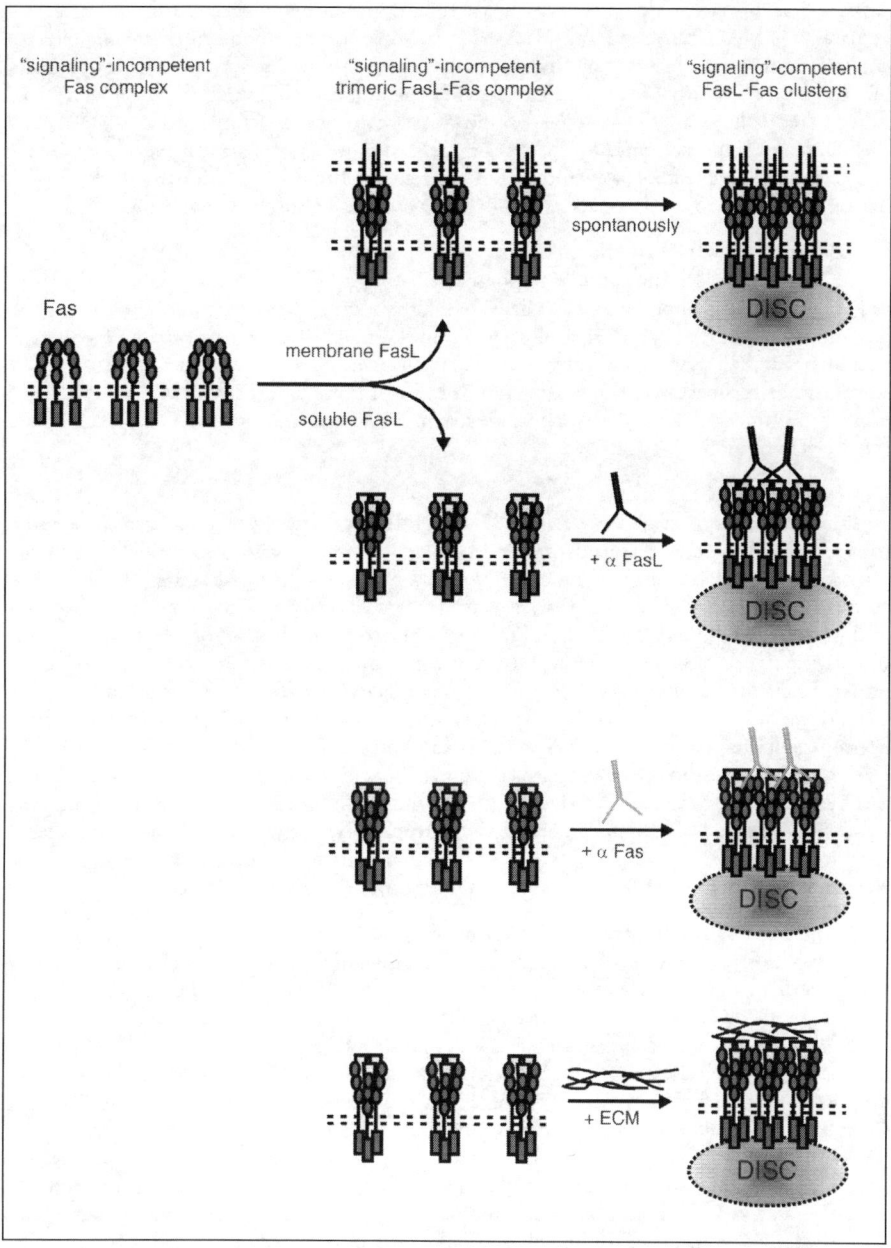

Figure 2. Mechanisms of Fas activation. Ligation of preassociated Fas complexes by membrane FasL or soluble FasL results in either case in "signaling"-incompetent trimeric FasL-Fas complexes. Initially formed membrane FasL-bound Fas complexes are capable of spontaneously inducing "signaling"-competent high molecular weight FasL-Fas clusters and DISC formation, whereas primary FasL-Fas complexes require exogenous oligomerization, e.g., by FasL- or Fas-antibodies to reach high activity. Immobilization of FasL by extracellular matrix components converts poorly active soluble FasL into highly active membrane FasL-like molecules. ECM = extracellular matrix.

caspase-8 an initiator caspase, which when activated in the apoptosome processes the effector caspase-3.[49] SMAC/DIABLO and HtrA2/Omi also contribute apoptosis by freeing effector caspases from the inhibitory molecules of the IAP family.[47] Fas can not only trigger apoptosis, but also necrosis, a form of caspase-independent programmed cell death.[50-52] Critically involved in the latter pathway are the serine/threonine kinase receptor interacting protein-1 (RIP1) and FADD,[53] but the mechanisms how these Fas-associated proteins generate reactive oxygen species and activate other effectors of necrotic cell death remain unresolved.[50] As caspase-8 cleaves and inactivates RIP necrosis takes place especially when caspase-8 is inhibited or absent.

Fas-Induced NFκB Activation

Cell death is not the only cellular response emanating from Fas activation. Fas is also capable to induce NFκB signaling. As caspases activated in the course of apoptosis inhibit NFκB signaling, stimulation of the latter is especially relevant in resistant cells. In Fas-mediated NFκB activation involving RIP, FADD and caspase-8 the enzymatic activity of the latter is dispensable.[54-57] In context of Fas-mediated NFκB activation, FLIP isoformes have a strong inhibitory effect.[54] Notably, $FLIP_L$ and caspase-8 have a positive role in NFκB activation via the T-cell receptor and the B-cell receptor.

Fas-Induced JNK Signaling

Initially, Fas-induced cJun N-terminal kinase (JNK) activation was recognized to be apoptosis-associated and either dependent or independent of caspase activation. In the first scenario, caspases cleave and activate components of the JNK pathway, e.g., the MAP3K MEKK1,[58-60] or cleave and inactivate regulators of JNK, e.g., $p21^{waf1/cip1}$.[61] Interfering with caspase activity results in abrogation of both JNK signaling and apoptosis, but exclusive blockade of JNK fails to prevent Fas-mediated cell death.[62,63] Therefore, JNK activation cannot be considered as a conditio sine qua non in Fas-mediated apoptosis, but might potentially act as an enhancer. In the second scenario, Fas-induced JNK activation occurs via a caspase-independent pathway by recruitment of death domain-associated protein 6 (DAXX) and the apoptosis signaling kinase-1 (ASK1, MAP3K5). DAXX binds directly to activated Fas at a site preceding the DD and additionally recruits ASK1, a MAP3K capable to activate JNK signaling. Fas-mediated JNK activation has also been observed under nonapoptotic conditions. In cardiac hypertrophy JNK activation plays a crucial role[64,65] as an initially protective mechanism that is blunted in vitro and in vivo when functional Fas is lacking.[65-67] A simplified overview of Fas signaling pathways in given in Figure 3.

FasL and Fas in Proliferation, Differentiation and Inflammation

Fas enhances proliferation of TCR-stimulated T-cells and thymocytes[68] and has costimulatory effects in thymocyte activation during positive selection.[69] Notably, FasL has also been implicated in T-cell activation through reverse signaling resulting in proliferation or cell cycle arrest.[70] Additionally, Fas exerts proliferative, but also apoptotic effects in human diploid fibroblasts[71-73] and Fas activation accelerates liver regeneration after partial hepatectomy.[74] Conversely, in healthy mice Fas activation results in massive apoptosis of hepatocytes. Fas can induce proinflammatory chemokine production by directly activating the NFκB pathway and might in addition enhance LPS- and IL-1-induced NFκB activation in macrophages and dendritic cells[75] and thus might have a supporting role in distinct inflammatory scenarios irrespective from its apoptotic functions.

FasL-induced T-cell killing has been proposed to be of special importance in immune priviledged sites such as the eye,[76] brain,[77,78] lung,[79] placenta and pregnant uterus.[80] Inflammation in these tissues is physiologically suppressed to avoid tissue destruction (see below). Bearing this concept in mind, exploitation of FasL as a tool of immunosuppression and generation of immune tolerance has been a promising attempt,[81] which, however, failed in many cases.[82,83]

The FasL-Fas System in Health and Disease

Investigations of the in vivo function of the FasL-Fas system rely mainly on mice bearing generalized lymphoproliferative disease (gld) and lymphoproliferation (lpr) mutations resulting in

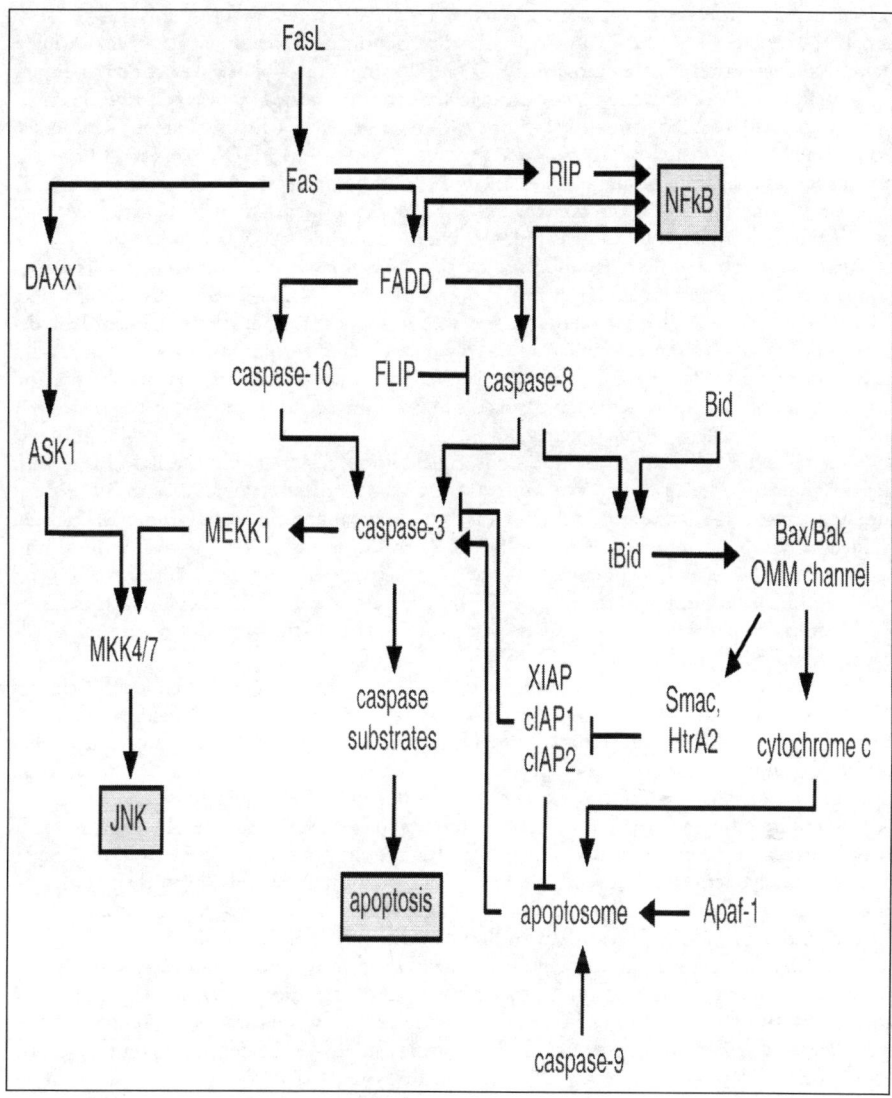

Figure 3. Fas signaling pathway. For details see text. OMM = outer mitochondrial membrane.

impaired FasL and Fas function, respectively.[84] FasL dysfunction in the gld phenotype is caused by a point mutation in the FasL gene. The Fas mutation in the lpr phenotype can either result from retroviral insertion and subsequent premature termination of transcription or a point mutation in the Fas death domain (the latter termed lpr-cg).[85]

Role of FasL and Fas in Immunobiology

FasL-Fas in T-Cell Activation and T-Cell Death

The T-cell immune response following antigen exposure can be subsectioned in three distinct events: clonal expansion of antigen specific T-cells, clearance of antigen and finally the contraction phase (peripheral deletion). In the beginning of an immune response, antigen specific T-cells are activated and proliferate, the number of reactive T-cells therefore spurts upwards. Fas signaling enhances T-cell receptor (TCR) driven proliferation of primary T-cells in vitro.[68,86] Interestingly, this effect disappeared after highdose anti-CD3 administration. As lpr or gld mice do not display major defects in T-cell activation in vitro and in vivo, the role of the FasL-Fas system seems to be nonessential and if at all of supportive nature. Although Fas itself is dispensable for T-cell activation, the opposite is true for Fas associated proteins. Absence of FADD or caspase-8 as well as presence of caspase inhibitors impede T-cell activation.[87-90] In these cases, even high-dose anti-CD3 stimulation is insufficient to overcome the activation blockade. In fact, there is increasing evidence that FADD and caspase-8 fulfill a Fas-independent function in T-cell signaling.

After antigen clearing, T-cell numbers quickly decline due to apoptosis, leaving a small number of memory T-cells. Early models suggested contributions of Fas and FasL in this process (for a review see ref. 91). Initially, several findings seemed to support this idea: Firstly, Fas or FasL defects cause marked lymphoaccumulation and often accelerated autoimmune disease;[92] secondly, activation induced cell death in T-cells after restimulation can be due to FasL-Fas interaction[91] and thirdly, aggravated lymphoaccumulation occurs in Bcl-2 transgenic mice.[93] However, these early findings were challenged by subsequent studies. Bcl-2 was shown to have no or an insignificant role in Fas-mediated T-cell death in another study.[94] In addition, accumulating T-cells in Fas or FasL deficient humans or mice are predominantly CD4⁻CD8⁻ T-cells that do not arise during normal immune responses. Most importantly, not Fas, but the proapoptotic protein Bim was reported to be essential for peripheral deletion of T-cells.[95] Thus, two models of apoptosis induction in activated T-cells during the contraction phase arose: activation induced cell death (AICD) and activated T-cell autonomous cell death (ACAD) (for review see ref. 96). Briefly, in the former TCR restimulation results in Fas-mediated apoptosis, whereas in the latter lack of survival signals triggers apoptosis.

Recently, three studies suggested that Fas and Bim cooperate in peripheral deletion of T-cells.[97-99] Hughes et al reported that Bim alone shuts down T-cell response after acute infection, but termination after more chronic infections requires both Fas and Bim.[97] It is tempting to speculate that controlling antigen presentation is the clue to the differences in Fas involvment.[100] After clearing an infection, antigen on antigen presenting cells (APCs) may either quickly become limited or persist. Limitation of antigen represents a withdrawal of survival factors for T-cells and might cause Bim accumulation and finally Bim-induced death. If antigen persists on APCs, T-cells might receive successive activation preventing Bim accumulation. But T-cells also express FasL, capable of killing either adjacent T-cells or APCs. This might again result in antigen limitation, survival factor withdrawal and thus in Fas-licensed Bim-dependent cell death (see Fig. 4).

Lpr (defective Fas) and gld (defective FasL) mice are prone to autoimmune disease displaying symptoms such as lymphadenopathy, production of autoantibodies, hypergammaglobulinemia and accumulation of CD4⁻CD8⁻ T-cells.[84] Development of a lupus-like autoimmune disease including glomerulonephritis, vasculitis and arthritis can also occur depending on the genetic background.[84,85,101] Furthermore, a role for the FasL-Fas system has been suggested in autoimmune thyroiditis, multiple sclerosis, experimental allergic encephalomyelitis (discussed in more detail below) and the pathogenesis of type-1 and -2 diabetes.[102-105]

Taken together, the pathologies listed above point to a lack in tolerance induction in B- and T-cells. Therefore, the FasL-Fas system is likely to hold a role in apoptosis and/or anergy induction in autoreactive cells. With respect to T-cell development, FasL-Fas have been reported to participate in thymic selection as well as in peripheral T-cell homeostasis. Observation of massive apoptosis during negative thymic selection was first attributed to Fas-mediated killing,[106,107] but lpr mice show normal thymic deletion of T-cells[108] thus arguing against a obligate involvement of Fas signaling.

The human equivalent to the gld and lpr phenotype is known as autoimmune lymphoproliferative syndrome (ALPS).[109] At least three major categories of ALPS can be distinguished according to the underlying molecular defects. Patients suffering from mutation in the Fas or FasL gene are classified as ALPS Ia and ALPS Ib, respectively. ALPS II is related to mutations in caspase-10 whereas

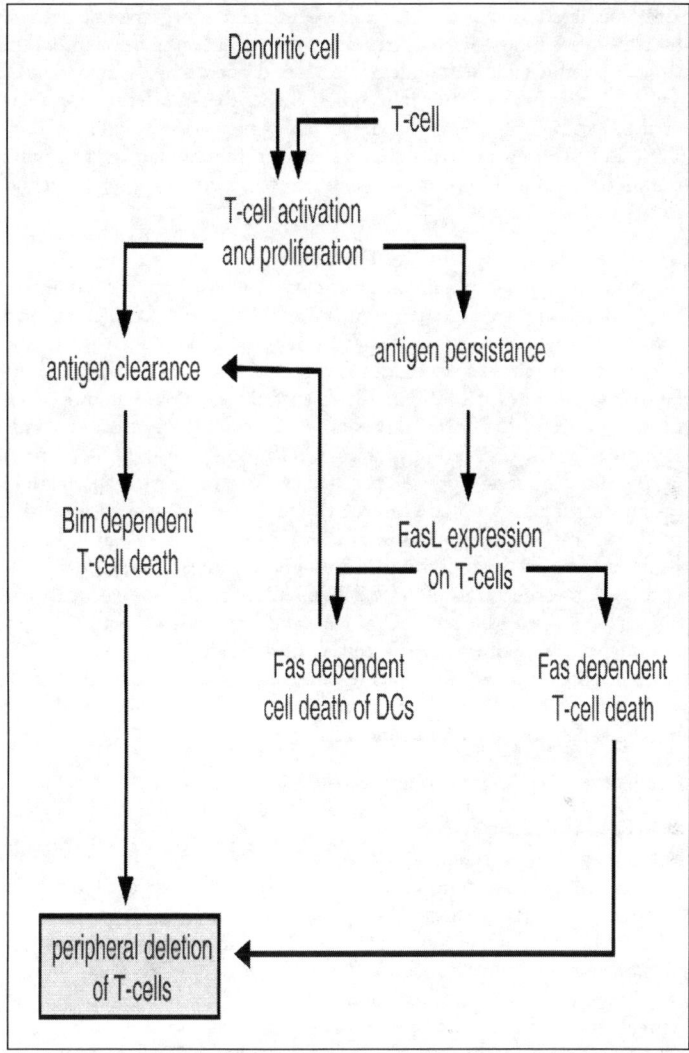

Figure 4. Role of Fas and Bim in peripheral deletion of T-cells. Rapid antigen clearance limits survival factors for T-cells, causes Bim accumulation and subsequent Bim-dependent T-cell death. In contrast, antigen persistence prevents Bim-accumulation, but results in FasL expression on T-cells, killing either adjacent T-cells or DCs. Killing of DCs in turn results in antigen limitation, survival-factor withdrawal and Bim-accumulation. DC = dendritic cell.

ALPS III is molecularly undefined.[109] Diagnostic criteria for ALPS necessarily include chronic nonmalignant lymphadenopathy and/or splenomegaly, peripheral expansion of CD4⁻CD8⁻ T-cells and impaired lymphocyte apoptosis.[110] Frequently associated and supportive of ALPS is presentation of family history, autoimmune disease and characteristic histopathology.[110]

Another pathology associated with the FasL-Fas system is toxic epidermal necrolysis (TEN). TEN is almost exclusively caused by adverse drug reactions and associated with a mortality of 30%. Clinical signs on the skin include among others separation of large sheets of epidermis from the dermis, bullae and generalized erythematous rash.[111] Hallmark of TEN is massive keratinocyte apoptosis mainly mediated by cytotoxic T-cells via the perforin/granzyme pathway and the FasL-Fas pathway.[111] In addition, keratinocytes from patients suffering from TEN express beside Fas lytically active FasL which is absent under normal conditions, thereby enabling Fas activation and apoptosis induction.[112] In this setting it becomes obvious that interfering with FasL-Fas interactions is a potential treatment strategy. Blocking of Fas by anti-Fas IgG contained in intravenous immune globulin (IVIG) abrogates FasL-mediated apoptosis in human keratinocytes in vitro[112] and administration of IVIG in TEN patients rapidly reverses disease progression and results in favorable outcome.[111,113]

Role of the FasL-Fas System in Immune Privilege

In certain organs and tissues the physiological immune response is suppressed since even minor inflammatory episodes might endanger their integrity and function. Beside brain, testis, ovary, pregnant uterus and placenta, the eye was the first established and is currently the best studied immune privileged site. This site-restricted immunosuppressed state allows, for example, corneal transplantation with success rates of 80-90% in the absence of systemic immunosuppressive therapy or tissue matching.[114] Recent studies revealed some of the complex mechanisms underlying the phenomena of immune privilege including physical mechanisms such as the blood-occular barrier as well as locally produced immunosuppressive cytokines, neuropeptides, NK-cell inhibitors, tight regulation of complement activation and limited expression of major histocompatibility class I and II.[114] In particular, FasL expression has been shown to play a key role by inducing apoptosis in Fas-sensitive inflammatory cells invading an immune privileged site. Contribution of FasL expression in preventing corneal transplant rejection and inflammation has been demonstrated in studies reporting (1) Fas-sensitive cells die from apoptosis induced by Fas on cultured corneas;[76,115] (2) intra-occular injection of wt or lpr T-cells in mice results in apoptosis versus survival;[116] (3) gld mice exhibit more severe occular inflammation after injection of herpes simplex virus or toxoplasma gondii than wt mice;[76,117] (4) significantly enhanced graft failure of allogeneic corneal transplants form FasL-defective mice compared to wt mice.[118]

FasL and Fas in the Cardiovascular System

Functions of FasL and Fas in the Heart

Within the last years there is accumulating evidence of Fas signaling in the heart under physiological and pathophysiological conditions. Chronic excessive afterload results in hypertrophy of the myocardium due to an initially beneficial adaptive response. However, persistent hypertrophy can ultimately lead to heart failure. In contrast to wt mice lpr mice present a blunted hypertrophic response to pressure overload induced by aortic banding.[66] In cultured cardiomyocytes FasL augments total protein synthesis and increases production of angiotensin II, endothelkin-I and atrial natriuretic factor all of which can be considered as molecular criteria of hypertrophic response.[66] Furthermore, biopsies of failing human hearts show Fas upregulation after volume overload.[119]

Increased mRNA levels of Fas and FasL are detected in human cardiac allografts during rejection.[120] Additionally, displaying a chimeric streptavidin-FasL (SA-FasL) protein artificially on cardiac vasculature prolongs graft survival in mice by selective deletion of alloreactive immune cells, predominantely CD4+ and CD8+ T-cells.[121] In sharp contrast to another study demonstrating accelerated graft rejection and polymorphonuclear infiltrates upon FasL overexpression in cardiac myocytes,[83] none of these features was present after immobilization of chimeric SA-FasL on cardiac vasculature endothelium.[121]

Further on, overexpression of FasL in endothelial cells attenuates ischemia-reperfusion injury in the heart[122] and results in a significant reduction in myocardial infarct size and neutrophil infiltration.[122] Recently, a link between the renin-angiotensin and FasL-Fas system in postinfarction hearts has been proposed.[123] Blockade of angiotensin II type I receptor (AT1) after myocardial infarction suppressed apoptosis in granulation tissue thereby attenuating left ventricular dilatation and dysfunction resulting in improved survival. Application of the AT1-blocker olmesartan reduced expression of DAXX and JNK activity in granulation tissue, whereas caspase-8 activity and FADD levels remained unaffected.[123] Thus, the negative regulatory effect of AT1 blockade on apoptosis might be due to interference with Fas-DAXX-ASK1 induced JNK activation.[123]

FasL has also been shown to regulate acute myocarditis induced by Trypanosoma cruzi infection (Chagas' disease). Chronic cardiopathic infection is associated with persistent inflammatory reaction of the myocardium, loss of cardiomyocytes and development of fibrosis.[124,125] In FasL-deficient mice, cardiac infiltration and cardiomyocyte destruction were significantly reduced[126] and in vivo blocking with a FasL-specific antibody elicited a similar effect.[127] Thus, parasitic activation of the host FasL-Fas system contributes to chagasic cardiomyopathy.

In a lipopolysacharide induced mouse model of sepsis blocking FasL with a soluble form of Fas showed significant cardioprotective effect. Transgenic mice with cardiac specific expression of soluble Fas revealed attenuated myocardial transcript levels of proinflammatory cytokines such as TNFα, interleukin-1ß (IL-1ß) and IL-6 after LPS-treatment compared to wt mice.[128]

The FasL-Fas System in Angiogenesis

A role of the FasL-Fas system in regulation of angiogenesis is becoming more and more apparent. Several inhibitors of angiogenesis including 2-methoxyestradiol, angiostatin, endostatin, thrombospondin-1 (TSP1) and pigment epithelium-derived factor (PEDF) function through FasL upregulation and Fas-mediated apoptosis in endothelial cells.[129-132] Interestingly, inducers of neovascularization (e.g., IL-8, bFGF and VEGF) enhance cell surface trafficking of Fas and facilitates TSP1- and PEDF-induced apoptosis.[129] In fact, TSP1- or PEDF-mediated inhibition of bFGF induced corneal neovascularization is reduced in lpr mice. Beside Fas, inducers of neovascularization also upregulate the antiapoptotic protein FLIP. This mechanism can be in turn opposed by inhibitors of angiogenesis by interfering with the Akt pathway.[133-135] Taken together, these data are supportive of a FasL-Fas regulated model of angiogenesis whereupon the extent of angiogenesis is determined by the interplay of angiogenesis inhibitor driven FasL expression on the one hand and angiogenesis inducer-mediated upregulation of Fas and FLIP on the other hand.

FasL and Fas Functions in Differentiation and Regeneration

Physiology and Pathophysiology of FasL and Fas in the Neurosystem

In the neurosystem the FasL-Fas system holds crucial roles in both physiological and pathophysiological settings. Fas and/or FasL expression has been demonstrated in neurons and glia cells (oligodendrocytes, astrocytes, microglia and Schwann cells),[136] particularly during development.[137,138] Although certain populations such as motoneurons are remarkably sensitive to Fas-mediated apoptosis,[139,140] physiological neuronal cell death does not appear to be usually mediated by the FasL-Fas system. Conversely, Fas engagement stimulates neurite outgrowth in vitro and enhances peripheral nerve regeneration in vivo by activation of ERK.[141,142] Furthermore, lpr mice display cognitive and sensomotoric defects, stria vascularis dysfunction, progressive atrophy of pyramidal neuron dendrites and delayed neurite regeneration.[143] Most neurological symptoms observed in lpr mice have been attributed to emerging autoimmune disease, but treatment with immunosuppressive drugs does not change the neurological phenotype which can even occur before onset of autoimmunity.[144-146] Thus, some of the neurological defects found in lpr mice might reflect loss of survival and regenerative functions of the FasL-Fas system. A prerequisite for a protective role of Fas signaling in neuronal homeostasis is circumvention of Fas-induced apoptosis. In addition to well known antiapoptotic proteins such as FLIP and Bcl-2 family proteins, the nervous system comes up with further remarkable death receptor regulatory molecules such as Lifeguard (LFG), phosphoprotein enriched in astrocytes-15kD (PEA-15) and Fas apoptotic inhibitory molecule (FAIM).[42,147-149] The latter exists in a long and a short isoform, $FAIM_L$ and $FAIM_S$, respectively. Whereas $FAIM_S$ is widely expressed and promotes neuronal differentiation and regeneration in the neurosystem, $FAIM_L$ is specifically found in neurons and can inhibit Fas-induced caspase-8 activation.[149]

Upregulation of Fas and FasL has further been implicated in spinal cord injury (SCI),[150-153] axotomy-induced motoneuron death[154] and brain damage caused by ischemia.[155-157] Two distinct signaling cascades are involved in Fas-mediated cell death in vitro:[139,140] Firstly, the DAXX-ASK1-p38-nNOS pathway and secondly the classical Fas-FADD-caspase-8 pathway.[158] Both branches seem to function in parallel. Trophic deprivation-induced Fas-mediated cell death is delayed in gld and lpr mice as well as in mice expressing dominant-negative FADD. However, it is unaltered in DAXX-DN transgenic mice.[158] Vice versa, neuronal NOS upregulation and NO production are abrogated in DAXX-DN mice, but are unchanged in FADD-DN transgenic mice.[158]

Fas-mediated apoptosis is a major determinant of secondary damage after SCI.[152] Moreover, in this setting, FasL neutralization promotes axonal regeneration and functional recovery.[150] Additionally, posttraumatic apoptosis was decreased in Fas-deficient mice and lack of Fas was associated with improved locomotor recovery.[151] Analyzing axotomy-induced apoptosis in facial and spinal motoneurons further confirms their sensitivity to Fas. Mouse strains defective in Fas signaling or transgenic mice expressing dominant-negative FADD display an increased number of surviving motoneurons after facial nerve transection compared to wt mice.[154] Remarkably, defective Fas signaling alone was insufficient for providing complete rescue, indicating involvement of further, independent pathways in apoptosis of motoneurons. Notably, stereotactical transplantation of human umbilical cord blood stem cells into the injury epicenter of rats after SCI has recently been reported to improve functional recovery by downregulation of Fas.[159] Fas and FasL are also key players in ischemic and traumatic brain injury where they are involved in tissue damage (for review see ref. 136 and refs. therein). Therapeutic neutralization of FasL attenuates brain damage in stroke by reducing recruitment of inflammatory cells in the penumbra.[156] Additionally, Fas deficient neonatal mice are resistant to hypoxic-ischemic brain damage.[157] Multiple sclerosis (MS) and the corresponding animal disease model experimental allergic encephalomyelitis (EAE) are characterized by organ-specific T-cell mediated tissue damage.[160-162] Herein, oligodendrocytes in inflammatory foci are destroyed by FasL expressing cytotoxic T-cells thereby rendering insulating myelin sheaths inoperative and impairing saltatory conduction along the axon.[163] Accordingly, disturbing the FasL-Fas system results in improved clinical signs of EAE.[136] As the FasL-Fas system is involved in both, T-cell fate and tissue damage, not only destructive, but also protective effects are observable.[164] Since recovery of EAE is associated with FasL-mediated T-cell apoptosis and/or AICD in the CNS, injection of antibodies raised against FasL impedes spontaneous remission[165,166] whereas injection of FasL improves clinical signs.[167,168] Thus, FasL dampens an augmented immune response against self antigens and therefore also constitutes a beneficial mechanism in EAE.

In conclusion, the FasL-Fas system acts as a double-edged sword in the neurosystem qualified to perform destructive and tutelary effects.

FasL and Fas in Homeostasis, Regeneration and Diseases of the Liver

Constitutive Fas expression is observed in almost all liver cell types, including hepatocytes,[169,170] cholangiocytes,[171] sinusoidal endothelial cells,[172] hepatic stellate cells[173] and Kupffer cells.[174] As all these cells are also susceptible to Fas-mediated apoptosis, the need for tight regulation of Fas and its ligand becomes obvious. Normally, only a small fraction of Fas can be found at the plasma membrane of liver cells, whereas the majority localizes to the Golgi complex and the trans Golgi network.[175,176] Upon stimulation, outward traffic of Fas-containing vesicles and subsequent fusion with the plasma membrane increases the initially low receptor densitiy at the cell surface.[176] Analogous to other cell types, Fas regulation by glycosylation and modulation at the transcriptional level has also been observed.[177,178] Logically, FasL expression is subjected to regulation, too. Healthy hepatocytes do not display FasL on their surface, although under pathological conditions such as alcoholic hepatitis and Wilson's disease it can be detected.[170] Furthermore, functional FasL expression has been observed in Kupffer cells.[179] The FasL-Fas system is critically involved in liver homeostasis and regeneration. Complete absence of Fas in mice results in liver hyperplasia, emphasizing a role of FasL-Fas in homeostasis of nonlymphoid tissue.[180] In patricular, Fas-deficient mice have a higher number of senescent hepatocytes pointing towards a key role of Fas in their removal.[180] Whereas proapoptotic effects of Fas seem to be mainly responsible for its role in liver homeostasis, the opposite counts for liver regeneration. After partial hepatectomy Fas engagement accelerates liver regeneration by enhancing cell proliferation via the ERK and NFκB pathway.[74,181]

In this scenario, hepatocytes switch the outcome of Fas signaling by augmented expression of antiapoptotic proteins (e.g., FLIP and Bcl-2) form apoptosis to proliferation.[74] Consequently, absence of Fas as seen in lpr mice results in delayed liver regeneration.[74] In liver pathophysiology, FasL-Fas-dependent regulation of hepatocyte cell death often goes awry. Both, excessive liver cell death as well as downregulation of apoptosis may result in liver disease (see Table 1). Increased or excessive hepatocyte apoptosis has not only instantaneous effects. Independent of its etiology, unbalanced hepatocyte cell death results in the long term in liver fibrosis and may subsequently progress to liver cirrhosis. Mechanistically, excessive apoptotic cell death overwhelms the clearance capacity of Kupffer and hepatic stellate cells.[182] Insufficient clearing of apoptotic bodies results in autolysis of the latter and release of pro-inflammatory molecules,[183,184] thereby recruiting mononuclear cells, exacerbating the inflammatory response and resulting in tissue damage.[185] Furthermore, activation of Kupffer cells and hepatic stellate cells enhances their expression of pro-fibrogenic genes and death ligands such as FasL,[182] thus again boosting hepatocyte cell death and mounting a feed-forward amplification loop.[182] Therefore, apoptosis can be considered as the nexus of liver injury and fibrosis.

The FasL-Fas System in Tumor Biology

Undermining the immune system and suppressing the anti-tumor response are essential events during carcinogenesis allowing tumor formation. In this context, the FasL-Fas system can elicit both tumorigenic and tumor suppressing roles in the pathogenesis of cancer.[186]

FasL and Fas in Tumor Immunosurveillance and Cancer Immunoediting

The immune system is capable of preventing development of tumors, a concept designated tumor immunosurveillance.[187,188] Mouse models and clinical data from patient established immunosurveillance as a effective tumor suppressor system mainly mediated by T-cells and NK-cells.[189] These cells use two independent mechanisms of tumor cell destruction: firstly, release of perforin and granzymes from granules and secondly apoptosis induction via FasL and TRAIL.[190,191] Beside cell death induction, both ligands also exert proinflammatory effects. Furthermore, not only T- or

Table 1. FasL-Fas in human liver disease

	Liver Disease	References
Enhanced Apoptosis	Autoimmune hepatitis	Hiraide A et al. Am J Gastroenterol 2005; 100:1322-1329 Fox CK et al. Liver 2001; 21:272-279
	Acute and chronic viral hepatitis	Kiyici M et al. Eur J Gastroenterol Hepatol 2003; 15:1079-1084. Rivero M et al. J Viral Hepat 2002; 9:107-113 Oksuz M et al. Eur J Gastroenterol Hepatol 2004; 16:341-345
	Acute hepatic failure	Leifeld L et al. Liver Int 2006; 26:872-879. Ryo K et al. Am J Gastroenterol 2000; 95:2047-2055
	Cholestatic disease	Miyoshi H et al. Gastroenterology 1999; 117:669-677
	Alcoholic hepatitis	Ribeiro PS et al. Am J Gastroenterol 2004; 99:1708-1717. Natori S et al. J Hepatol 2001; 34:248-253
	Non alcoholic steatohepatitis	Ribeiro PS et al. Am J Gastroenterol 2004; 99:1708-1717. Feldstein AE et al. Gastroenterology 2003; 125:437-443
	Wilson's disease	Strand S et al. Nat Med 1998; 4:588-593
	Graft rejection	Rivero M et al. Am J Gastroenterol 2002; 97:1501-1506
Reduced Apoptosis	Hepatocarcinoma	Lee SH et al. Human Pathology 2001; 32:250-256 Nagao M et al. Hepatology 1999; 30:413-421. Okano H et al. Lab Invest 2003; 83:1033-1043

NK-cells might express FasL, but also tumor cells themselves. This, in effect, raises a secondary, site-restricted antitumoral immune response cooperatively mounted by the immune system and the tumor. Involvement of the FasL-Fas system in tumor surveillance becomes evident as occurrence of plasmacytoid tumors in older lpr and gld mice is increased.[192] Additionally, cross-breading of Fas or FasL deficient mice with tumor susceptible mice significantly boosted tumor development.[193,194] Finally, genetic polymorphisms of Fas and FasL have been implicated in cervical carcinogenesis[143] and increased risk of breast cancer.[195] Obviously tumor surveillance by the immune system delivers selection pressure upon the developing tumor, thereby actively determining tumor shape and dignity.[187] This dynamic process, known as immunoediting, consists of three stages: elimination, equilibrium and escape.[196] Elimination describes destruction of premalignant or early stage malignant cells by immune-mediated tumor surveillance, equilibrium denotes latency after incomplete removal of transformed cells and escape refers to the final breakthrough of tumor growth.[187]

Tumor Immune Privilege, Fas Counterattack and Pro-Inflammatory Properties of the FasL-Fas System

Evasion of the hosts immune system and establishing an "immune privileged" tumor environment is a vital achievement of cancer cells. The FasL-Fas system has been identified among others as a major player in creating immune privilege (for review see 197 and refs. therein). Initially, FasL expression on SW620 cells was reported to induce apoptosis in Fas-sensitive lymphoid cells in vitro.[198] To date, functional FasL expression has been verified in various tumors of different origins[186,199-203] and apoptosis of tumor-infiltrating lymphocytes (TIL) in FasL expressing tumors has been observed in situ.[204-207] Consequently, FasL expressing tumor cells might undermine host tumor surveillance by apoptosis induction in TILs, a concept often termed "Fas counterattack". Beside cytotoxicity for tumor infiltrating T-cells, expression of FasL offers further benefits for the tumor. FasL impairs antibody production in B-cells[208] and negatively affects T-cell activation.[209] Considering co-expression of Fas and FasL in many tumors, autocrine or juxtacrine interactions may confer in addition to immunoprotection proliferation signals.[210,211]

As already discussed in context with protective roles of FasL-Fas in the neurosystem, FasL expression of cancer cells requires their protection from Fas-mediated cell death.[212] Molecular mechanisms rendering tumor cells relatively resistant to Fas-mediated apoptosis occur at various stages of Fas signaling including secretion of soluble decoy receptors,[213] regulation of Fas surface expression[214,215] and signal modulation at the DISC level or downstream by modulating the expression of e.g., FLIP, FADD, XIAP and caspase-8.[216-220] However, the concept of Fas counterattack remains controversial as some ambiguous results were observed in animal models.[221-225] Curiously, tumor survival was negatively affected in some studies by ectopic overexpression of FasL.[223,226] Recently, a proinflammatory rather than counterattack role of FasL in a tumor prone mouse model lacking functional FasL was suggested.[227] Although tumor number was higher in these animals, tumor infiltrating T-cell count was comparable to controls expressing functional FasL.[227] Unexpectedly, a decreased number of neutrophils in the tumor was observed in absence of functional FasL. Additionally, in these mice decreased neutrophil recruitment correlated with higher tumor multiplicity.[227] Thus, in this setting, neutrophils recruited by direct or indirect chemotactic activity of FasL seemingly exert tumor suppressive effects. These findings are in sharp contrast to the tumorigenic role attributed to inflammatory cells. However, tumors investigated in this study were early stage whereas the majority of studies supporting inflammation-mediated tumor progression were conducted in full-blown malignant diseases.[227] It is tempting to speculate that this discrepancy is due to the acquired ability of late stage tumors to transform the host immune response into tumor growth, whereupon early state tumors or premalignant cells lack this feature.[227]

As already insinuated above, the FasL-Fas system also holds pro-inflammatory properites, but the exact role of FasL in leukocyte recruitment remains to be resolved. Multiple in vivo and in vitro studies confirmed association of FasL expression and inflammatory influx,[228-230] raising the question if FasL itself presents the chemotactic stimulus or if leukycote migration depends on secretion of chemotactic factors from dying cells. On the one hand, chemotaxis of leukocytes in response to increasing gradients of soluble FasL in vitro points towards a direct chemotactic effect of FasL.[32,33] On the other hand, membrane-bound FasL is capable of inducing apoptosis, pro-inflammatory cytokine production in monocytes and macrophages[228,231] and a more robust inflammatory influx which was diminished by proteolytically shed soluble FasL.[229] Thus, inflammation and neutrophil recruitment observed in systems ectopically overexpressing FasL might result from triggering excessive apoptosis and subsequent release of chemotactic factors[232] which tumors probably circumvent by expressing both, membrane FasL and soluble FasL.[233] Despite accumulating evidence of FasL-Fas in immune privilege, Fas counterattack and inflammation, the molecular conditions determining the balance between these responses remain to be identified.

Therapeutic Concepts Targeting the FasL-Fas System

Therapeutic modulation of the FasL-Fas system can have two fundamentally different goals: Firstly, in cases where the activity of the FasL-Fas system contributes to the pathology of a disease, inhibition of the FasL-Fas interaction might be beneficial. In contrast, exogenous stimulation of Fas can offer a promising treatment option if the activity of the FasL-Fas system is expected to antagonize the devastating effects of a particular disease. Therapeutic inhibition of the FasL-Fas system can be achieved straight forward in a classical way by blocking with FasL- or Fas-specific antibodies or neutralizing soluble receptors. On the contrary, concepts aiming to therapeutically exploit Fas activation are more challenging as they have to circumvent the severe side effects associated with systemic Fas activation. Functional modulation of the FasL-Fas system can be achieved by directly targeting the conveniently accessible extracellular domains of these molecules, but might also be realized in an indirect, less specific manner by interference with Fas-associated signaling pathways or FasL-Fas expression. In fact, the antitumoral effect of some chemotherapeutic drugs relies in part on upregulation of Fas and/or FasL and subsequent apoptosis induction.[234-236] Inhibition of components of the extrinsic apoptotic signaling pathway also blocks Fas-induced effects.[237-239] In the following, we focus on reagents and concepts directly targeting FasL or Fas.

Soluble Fas Variants

To obtain soluble decoy receptors of members of the TNF receptor superfamily, it is an established strategy to link the extracellular domain of a particular TNF receptor to the constant region of immunoglobulin G (Fc). In case of TNFR2 the resulting dimeric fusion protein is of high clinical importance for the treatment of TNF-driven autoimmune diseases, such as rheumatoid arthritis. Corresponding Fc fusion proteins of RANK and TACI are in phase I and III clinical trials.[240-242] The Fc fusion proteins of murine and human Fas have, compared to the TNF-TNFR2 interaction, a relatively low affinity for their cognate ligand, FasL and are accordingly significantly less efficient in inhibiting of FasL-induced cell death than neutralizing anti-Fas antibodies.[26,243,244] Nevertheless Fas-Fc fusion proteins have been successfully used in experimental in vivo models to antagonize the deleterious Fas-mediated effects in hepatitis, graft versus host disease and cyclophosphamide-induced diabetes.

Based on the X-ray crystal structure of several ligand-bound receptors of the TNF receptor superfamily and homology considerations, it is commonly accepted that a FasL trimer interacts with three molecules of Fas, each of them binding to the interface of two subunits of the ligand trimer.[20] As the Fas-Fc fusion protein only occupies two of the three binding sites of FasL, it appears possible to obtain soluble Fas variants with higher neutralization capacity by increasing the number of the receptor domains within the neutralizing molecule. In fact, oligomerizaton of Fas-Fc using Protein A results in more efficient FasL inhibition and trimeric as well as pentameric Fas variants that have been generated by genetic fusion with heterologous trimerization and pentamerization domains from Tenascin-C and the cartilage oligomeric matrix protein (COMP) also showed significantly enhanced inhibition of the FasL.[245,246] With respect to the in vivo neutralization capacity of the various Fas variants, however, one should also take into consideration that the effect of Fas-Fc not only relies on simple neutralization of FasL, but might also require recruitment of effector cells to FasL expressing cells by the Fc part of the molecule. Furthermore, there is evidence that membrane FasL engages in intracellular signaling pathways (retrograde signaling) upon binding of oligomerized Fas.[70] It is therefore tempting to speculate that in an in vivo situation soluble variants of FasL differ in their capability to stimulate retrograde FasL signaling depending on the degree of oligomerization. In fact, there is evidence that a naturally appearing soluble Fas variant lacking the transmembrane domain of the molecule induces cell death in FasL expressing cells.[247] Another naturally occurring inhibitory receptor for FasL is decoy receptor-3 (DcR3), a soluble member of the TNF receptor family. Beside FasL DcR3 also binds also the immunostimulatory TNF ligands LIGHT and TL1α.[213,248,249] Notably, this decoy receptor looses its ability to inhibit FasL, but not LIGHT and TL1α, by thrombin mediated cleavage between the cysteine rich domains of the molecule and an extended C-terminal domain of yet poorly understood function.[250,251] Recombinant, noncleavable variants of DcR3 have, in fact, been used successfully in an in vivo model to attenuate FasL-driven lung damage.[251] The activity of the FasL-Fas system might also be inhibited by blocking FasL-specific antibodies or treatment with antagonistic Fas specific antibodies. Several of such antibodies have been described.[26,243,252-254] Long term treatment with antagonizing Fas specific antibodies has to be carefully reviewed as it triggers host immune response and antibody production. Thus, producing cross-linking antibodies could convert initially antagonistic antibodies towards agonistic reagents. This is illustrated by the finding that the Fas-specific antibody ZB4, which is a potent antagonist without cross-linking, strongly induces cell death upon oligomerization. Notably, some Fas-specific antibodies elicit agonistic as well as antagonistic effects depending on which particular cell type is regarded. For example, the human Fas-specific IgM antibody CH11, a popular experimental tool for Fas activation, antagonizes the action of FasL in peripheral T-cells.[255] Further on, Fas activation may also be mediated by synergistic action of non-agonistic antibodies and soluble FasL trimers.[256]

Systemic Fas activation rapidly results in hepatocyte apoptosis and deadly liver failure. Therapeutic concepts based on exogenous activation of Fas must therefore allow cell type, tissue or organ restricted Fas activation in vivo. One might expect that this requirement forbids the systemic application of agonistic Fas antibodies. However, there is experimental evidence that Fas-sensitive cell types respond quite different to agonistic antibodies. The hamster anti-mouse Fas monoclonal antibodies (mAb) Jo2 and RK-8 both strongly induce cell death in vitro in thymocytes, but only Jo2 is toxic on cultured primary hepatocytes.[257-259] The surprisingly different activities of Jo2 and RK-8 also translate in different in vivo effects. While Jo2 triggers severe liver damage, RK-8 application is free of this adverse response, but is still able to induce apoptosis in thymocytes leading to thymic atrophy.[257-259] In fact, administration of RK-8 can be used to antagonize the lymphadenopathy and splenomegaly occuring in FasL-deficient gld mice. Moreover, a therapeutic effect related to the RK-8-mediated depletion of autoreactive T-cells has been demonstrated in a collagen-induced type II arthritis model.[258,260] Thymocytes have been classified as type I cells, whereas the hepatocytes have been assigned to the type II cell category.[46] Thus, the distinct molecular mechanisms of Fas activation proposed to work in type I and type II cells might be differently engaged by some agonistic Fas antibodies. This in turn leads to selective bioactivity as observed for the RK-8 antibody. By immunizing Fas-deficient mice with human Fas a anti-Fas monoclonal antibody has been generated recognizing Fas from different species including men and mice.[261] This antibody as well as a humanized variant derived thereof show similar properties as the RK-8 antibody.[262] Accordingly, these antibodies have been successfully used to trigger apoptosis in melanoma xenotransplants and to prevent graft versus host disease in a SCID mouse model with human Fas transgenic splenocytes.[263,264]

Cell Surface Antigen-Restricted Activation of Fas

It has been shown that soluble, poorly active FasL trimers gain high activity upon binding to fibronectin, a compound of the extracellular matrix via a motif immediately preceding the THD of the molecule.[31] This observation gave first evidence for the idea that spatial fixation of soluble FasL trimers is sufficient to convert them into molecules displaying membrane FasL-like activity. In accordance with this hypothesis, we and others showed that fusion proteins composed of an

N-terminal cell surface antigen-recognizing single chain fragment (scFv) and soluble FasL exert on antigen positive cells a several order of magnitude higher activity than on antigen negative cells.[265-267] Thus, cell surface retention of scFv-FasL fusion proteins by interaction with their cognate cell surface antigens constitutes pseudo-membrane FasL (see Fig. 5). It is obvious that the use of scFv recognizing appropriate tumor markers allows construction of Fas agonists with tumor localized action. The feasibility of this principle has been demonstrated with a scFv-FasL fusion protein recognizing FAP (fibroblast activation protein; anti-FAP-FasL). FAP is a transmembrane protein and is restrictedly expressed during angiogenesis and on activated fibroblasts occurring in wound healing or in the stroma of epithelial cancer.[268,269] In vitro this anti-FAP-FasL fusion protein showed on transfectants stably expressing FAP a comparable or even higher activity than oligomerized soluble FasL, but required in the corresponding FAP-negative cell line a one thousand fold higher concentration to induce cell death.[265] In accordance with the proposed mode of action, antibodies that interfere with the binding of the anti-FAP-FasL fusion protein to FAP rescued FAP-expressing cells from apoptosis induction.[265] More important, administration of even high amounts of the anti-FAP-FasL fusion protein was nontoxic in mice and prevented the development of FAP-positive, but not of FAP-negative xenotransplants.[265] Cell surface antigen-dependent enhancement of Fas activation has also been demonstrated for scFv-FasL fusion proteins recognizing CD7[267] and CD20.[266] Notably, cell surface retention-dependent activation of Fas not only works with single chain-FasL fusion proteins, but also with other types of FasL variants, provided they interact with a cell associated structure. Especially, this allows the construction of bifunctional molecules containing besides FasL a second domain with a potentially anti-tumoral effect. For example, a fusion protein consisting of the N-terminal extracellular domain of CD40 and the C-terminal THD of FasL not only robustly activates Fas after binding to membrane CD40L, but also concomitantly interrupts autocrine antiapoptotic CD40-CD40L signaling in T47D breast cancer cells.[270] Accordingly, the CD40-FasL fusion protein displayed much higher apoptotic activity on these tumor cells than oligomerized FasL which only activates Fas. Notably, bispecific antibodies composed of a non-agonistic Fas specific antibody fragment and a second antibody fragment recognizing a tumor marker displayed a similar antigen-dependent mode of Fas activation as described for the genetically engineered FasL fusion proteins.[271,272] With respect to the safeness of the various FasL fusion proteins, one has to take into consideration that their repeated administration might lead to an immune response generating antibodies leading to oligomeriziation of the corresponding fusion protein and thus its antigen-independent activation. As secondary oligomerization of FasL trimers results in high activity, targeting domains that trigger the formation of higher order FasL oligomers are also not useful for cell surface immobilization-dependent Fas activation. Antigen-dependent activation of TNFR2, TRAILR2 and OX40 have also been described for scFv fusion proteins of their corresponding ligands (TNF, TRAIL, OX40L) indicating that receptor activation by cell surface retention of appropriately designed ligand fusion proteins is a broadly applicable mechanism in the TNF ligand family.[273-278]

FasL Prodrugs

It has been recently shown that in principle it is possible to generate FasL prodrugs that are only activated after antibody-directed retention on tumor cells and subsequent processing by tumor-associated proteases, e.g., matrix metalloproteases (MMPs) and urokinase plasminogen activator (uPA).[246] Besides the THD of FasL, the FasL prodrug contains three functional relevant parts: Firstly, the extracellular domain of Fas, for intra- and/or intermolecular inhibition of the FasL part of the prodrug. Secondly, a scFv mediating cell surface retention of the prodrug and thirdly a linker containing recognition sites for tumor-associated proteases that separates the inhibitory Fas domain from the scFv-FasL part of the molecule (see Fig. 6).[246] In vitro, the FasL prodrug was practically inactive and remained intact when applied to antigen-negative, MMP- and uPA-expressing tumor cells whereas antigen-positive tumor cells were readily killed. Notably, prodrug processing preceded antigen-dependent Fas activation by the FasL prodrug. Thus, the FasL prodrug is first retained on the cell surface by antigen binding via its scFv domain. Cell surface

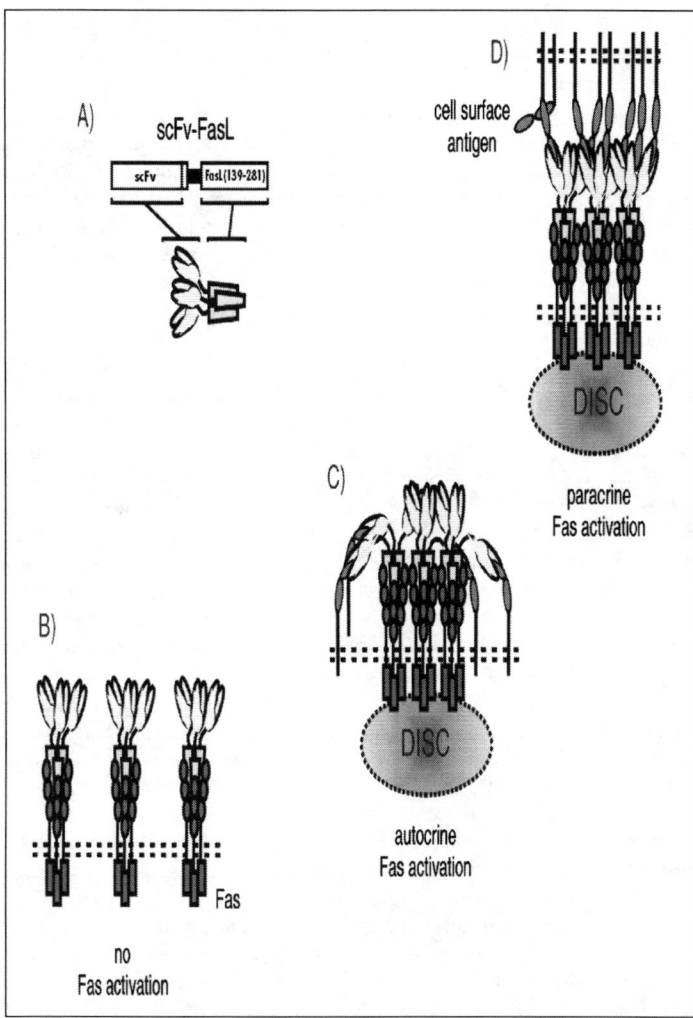

Figure 5. Cell surface antigen-restricted activation of Fas. A) Schematic representation of scFv-FasL. B) Fas binding of scFv-FasL on antigen negative does not result in Fas activation. Thus, scFv-FasL acts like soluble FasL. C) Binding of the single chain domain of scFv-FasL to antigen positive Fas expressing cells enables autocrine Fas activation. D) scFv-FasL binding to antigen positive cells also induces paracrine Fas activation. For details see text. scFv = single chain fragment.

retention is a prerequisite for subsequent processing by cell-associated proteases.[246] After release of the inhibitory Fas domain the FasL part of the prodrug is now able to activate Fas. So, Fas triggering by the FasL prodrug needs FAP expression as well as the action of appropriate tumor-associated proteases. First in vivo proof of principle for the feasibility of the FasL prodrug concept has been demonstrated in a xenotransplantation model in which a FasL prodrug only reduced the growth of FAP-expressing but not FAP-negative HT1080 tumor cells.[246] Due to the autoinhibitory Fas domain of the FasL prodrug, cell surface binding alone does not lead to activation of the prodrug. Thus, in this approach it appears possible to use immobilization domains targeting structures that are not selectively expressed on tumor cells.

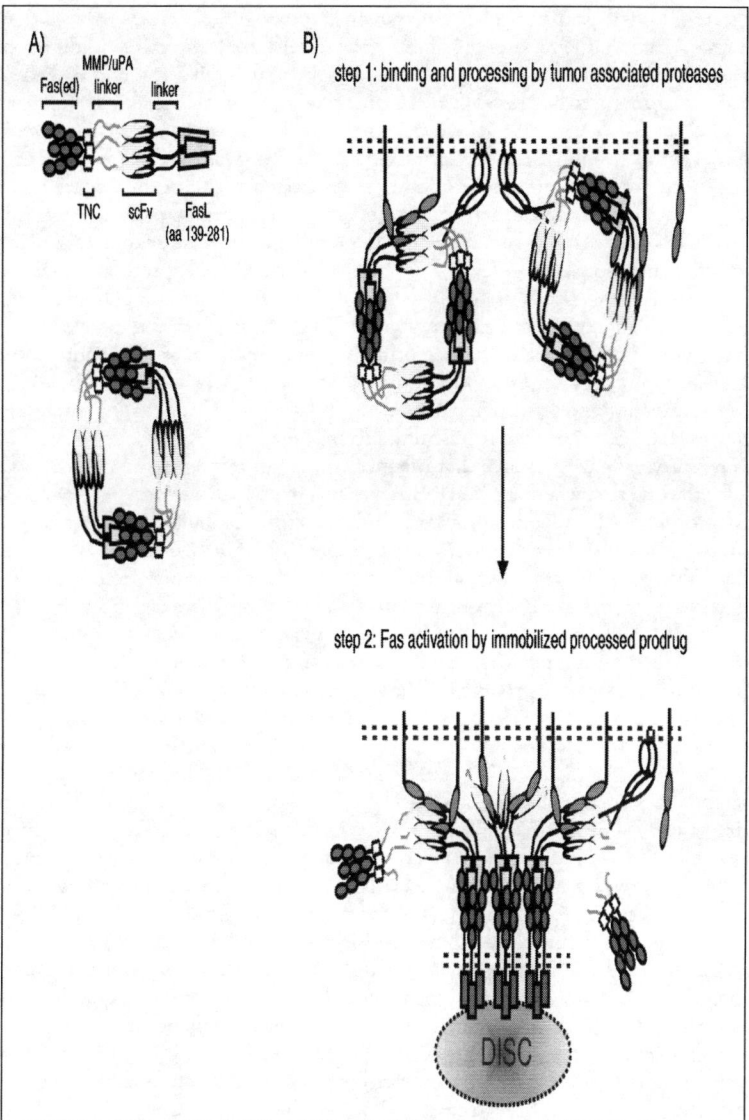

Figure 6. Tumor associated protease-licensed Fas activation. A) Domain architecture of a FasL prodrug (above) and spontaneous head-to-tail assembly of prodrug molecules (below). B) Prodrug activation requires antigen binding and subsequent processing by tumor associated proteases (step 1). After removal of the inhibitory Fas domain the remaining cell surface antigen-bound scFv-FasL part of the molecule acts like membrane FasL (step 2).

FasL in Gene Therapy

Therapeutic approaches using FasL gene therapy reflect the function of this molecule in tumor surveillance and immune privilege. There are attempts to use FasL expression to protect transplants from rejection by the immune system, but there are also concepts employing FasL encoding viral vectors to induce apoptosis in tumor cells. Early on after the realization that activated T-cells are highly susceptible towards Fas-induced apoptosis, there were attempts to utilize ectopic FasL expression to confer immune privilege to transplants. Although in some studies FasL-transfected transplants showed lower rejection due to killing of infiltrating T-cells, there were also studies coming up with the surprising observation that FasL expression accelerates graft rejection.[7] FasL-dependent graft rejection was found to be caused by recruitment of immune cells, especially neutrophils.[7,191] In accordance, mice deficient for MIP1a, an important chemoattractant for neutrophils, show strongly reduced rejection of FasL-expressing tumor cells.[279] Several mechanisms that might be responsible for the production of neutrophil chemoattractants have been identified and might act in a redundant fashion. Fas can activate pro-inflammatory signaling pathways resulting in the activation of NFκB and MAP kinases and accordingly upregulate inflammation related cytokines and chemokines, including IL-8 and MIP1a.[7,191] In particular, Fas can upregulate IL-1α, which in turn again induces chemoattractant proteins.[280] Further on, some studies found that soluble FasL itself can act as a chemoattractant factor for neutrophils,[32,33] but other studies failed to reconcile this observation.[30,229,281,282] Instead, they demonstrated that membrane FasL in contrast to soluble FasL is sufficient to trigger neutrophil infiltration. As caspases activated in course of apoptosis inhibit NFκB activation and protein translation, pro-inflammatory Fas signaling barely takes place in Fas-sensitive cells, but is instead readily induced in some Fas-resistant cell types.[7,191] Notably, studies in recent years gave evidence that the mechanism conferring Fas resistance is of crucial relevance for the question whether Fas activation results in pro-inflammatory signaling. The long and short isoform of FLIP not only inhibit Fas-induced apoptosis, but also prevent NFκB activation.[7,191] In contrast, cells gaining Fas resistance by expression of Bcl-2 or BclxL exhibit a strongly increased capability to activate NFκB and to produce pro-inflammatory factors. It is therefore tempting to speculate that the mechanisms protecting FasL positive transplants and/or its neighboring cells are a major parameter deciding between graft acceptance and graft rejection. How the aforementioned mechanisms play together in making this decision warrants further experimental verification. Thus, it is still not possible to reliably predict the overall consequences of FasL gene transfer approaches. In fact, even closely related FasL gene therapy experiments came up with opposite results. For example several reports investigated in mouse models the engraftment of islets of Langerhans expressing wild type FasL under the control of the insulin promoter. In these studies a rapid onset of diabetes was observed and FasL-positive islets grafts from nondiabetic and NOD mice elicited a strong immune reaction.[82,283-285] In contrast, islets grafts cotransplanted with FasL expressing myoblasts or FasL-decorated splenocytes showed durable protection against graft rejection.[286,287] Noteworthy, a cleavage resistant FasL isoform sustained islets allograft survival in this model pointing to a crucial role of the chemoattractant function of soluble FasL in this setting.[287] Furthermore, long term acceptance of allogeneic islets has been achieved by cotransplantation of FasL expressing testicular cell aggregates suggesting that ectopic FasL expression can lead to immune hyporesponsiveness in an antigen dependent fashion.[288] The major benefit of the protection of grafts by artificial FasL expression lies in the alloantigen specificity of the immunosuppressive effect leaving the immune competence for other antigens intact.

Systemic effects of FasL, especially liver toxicity might be no major problem in transplantation setting to distant locations, but have to be taken into account when FasL encoding viral vectors are used. Indeed, intravenous administration of adenovirus encoding membrane FasL under the control of a constitutive active promoter induces the characteristic signs of liver damage that can also be observed after intravenous injection of agonistic Fas antibodies or oligomerized FasL. However, it is possible to restrict FasL expression by injection of replication defective viral vectors locally, for example in arthritic joints or salivary glands. In fact, FasL gene transfer into arthritic joints results in apoptosis of synovial cells in collagen induced arthritis without eliciting systemic toxicity.[289-291] Likewise, local FasL gene transfer into salivary glands reduces the number of infiltrating immune cells in a murine model of chronic sialadenitis, again without adverse systemic side effects.[292] Local activity of FasL in gene therapy has also been achieved with cell type-specific promoters as well as with a tetracycline regulated promoter.[293-299]

References

1. Yonehara S, Ishii A, Yonehara M. A cell-killing monoclonal antibody (anti-Fas) to a cell surface antigen codownregulated with the receptor of tumor necrosis factor. J Exp Med 1989; 169:1747-1756.
2. Trauth BC, Klas C, Peters AM et al. Monoclonal antibody-mediated tumor regression by induction of apoptosis. Science 1989; 245:301-305.
3. Itoh N, Yonehara S, Ishii A et al. The polypeptide encoded by the cDNA for human cell surface antigen Fas can mediate apoptosis. Cell 1991; 66:233-243.
4. Suda T, Takahashi T, Golstein P et al. Molecular cloning and expression of the Fas ligand, a novel member of the tumor necrosis factor family. Cell 1993; 75:1169-1178.
5. Takahashi T, Tanaka M, Inazawa J et al. Human Fas ligand: gene structure, chromosomal location and species specificity. Int Immunol 1994; 6:1567-1574.
6. Cheng J, Liu C, Koopman WJ et al. Characterization of human Fas gene. Exon/intron organization and promoter region. J Immunol 1995; 154:1239-1245.
7. Wajant H, Pfizenmaier K, Scheurich P. Non-apoptotic Fas signaling. Cytokine Growth Factor Rev 2003; 14:53-66.
8. Cheng J, Zhou T, Liu C et al. Protection from Fas-mediated apoptosis by a soluble form of the Fas molecule. Science 1994; 263:1759-1762.
9. Locksley RM, Killeen N, Lenardo MJ. The TNF and TNF receptor superfamilies: Integrating mammalian biology. Cell 2001; 104:487-501.
10. Zhang G. Tumor necrosis factor family ligand-receptor binding. Curr Opin Struct Biol 2004; 14:154-160.
11. Orlinick JR, Vaishnaw A, Elkon KB et al. Requirement of cysteine-rich repeats of the Fas receptor for binding by the Fas ligand. J Biol Chem 1997; 272:28889-28894.
12. Starling GC, Bajorath J, Emswiler J et al. Identification of amino acid residues important for ligand binding to Fas. J Exp Med 1997; 185:1487-1492.
13. Papoff G, Hausler P, Eramo A et al. Identification and characterization of a ligand-independent oligomerization domain in the extracellular region of the CD95 death receptor. J Biol Chem 1999; 274:38241-38250.
14. Siegel RM, Frederiksen JK, Zacharias DA et al. Fas preassociation required for apoptosis signaling and dominant inhibition by pathogenic mutations. Science 2000; 288:2354-2357.
15. Itoh N, Nagata S. A novel protein domain required for apoptosis. Mutational analysis of human Fas antigen. J Biol Chem 1993; 268:10932-10937.
16. Chan FK, Chun HJ, Zheng L et al. A domain in TNF receptors that mediates ligand-independent receptor assembly and signaling. Science 2000; 288:2351-2354.
17. Fesik SW. Insights into programmed cell death through structural biology. Cell 2000; 103:273-282.
18. Stahnke K, Hecker S, Kohne E et al. CD95 (APO-1/FAS)-mediated apoptosis in cytokine-activated hematopoietic cells. Exp Hematol 1998; 26:844-850.
19. Orlinick JR, Elkon KB, Chao MV. Separate domains of the human Fas ligand dictate self-association and receptor binding. J Biol Chem 1997; 272:32221-32229.
20. Bodmer JL, Schneider P, Tschopp J. The molecular architecture of the TNF superfamily. Trends Biochem Sci 2002; 27:19-26.
21. Gruss HJ, Dower SK. Tumor necrosis factor ligand superfamily: involvement in the pathology of malignant lymphomas. Blood 1995; 85:3378-3404.
22. Wenzel J, Sanzenbacher R, Ghadimi M et al. Multiple interactions of the cytosolic polyproline region of the CD95 ligand: Hints for the reverse signal transduction capacity of a death factor. FEBS Lett 2001; 509:255-262.
23. Blott EJ, Bossi G, Clark R et al. Fas ligand is targeted to secretory lysosomes via a proline-rich domain in its cytoplasmic tail. J Cell Sci 2001; 114:2405-2416.
24. Janssen O, Qian J, Linkermann A et al. CD95 ligand—Death factor and costimulatory molecule? Cell Death Differ 2003; 10:1215-1225.
25. Wetzel M, Li L, Harms KM et al. Tissue inhibitor of metalloproteinases-3 facilitates Fas-mediated neuronal cell death following mild ischemia. Cell Death Differ 2007; 15:143-151.
26. Kayagaki N, Kawasaki A, Ebata T et al. Metalloproteinase-mediated release of human Fas ligand. J Exp Med 1995; 182:1777-1783.
27. Mitsiades N, Yu WH, Poulaki V et al. Matrix metalloproteinase-7-mediated cleavage of Fas ligand protects tumor cells from chemotherapeutic drug cytotoxicity. Cancer Res 2001; 61:577-581.
28. Tanaka M, Itai T, Adachi M et al. Downregulation of Fas ligand by shedding. Nat Med 1998; 4:31-36.
29. Schneider P, Holler N, Bodmer JL et al. Conversion of membrane-bound Fas(CD95) ligand to its soluble form is associated with downregulation of its proapoptotic activity and loss of liver toxicity. J Exp Med 1998; 187:1205-1213.

30. Shudo K, Kinoshita K, Imamura R et al. The membrane-bound but not the soluble form of human Fas ligand is responsible for its inflammatory activity. Eur J Immunol 2001; 31:2504-2511.
31. Aoki K, Kurooka M, Chen JJ et al. Extracellular matrix interacts with soluble CD95L: Retention and enhancement of cytotoxicity. Nat Immunol 2001; 2:333-337.
32. Ottonello L, Tortolina G, Amelotti M et al. Soluble Fas ligand is chemotactic for human neutrophilic polymorphonuclear leukocytes. J Immunol 1999; 162:3601-3606.
33. Seino K, Iwabuchi K, Kayagaki N et al. Chemotactic activity of soluble Fas ligand against phagocytes. J Immunol 1998; 161:4484-4488.
34. Lee KH, Feig C, Tchikov V et al. The role of receptor internalization in CD95 signaling. EMBO J 2006; 25:1009-1023.
35. Algeciras-Schimnich A, Shen L, Barnhart BC et al. Molecular ordering of the initial signaling events of CD95. Mol Cell Biol 2002; 22:207-220.
36. Legembre P, Daburon S, Moreau P et al. Cutting Edge: modulation of Fas-mediated apoptosis by lipid rafts in T lymphocytes. J Immunol 2006; 176:716-720.
37. Eramo A, Sargiacomo M, Ricci-Vitiani L et al. CD95 death-inducing signaling complex formation and internalization occur in lipid rafts of type I and type II cells. Eur J Immunol 2004; 34:1930-1940.
38. Henkler F, Behrle E, Dennehy KM et al. The extracellular domains of FasL and Fas are sufficient for the formation of supramolecular FasL-Fas clusters of high stability. J Cell Biol 2005; 168:1087-1098.
39. Siegel RM, Muppidi JR, Sarker M et al. SPOTS: signaling protein oligomeric transduction structures are early mediators of death receptor-induced apoptosis at the plasma membrane. J Cell Biol 2004; 167:735-744.
40. Muzio M, Chinnaiyan AM, Kischkel FC et al. FLICE, a novel FADD-homologous ICE/CED-3-like protease, is recruited to the CD95 (Fas/APO-1) death-inducing signaling complex. Cell 1996; 85:817-827.
41. Chinnaiyan AM, O'Rourke K, Tewari M et al. FADD, a novel death domain-containing protein, interacts with the death domain of Fas and initiates apoptosis. Cell 1995; 81:505-512.
42. Boldin MP, Varfolomeev EE, Pancer Z et al. A novel protein that interacts with the death domain of Fas/APO1 contains a sequence motif related to the death domain. J Biol Chem 1995; 270:7795-7798.
43. Donepudi M, Mac SA, Briand C et al. Insights into the regulatory mechanism for caspase-8 activation. Mol Cell 2003; 11:543-549.
44. Boatright KM, Renatus M, Scott FL et al. A unified model for apical caspase activation. Mol Cell 2003; 11:529-541.
45. Peter ME, Krammer PH. The CD95(APO-1/Fas) DISC and beyond. Cell Death Differ 2003; 10:26-35.
46. Barnhart BC, Alappat EC, Peter ME. The CD95 type I/type II model. Semin Immunol 2003; 15:185-193.
47. Vaux DL, Silke J. Mammalian mitochondrial IAP binding proteins. Biochem Biophys Res Commun 2003; 304:499-504.
48. Vande WL, Lamkanfi M, Vandenabeele P. The mitochondrial serine protease HtrA2/Omi: An overview. Cell Death Differ 2008;
49. Riedl SJ, Salvesen GS. The apoptosome: Signalling platform of cell death. Nat Rev Mol Cell Biol 2007; 8:405-413.
50. Holler N, Zaru R, Micheau O et al. Fas triggers an alternative, caspase-8-independent cell death pathway using the kinase RIP as effector molecule. Nat Immunol 2000; 1:489-495.
51. Matsumura H, Shimizu Y, Ohsawa Y et al. Necrotic death pathway in Fas receptor signaling. J Cell Biol 2000; 151:1247-1256.
52. Vercammen D, Brouckaert G, Denecker G et al. Dual signaling of the Fas receptor: Initiation of both apoptotic and necrotic cell death pathways. J Exp Med 1998; 188:919-930.
53. Berghe TV, van Loo G, Saelens X et al. Differential signaling to apoptotic and necrotic cell death by Fas-associated death domain protein FADD. J Biol Chem 2004; 279:7925-7933.
54. Kreuz S, Siegmund D, Rumpf JJ et al. NFkappaB activation by Fas is mediated through FADD, caspase-8 and RIP and is inhibited by FLIP. J Cell Biol 2004; 166:369-380.
55. Hu WH, Johnson H, Shu HB. Activation of NF-kappaB by FADD, Casper and caspase-8. J Biol Chem 2000; 275:10838-10844.
56. Wajant H, Haas E, Schwenzer R et al. Inhibition of death receptor-mediated gene induction by a cycloheximide-sensitive factor occurs at the level of or upstream of Fas-associated death domain protein (FADD). J Biol Chem 2000; 275:24357-24366.
57. Chaudhary PM, Eby MT, Jasmin A et al. Activation of the NF-kappaB pathway by caspase 8 and its homologs. Oncogene 2000; 19:4451-4460.
58. Cardone MH, Salvesen GS, Widmann C et al. The regulation of anoikis: MEKK-1 activation requires cleavage by caspases. Cell 1997; 90:315-323.

59. Widmann C, Gerwins P, Johnson NL et al. MEK kinase 1, a substrate for DEVD-directed caspases, is involved in genotoxin-induced apoptosis. Mol Cell Biol 1998; 18:2416-2429.
60. Widmann C, Johnson NL, Gardner AM et al. Potentiation of apoptosis by low dose stress stimuli in cells expressing activated MEK kinase 1. Oncogene 1997; 15:2439-2447.
61. Ham YM, Choi JS, Chun KH et al. The c-Jun N-terminal kinase 1 activity is differentially regulated by specific mechanisms during apoptosis. J Biol Chem 2003; 278:50330-50337.
62. Low W, Smith A, Ashworth A et al. JNK activation is not required for Fas-mediated apoptosis. Oncogene 1999; 18:3737-3741.
63. Lenczowski JM, Dominguez L, Eder AM et al. Lack of a role for Jun kinase and AP-1 in Fas-induced apoptosis. Mol Cell Biol 1997; 17:170-181.
64. Esposito G, Prasad SV, Rapacciuolo A et al. Cardiac overexpression of a G(q) inhibitor blocks induction of extracellular signal-regulated kinase and c-Jun NH(2)-terminal kinase activity in in vivo pressure overload. Circulation 2001; 103:1453-1458.
65. Choukroun G, Hajjar R, Fry S et al. Regulation of cardiac hypertrophy in vivo by the stress-activated protein kinases/c-Jun NH(2)-terminal kinases. J Clin Invest 1999; 104:391-398.
66. Badorff C, Ruetten H, Mueller S et al. Fas receptor signaling inhibits glycogen synthase kinase 3 beta and induces cardiac hypertrophy following pressure overload. J Clin Invest 2002; 109:373-381.
67. Cross DA, Alessi DR, Cohen P et al. Inhibition of glycogen synthase kinase-3 by insulin mediated by protein kinase B. Nature 1995; 378:785-789.
68. Alderson MR, Armitage RJ, Maraskovsky E et al. Fas transduces activation signals in normal human T-lymphocytes. J Exp Med 1993; 178:2231-2235.
69. Kurasawa K, Hashimoto Y, Kasai M et al. The Fas antigen is involved in thymic T-cell development as a costimulatory molecule, but not in the deletion of neglected thymocytes. J Allergy Clin Immunol 2000; 106:S19-S31.
70. Sun M, Fink PJ. A new class of reverse signaling costimulators belongs to the TNF family. J Immunol 2007; 179:4307-4312.
71. Aggarwal BB, Singh S, LaPushin R et al. Fas antigen signals proliferation of normal human diploid fibroblast and its mechanism is different from tumor necrosis factor receptor. FEBS Lett 1995; 364:5-8.
72. Freiberg RA, Spencer DM, Choate KA et al. Fas signal transduction triggers either proliferation or apoptosis in human fibroblasts. J Invest Dermatol 1997; 108:215-219.
73. Ahn JH, Park SM, Cho HS et al. Non-apoptotic signaling pathways activated by soluble Fas ligand in serum-starved human fibroblasts. Mitogen-activated protein kinases and NF-kappaB-dependent gene expression. J Biol Chem 2001; 276:47100-47106.
74. Desbarats J, Newell MK. Fas engagement accelerates liver regeneration after partial hepatectomy. Nat Med 2000; 6:920-923.
75. Ma Y, Liu H, Tu-Rapp H et al. Fas ligation on macrophages enhances IL-1R1-Toll-like receptor 4 signaling and promotes chronic inflammation. Nat Immunol 2004; 5:380-387.
76. Griffith TS, Brunner T, Fletcher SM et al. Fas ligand-induced apoptosis as a mechanism of immune privilege. Science 1995; 270:1189-1192.
77. Sabelko-Downes KA, Cross AH, Russell JH. Dual role for Fas ligand in the initiation of and recovery from experimental allergic encephalomyelitis. J Exp Med 1999; 189:1195-1205.
78. Suvannavejh GC, Dal Canto MC, Matis LA et al. Fas-mediated apoptosis in clinical remissions of relapsing experimental autoimmune encephalomyelitis. J Clin Invest 2000; 105:223-231.
79. Gochuico BR, Miranda KM, Hessel EM et al. Airway epithelial Fas ligand expression: potential role in modulating bronchial inflammation. Am J Physiol Lung Cell Mol Physiol 1998; 274:L444-L449.
80. Hunt JS, Vassmer D, Ferguson TA et al. Fas ligand is positioned in mouse uterus and placenta to prevent trafficking of activated leukocytes between the mother and the conceptus. J Immunol 1997; 158:4122-4128.
81. Bohana-Kashtan O, Civin CI. Fas ligand as a tool for immunosuppression and generation of immune tolerance. Stem Cells 2004; 22:908-924.
82. Kang SM, Schneider DB, Lin Z et al. Fas ligand expression in islets of langerhans does not confer immune privilege and instead targets them for rapid destruction. Nat Med 1997; 3:738-743.
83. Takeuchi T, Ueki T, Nishimatsu H et al. Accelerated rejection of Fas ligand-expressing heart grafts. J Immunol 1999; 162:518-522.
84. Cohen PL, Eisenberg RA. Lpr and gld: single gene models of systemic autoimmunity and lymphoproliferative disease. Annu Rev Immunol 1991; 9:243-269.
85. Watanabe-Fukunaga R, Brannan CI, Copeland NG et al. Lymphoproliferation disorder in mice explained by defects in Fas antigen that mediates apoptosis. Nature 1992; 356:314-317.
86. Kennedy NJ, Kataoka T, Tschopp J et al. Caspase activation is required for T-cell proliferation. J Exp Med 1999; 190:1891-1896.

87. Alam A, Cohen LY, Aouad S et al. Early activation of caspases during T-lymphocyte stimulation results in selective substrate cleavage in nonapoptotic cells. J Exp Med 1999; 190:1879-1890.

88. Mack A, Hacker G. Inhibition of caspase or FADD function blocks proliferation but not MAP kinase-activation and interleukin-2-production during primary stimulation of T-cells. Eur J Immunol 2002; 32:1986-1992.

89. Beisner DR, Chu IH, Arechiga AF et al. The requirements for Fas-associated death domain signaling in mature T-cell activation and survival. J Immunol 2003; 171:247-256.

90. Chun HJ, Zheng L, Ahmad M et al. Pleiotropic defects in lymphocyte activation caused by caspase-8 mutations lead to human immunodeficiency. Nature 2002; 419:395-399.

91. Green DR, Droin N, Pinkoski M. Activation-induced cell death in T-cells. Immunol Rev 2003; 193:70-81.

92. Rieux-Laucat F, Le Deist F, Fischer A. Autoimmune lymphoproliferative syndromes: Genetic defects of apoptosis pathways. Cell Death Differ 2003; 10:124-133.

93. Reap EA, Felix NJ, Wolthusen PA et al. bcl-2 transgenic Lpr mice show profound enhancement of lymphadenopathy. J Immunol 1995; 155:5455-5462.

94. Strasser A, Harris AW, Huang DC et al. Bcl-2 and Fas/APO-1 regulate distinct pathways to lymphocyte apoptosis. EMBO J 1995; 14:6136-6147.

95. Hildeman DA, Zhu Y, Mitchell TC et al. Activated T-cell death in vivo mediated by proapoptotic bcl-2 family member bim. Immunity 2002; 16:759-767.

96. Lu B, Finn OJ. T-cell death and cancer immune tolerance. Cell Death Differ 2007; 15:70-79.

97. Hughes PD, Belz GT, Fortner KA et al. Apoptosis regulators Fas and bim cooperate in shutdown of chronic immune responses and prevention of autoimmunity. Immunity 2008; 28:197-205.

98. Hutcheson J, Scatizzi JC, Siddiqui AM et al. Combined deficiency of proapoptotic regulators bim and Fas results in the early onset of systemic autoimmunity. Immunity 2008; 28:206-217.

99. Weant AE, Michalek RD, Khan IU et al. Apoptosis regulators bim and fas function concurrently to control autoimmunity and CD8(+) T-cell contraction. Immunity 2008; 28:218-230.

100. Green DR. Fas Bim Boom. Immunity 2008; 28:141-143.

101. Takahashi T, Tanaka M, Brannan CI et al. Generalized lymphoproliferative disease in mice, caused by a point mutation in the Fas ligand. Cell 1994; 76:969-976.

102. Siegel RM, Chan FK, Chun HJ et al. The multifaceted role of Fas signaling in immune cell homeostasis and autoimmunity. Nat Immunol 2000; 1:469-474.

103. Schumann DM, Maedler K, Franklin I et al. The Fas pathway is involved in pancreatic beta cell secretory function. Proc Natl Acad Sci USA 2007; 104:2861-2866.

104. Maedler K, Spinas GA, Lehmann R et al. Glucose induces {beta}-cell apoptosis via upregulation of the Fas receptor in human islets. Diabetes 2001; 50:1683-1690.

105. Donath MY, Storling J, Maedler K et al. Inflammatory mediators and islet beta-cell failure: A link between type 1 and type 2 diabetes. J Mol Med 2003; 81:455-470.

106. Surh CD, Sprent J. T-cell apoptosis detected in situ during positive and negative selection in the thymus. Nature 1994; 372:100-103.

107. Castro JE, Listman JA, Jacobson BA et al. Fas modulation of apoptosis during negative selection of thymocytes. Immunity 1996; 5:617-627.

108. Singer GG, Abbas AK. The Fas antigen is involved in peripheral but not thymic deletion of T-lympho-cytes in T-cell receptor transgenic mice. Immunity 1994; 1:365-371.

109. Bidere N, Su HC, Lenardo MJ. Genetic disorders of programmed cell death in the immune system. Annu Rev Immunol 2006; 24:321-352.

110. Sneller MC, Dale JK, Straus SE. Autoimmune lymphoproliferative syndrome. Curr Opin Rheumatol 2003; 15:417-421.

111. Pereira FA, Mudgil AV, Rosmarin DM. Toxic epidermal necrolysis. J Am Acad Dermatol 2007; 56:181-200.

112. Viard I, Wehrli P, Bullani R et al. Inhibition of toxic epidermal necrolysis by blockade of cd95 with human intravenous immunoglobulin. Science 1998; 282:490-493.

113. Paquet P, Pierard GE, Quatresooz P. Novel treatments for drug-induced toxic epidermal necrolysis (Lyell's syndrome). Int Arch Allergy Immunol 2005; 136:205-216.

114. Ferguson TA, Griffith TS. A vision of cell death: Fas ligand and immune privilege 10 years later. Immunol Rev 2006; 213:228-238.

115. Stuart PM, Griffith TS, Usui N et al. CD95 ligand (FasL)-induced apoptosis is necessary for corneal allograft survival. J Clin Invest 1997; 99:396-402.

116. Griffith TS, Yu X, Herndon JM et al. CD95-induced apoptosis of lymphocytes in an immune privileged site induces immunological tolerance. Immunity 1996; 5:7-16.

117. Hu MS, Schwartzman JD, Yeaman GR et al. Fas-FasL interaction involved in pathogenesis of ocular toxoplasmosis in mice. Infect Immun 1999; 67:928-935.

118. Yamagami S, Kawashima H, Tsuru T et al. Role of Fas-Fas ligand interactions in the immunorejection of allogeneic mouse corneal transplants. Transplantation 1997; 64:1107-1111.
119. Filippatos G, Leche C, Sunga R et al. Expression of FAS adjacent to fibrotic foci in the failing human heart is not associated with increased apoptosis. Am J Physiol 1999; 277:H445-H451.
120. Perez EC, Shulzhenko N, Morgun A et al. Expression of Fas, Fasl and soluble Fas mrna in endomyocardial biopsies of human cardiac allografts. Human Immunology 2006; 67:22-26.
121. Askenasy N, Yolcu ES, Wang Z et al. Display of Fas ligand protein on cardiac vasculature as a novel means of regulating allograft rejection. Circulation 2003; 107:1525-1531.
122. Yang J, Jones SP, Suhara T et al. Endothelial cell overexpression of Fas ligand attenuates ischemia-reperfusion injury in the heart. J Biol Chem 2003; 278:15185-15191.
123. Kanamori H, Takemura G, Li Y et al. Inhibition of Fas-associated apoptosis in granulation tissue cells accompanies attenuation of postinfarction left ventricular remodeling by olmesartan. Am J Physiol Heart Circ Physiol 2007; 292:H2184-H2194.
124. Higuchi MD, Ries MM, Aiello VD et al. Association of an increase in CD8[+] T-cells with the presence of Trypanosoma cruzi antigens in chronic, human, chagasic myocarditis. Am J Trop Med Hyg 1997; 56:485-489.
125. Tostes S Jr, Bertulucci Rocha-Rodrigues D, de Araujo PG et al. Myocardiocyte apoptosis in heart failure in chronic Chagas' disease. Int J Cardiol 2005; 99:233-237.
126. de Oliveira GM, Diniz RL, Batista W et al. Fas ligand-dependent inflammatory regulation in acute myocarditis induced by Trypanosoma cruzi infection. Am J Pathol 2007; 171:79-86.
127. Guillermo LV, Silva EM, Ribeiro-Gomes FL et al. The Fas death pathway controls coordinated expansions of type 1 CD8 and type 2 CD4 T-cells in Trypanosoma cruzi infection. J Leukoc Biol 2007; 81:942-951.
128. Niu J, Azfer A, Kolattukudy PE. Protection against lipopolysacharide-induced myocardial dysfunction in mice by cardiac-specific expression of soluble Fas. J Mol Cell Cardiol 2008; 44:160-169.
129. Volpert OV, Zaichuk T, Zhou W et al. Inducer-stimulated Fas targets activated endothelium for destruction by anti-angiogenic thrombospondin-1 and pigment epithelium-derived factor. Nat Med 2002; 8:349-357.
130. Lucas R, Holmgren L, Garcia I et al. Multiple forms of angiostatin induce apoptosis in endothelial cells. Blood 1998; 92:4730-4741.
131. Jimenez B, Volpert OV, Crawford SE et al. Signals leading to apoptosis-dependent inhibition of neovascularization by thrombospondin-1. Nat Med 2000; 6:41-48.
132. Stellmach V, Crawford SE, Zhou W et al. Prevention of ischemia-induced retinopathy by the natural ocular antiangiogenic agent pigment epithelium-derived factor. Proc Natl Acad Sci USA. 2001; 98:2593-2597.
133. Zaichuk TA, Shroff EH, Emmanuel R et al. Nuclear factor of activated T-cells balances angiogenesis activation and inhibition. J Exp Med 2004; 199:1513-1522.
134. Kamphaus GD, Colorado PC, Panka DJ et al. Canstatin, a novel matrix-derived inhibitor of angiogenesis and tumor growth. J Biol Chem 2000; 275:1209-1215.
135. Panka DJ, Mier JW. Canstatin inhibits Akt activation and induces Fas-dependent apoptosis in endothelial cells. J Biol Chem 2003; 278:37632-37636.
136. Choi C, Benveniste EN. Fas ligand/Fas system in the brain: regulator of immune and apoptotic responses. Brain Res Rev 2004; 44:65-81.
137. Shin DH, Lee E, Kim HJ et al. Fas ligand mRNA expression in the mouse central nervous system. Journal of Neuroimmunology 2002; 123:50-57.
138. Park C, Sakamaki K, Tachibana O et al. Expression of Fas Antigen in the Normal Mouse Brain. Biochem Biophys Res Commun 1998; 252:623-628.
139. Raoul C, Henderson CE, Pettmann B. Programmed cell death of embryonic motoneurons triggered through the Fas death receptor. J Cell Biol 1999; 147:1049-1062.
140. Raoul C, Estevez AG, Nishimune H et al. Motoneuron death triggered by a specific pathway downstream of Fas. potentiation by ALS-linked SOD1 mutations. Neuron 2002; 35:1067-1083.
141. Desbarats J, Birge RB, Mimouni-Rongy M et al. Fas engagement induces neurite growth through ERK activation and p35 upregulation. Nat Cell Biol 2003; 5:118-125.
142. Pettmann B, Henderson CE. Killer wiles: Growing interest in Fas. Nat Cell Biol 2003; 5:91-92.
143. Lambert C, Landau AM, Desbarats J. Fas-beyond death: A regenerative role for Fas in the nervous system. Apoptosis 2003; 8:551-562.
144. Ruckenstein MJ, Milburn M, Hu L. Strial dysfunction in the MRL-Fas mouse. Otolaryngol Head Neck Surg 1999; 121:452-456.
145. Ruckenstein MJ, Sarwar A, Hu L et al. Effects of immunosuppression on the development of cochlear disease in the MRL-Fas(lpr) mouse. Laryngoscope 1999; 109:626-630.

146. Hess DC, Taormina M, Thompson J et al. Cognitive and neurologic deficits in the MRL/lpr mouse: a clinicopathologic study. J Rheumatol 1993; 20:610-617.
147. Fernandez M, Segura MF, Sole C et al. Lifeguard/neuronal membrane protein 35 regulates Fas ligand-mediated apoptosis in neurons via microdomain recruitment. J Neurochem 2007; 103:190-203.
148. Somia NV, Schmitt MJ, Vetter DE et al. LFG: An anti-apoptotic gene that provides protection from Fas-mediated cell death. Proc Natl Acad Sci USA1999; 96:12667-12672.
149. Segura MF, Sole C, Pascual M et al. The long form of Fas apoptotic inhibitory molecule is expressed specifically in neurons and protects them against death receptor-triggered apoptosis. J Neurosci 2007; 27:11228-11241.
150. Demjen D, Klussmann S, Kleber S et al. Neutralization of CD95 ligand promotes regeneration and functional recovery after spinal cord injury. Nat Med 2004; 10:389-395.
151. Casha S, Yu WR, Fehlings MG. FAS deficiency reduces apoptosis, spares axons and improves function after spinal cord injury. Exp Neurol 2005; 196:390-400.
152. Yoshino O, Matsuno H, Nakamura H et al. The role of Fas-mediated apoptosis after traumatic spinal cord injury. Spine 2004; 29:1394-1404.
153. Ackery A, Robins S, Fehlings MG. Inhibition of Fas-mediated apoptosis through administration of soluble Fas receptor improves functional outcome and reduces posttraumatic axonal degeneration after acute spinal cord injury. J Neurotrauma 2006; 23:604-616.
154. Ugolini G, Raoul C, Ferri A et al. Fas/tumor necrosis factor receptor death signaling is required for axotomy-induced death of motoneurons in vivo. J Neurosci 2003; 23:8526-8531.
155. Martin-Villalba A, Herr I, Jeremias I et al. CD95 Ligand (Fas-L/APO-1L) and tumor necrosis factor-related apoptosis-inducing ligand mediate ischemia-induced apoptosis in neurons. J Neurosci 1999; 19:3809-3817.
156. Martin-Villalba A, Hahne M, Kleber S et al. Therapeutic neutralization of CD95-ligand and TNF attenuates brain damage in stroke. Cell Death Differ 2001; 8:679-686.
157. Graham EM, Sheldon RA, Flock DL et al. Neonatal mice lacking functional Fas death receptors are resistant to hypoxic-ischemic brain injury. Neurobiol Dis 2004; 17:89-98.
158. Raoul C, Barthelemy C, Couzinet A et al. Expression of a dominant negative form of Daxx in vivo rescues motoneurons from Fas (CD95)-induced cell death. J Neurobiol 2005; 62:178-188.
159. Dasari VR, Spomar DG, Li L et al. Umbilical cord blood stem cell mediated downregulation of Fas improves functional recovery of rats after spinal cord injury. Neurochem Res 2008; 33:134-149.
160. McFarland HF, Martin R. Multiple sclerosis: A complicated picture of autoimmunity. Nat Immunol 2007; 8:913-919.
161. Diem R, Sattler MB, Bahr M. Neurodegeneration and -protection in autoimmune CNS inflammation. J Neuroimmunol 2007; 184:27-36.
162. Fox EJ. Immunopathology of multiple sclerosis. Neurology 2004; 63:S3-S7.
163. Hemmer B, Archelos JJ, Hartung HP. New concepts in the immunopathogenesis of multiple sclerosis. Nat Rev Neurosci 2002; 3:291-301.
164. Aktas O, Prozorovski T, Zipp F. Death ligands and autoimmune demyelination. Neuroscientist 2006; 12:305-316.
165. Wildbaum G, Westermann J, Maor G et al. A targeted DNA vaccine encoding Fas ligand defines its dual role in the regulation of experimental autoimmune encephalomyelitis. J Clin Invest 2000; 106:671-679.
166. Okuda Y, Sakoda S, Fujimura H et al. Intrathecal administration of neutralizing antibody against Fas ligand suppresses the progression of experimental autoimmune encephalomyelitis. Biochem Biophys Res Commun 2000; 275:164-168.
167. Ciusani E, Gelati M, Frigerio S et al. Modulation of experimental allergic encephalomyelitis in Lewis rats by administration of a peptide of Fas ligand. J Autoimmun 2001; 17:273-280.
168. Zhu B, Luo L, Chen Y et al. Intrathecal Fas ligand infusion strengthens immunoprivilege of central nervous system and suppresses experimental autoimmune encephalomyelitis. J Immunol 2002; 169:1561-1569.
169. Ni R, Tomita Y, Matsuda K et al. Fas-mediated apoptosis in primary cultured mouse hepatocytes. Exp Cell Res 1994; 215:332-337.
170. Galle PR, Hofmann WJ, Walczak H et al. Involvement of the CD95 (APO-1/Fas) receptor and ligand in liver damage. J Exp Med 1995; 182:1223-1230.
171. Ueno Y, Ishii M, Yahagi K et al. Fas-mediated cholangiopathy in the murine model of graft versus host disease. Hepatology 2000; 31:966-974.
172. Cardier JE, Schulte T, Kammer H et al. Fas (CD95, APO-1) antigen expression and function in murine liver endothelial cells: implications for the regulation of apoptosis in liver endothelial cells. FASEB J 1999; 13:1950-1960.

173. Saile B, Knittel T, Matthes N et al. CD95/CD95L-mediated apoptosis of the hepatic stellate cell. A mechanism terminating uncontrolled hepatic stellate cell proliferation during hepatic tissue repair. Am J Pathol 1997; 151:1265-1272.

174. Muschen M, Warskulat U, Douillard P et al. Regulation of CD95 (APO-1/Fas) receptor and ligand expression by lipopolysaccharide and dexamethasone in parenchymal and nonparenchymal rat liver cells. Hepatology 1998; 27:200-208.

175. Bennett M, Macdonald K, Chan SW et al. Cell surface trafficking of Fas: A rapid mechanism of p53-mediated apoptosis. Science 1998; 282:290-293.

176. Sodeman T, Bronk SF, Roberts PJ et al. Bile salts mediate hepatocyte apoptosis by increasing cell surface trafficking of Fas. Am J Physiol Gastrointest Liver Physiol 2000; 278:G992-G999.

177. Chan H, Bartos DP, Owen-Schaub LB. Activation-dependent transcriptional regulation of the human Fas promoter requires NF-kappaB p50-p65 recruitment. Mol Cell Biol 1999; 19:2098-2108.

178. Peter ME, Hellbardt S, Schwartz-Albiez R et al. Cell surface sialylation plays a role in modulating sensitivity towards APO-1-mediated apoptotic cell death. Cell Death Differ 1995; 2:163-171.

179. Sun Z, Wada T, Maemura K et al. Hepatic allograft-derived Kupffer cells regulate T-cell response in rats. Liver Transpl 2003; 9:489-497.

180. Adachi M, Suematsu S, Kondo T et al. Targeted mutation in the Fas gene causes hyperplasia in peripheral lymphoid organs and liver. Nat Genet 1995; 11:294-300.

181. Kataoka T, Budd RC, Holler N et al. The caspase-8 inhibitor FLIP promotes activation of NF-kappaB and Erk signaling pathways. Curr Biol 2000; 10:640-648.

182. Canbay A, Friedman S, Gores GJ. Apoptosis: The nexus of liver injury and fibrosis. Hepatology 2004; 39:273-278.

183. Canbay A, Higuchi H, Bronk SF et al. Fas enhances fibrogenesis in the bile duct ligated mouse: A link between apoptosis and fibrosis. Gastroenterology 2002; 123:1323-1330.

184. Canbay A, Taimr P, Torok N et al. Apoptotic body engulfment by a human stellate cell line is profibrogenic. Lab Invest 2003; 83:655-663.

185. Platt N, da Silva RP, Gordon S. Recognizing death: The phagocytosis of apoptotic cells. Trends Cell Biol 1998; 8:365-372.

186. Houston A, O'Connell J. The Fas signalling pathway and its role in the pathogenesis of cancer. Curr Opin Pharmacol 2004; 4:321-326.

187. Stagg J, Johnstone RW, Smyth MJ. From cancer immunosurveillance to cancer immunotherapy. Immunol Rev 2007; 220:82-101.

188. Swann JB, Smyth MJ. Immune surveillance of tumors. J Clin Invest 2007; 117:1137-1146.

189. Smyth MJ, Dunn GP, Schreiber RD. Cancer immunosurveillance and immunoediting: the roles of immunity in suppressing tumor development and shaping tumor immunogenicity. Adv Immunol 2006; 90:1-50.

190. Wajant H, Pfizenmaier K, Scheurich P. TNF-related apoptosis inducing ligand (TRAIL) and its receptors in tumor surveillance and cancer therapy. Apoptosis 2002; 7:449-459.

191. Wajant H CD95L/FasL and TRAIL in tumour surveillance and cancer therapy. Cancer Treat Res 2006; 130:141-65.:141-165.

192. Davidson WF, Giese T, Fredrickson TN. Spontaneous development of plasmacytoid tumors in mice with defective Fas-Fas ligand interactions. J Exp Med 1998; 187:1825-1838.

193. Zornig M, Grzeschiczek A, Kowalski MB et al. Loss of Fas/Apo-1 receptor accelerates lymphomagenesis in E mu L-MYC transgenic mice but not in animals infected with MoMuLV. Oncogene 1995; 10:2397-2401.

194. Peng SL, Robert ME, Hayday AC et al. A tumor-suppressor function for Fas (CD95) revealed in T-cell-deficient mice. J Exp Med 1996; 184:1149-1154.

195. Zhang B, Sun T, Xue L et al. Functional polymorphisms in FAS and FASL contribute to increased apoptosis of tumor infiltration lymphocytes and risk of breast cancer. Carcinogenesis 2007; 28:1067-1073.

196. Dunn GP, Old LJ, Schreiber RD. The three Es of cancer immunoediting. Annu Rev Immunol 2004; 22:329-360.

197. Mellor AL, Munn DH. Creating immune privilege: Active local suppression that benefits friends, but protects foes. Nat Rev Immunol 2008; 8:74-80.

198. O'Connell J, O'Sullivan GC, Collins JK et al. The Fas counterattack: Fas-mediated T-cell killing by colon cancer cells expressing Fas ligand. J Exp Med 1996; 184:1075-1082.

199. Ryan AE, Lane S, Shanahan F et al. Fas ligand expression in human and mouse cancer cell lines; a caveat on over-reliance on mRNA data. J Carcinog 2006; 5:5.

200. Yu JS, Lee PK, Ehtesham M et al. Intratumoral T-cell subset ratios and Fas ligand expression on brain tumor endothelium. J Neurooncol 2003; 64:55-61.

201. Ho SY, Guo HR, Chen HH et al. Prognostic implications of Fas-ligand expression in nasopharyngeal carcinoma. Head Neck 2004; 26:977-983.

202. Krishnakumar S, Kandalam M, Mohan A et al. Expression of Fas ligand in retinoblastoma. Cancer 2004; 101:1672-1676.
203. Ryan AE, Shanahan F, O'Connell J et al. Fas ligand promotes tumor immune evasion of colon cancer in vivo. Cell Cycle 2006; 5:246-249.
204. Okada K, Komuta K, Hashimoto S et al. Frequency of apoptosis of tumor-infiltrating lymphocytes induced by Fas counterattack in human colorectal carcinoma and its correlation with prognosis. Clin Cancer Res 2000; 6:3560-3564.
205. Bennett MW, O'Connell J, O'Sullivan GC et al. The Fas counterattack in vivo: Apoptotic depletion of tumor-infiltrating lymphocytes associated with Fas ligand expression by human esophageal carcinoma. J Immunol 1998; 160:5669-5675.
206. Vogel A, Aslan JE, Willenbring H et al. Sustained phosphorylation of Bid is a marker for resistance to Fas-induced apoptosis during chronic liver diseases. Gastroenterology 2006; 130:104-119.
207. Chida Y, Sudo N, Takaki A et al. The hepatic sympathetic nerve plays a critical role in preventing Fas induced liver injury in mice. Gut 2005; 54:994-1002.
208. Stohl W, Xu D, Starling GC et al. Promotion of activated human B-cell apoptosis and inhibition of Ig production by soluble CD95 ligand: CD95-based downregulation of Ig production need not culminate in activated B-cell death. Cell Immunol 2000; 203:1-11.
209. Lepple-Wienhues A, Belka C, Laun T et al. Stimulation of CD95 (Fas) blocks T-lymphocyte calcium channels through sphingomyelinase and sphingolipids. Proc Natl Acad Sci USA. 1999; 96:13795-13800.
210. Li H, Cai X, Fan X et al. Fas Ag-FasL coupling leads to ERK1/2-mediated proliferation of gastric mucosal cells. Am J Physiol Gastrointest Liver Physiol 2008; 294:G263-G275.
211. Mitsiades CS, Poulaki V, Fanourakis G et al. Fas signaling in thyroid carcinomas is diverted from apoptosis to proliferation. Clin Cancer Res 2006; 12:3705-3712.
212. Houston A, Waldron-Lynch FD, Bennett MW et al. Fas ligand expressed in colon cancer is not associated with increased apoptosis of tumor cells in vivo. Int J Cancer 2003; 107:209-214.
213. Pitti RM, Marsters SA, Lawrence DA et al. Genomic amplification of a decoy receptor for Fas ligand in lung and colon cancer. Nature 1998; 396:699-703.
214. Peshes-Yaloz N, Rosen D, Sondel PM et al. Up-regulation of Fas (CD95) expression in tumour cells in vivo. Immunology 2007; 120:502-511.
215. Ivanov VN, Lopez BP, Maulit G et al. FAP-1 association with Fas (Apo-1) inhibits Fas expression on the cell surface. Mol Cell Biol 2003; 23:3623-3635.
216. Huerta S, Heinzerling JH, Anguiano-Hernandez YM et al. Modification of gene products involved in resistance to apoptosis in metastatic colon cancer cells: roles of Fas, Apaf-1, NFkappaB, IAPs, Smac/DIABLO and AIF. J Surg Res 2007; 142:184-194.
217. Wang L, Azad N, Kongkaneramit L et al. The Fas death signaling pathway connecting reactive oxygen species generation and FLICE inhibitory protein down-regulation. J Immunol 2008; 180:3072-3080.
218. Irmler M, Thome M, Hahne M et al. Inhibition of death receptor signals by cellular FLIP. Nature 1997; 388:190-195.
219. Tourneur L, Mistou S, Michiels FM et al. Loss of FADD protein expression results in a biased Fas-signaling pathway and correlates with the development of tumoral status in thyroid follicular cells. Oncogene 2003; 22:2795-2804.
220. Fulda S, Kufer MU, Meyer E et al. Sensitization for death receptor- or drug-induced apoptosis by re-expression of caspase-8 through demethylation or gene transfer. Oncogene 2001; 20:5865-5877.
221. Hahne M, Rimoldi D, Schroter M et al. Melanoma cell expression of Fas(Apo-1/CD95) ligand: implications for tumor immune escape. Science 1996; 274:1363-1366.
222. Seino K, Kayagaki N, Okumura K et al. Antitumor effect of locally produced CD95 ligand. Nat Med 1997; 3:165-170.
223. Arai H, Gordon D, Nabel EG et al. Gene transfer of Fas ligand induces tumor regression in vivo. Proc Natl Acad Sci USA. 1997; 94:13862-13867.
224. Igney FH, Behrens CK, Krammer PH. CD95L mediates tumor counterattack in vitro but induces neutrophil-independent tumor rejection in vivo. Int J Cancer 2005; 113:78-87.
225. Ryan AE, Shanahan F, O'Connell J et al. Addressing the "Fas counterattack" controversy: blocking Fas ligand expression suppresses tumor immune evasion of colon cancer in vivo. Cancer Res 2005; 65:9817-9823.
226. Seino K, Kayagaki N, Fukao K et al. Rejection of Fas ligand-expressing grafts. Transplant Proc 1997; 29:1092-1093.
227. Fingleton B, Carter KJ, Matrisian LM. Loss of functional Fas ligand enhances intestinal tumorigenesis in the min mouse model. Cancer Res 2007; 67:4800-4806.

228. Hohlbaum AM, Gregory MS, Ju ST et al. Fas ligand engagement of resident peritoneal macrophages in vivo induces apoptosis and the production of neutrophil chemotactic factors. J Immunol 2001; 167:6217-6224.
229. Hohlbaum AM, Moe S, Marshak-Rothstein A. Opposing effects of transmembrane and soluble Fas ligand expression on inflammation and tumor cell survival. J Exp Med 2000; 191:1209-1220.
230. Seino K, Ogino T, Fukunaga K et al. Attempts to reveal the mechanism of CD95-ligand-mediated inflammation. Transplant Proc 1999; 31:1942-1943.
231. Park DR, Thomsen AR, Frevert CW et al. Fas (CD95) induces proinflammatory cytokine responses by human monocytes and monocyte-derived macrophages. J Immunol 2003; 170:6209-6216.
232. O'Connell J, Houston A, Bennett MW et al. Immune privilege or inflammation? Insights into the Fas ligand enigma. Nat Med 2001; 7:271-274.
233. Abrahams VM, Straszewski SL, Kamsteeg M et al. Epithelial ovarian cancer cells secrete functional Fas ligand. Cancer Res 2003; 63:5573-5581.
234. Friesen C, Herr I, Krammer PH et al. Involvement of the CD95 (APO-1/FAS) receptor/ligand system in drug-induced apoptosis in leukemia cells. Nat Med 1996; 2:574-577.
235. Fulda S, Sieverts H, Friesen C et al. The CD95 (APO-1/Fas) system mediates drug-induced apoptosis in neuroblastoma cells. Cancer Res 1997; 57:3823-3829.
236. Muller M, Strand S, Hug H et al. Drug-induced apoptosis in hepatoma cells is mediated by the CD95 (APO-1/Fas) receptor/ligand system and involves activation of wild-type p53. J Clin Invest 1997; 99:403-413.
237. Zender L, Hutker S, Liedtke C et al. Caspase 8 small interfering RNA prevents acute liver failure in mice. Proc Natl Acad Sci USA 2003; 100:7797-7802.
238. Contreras JL, Vilatoba M, Eckstein C et al. Caspase-8 and caspase-3 small interfering RNA decreases ischemia/reperfusion injury to the liver in mice. Surgery 2004; 136:390-400.
239. Song E, Lee SK, Wang J et al. RNA interference targeting Fas protects mice from fulminant hepatitis. Nat Med 2003; 9:347-351.
240. Wong M, Ziring D, Korin Y et al. TNF alpha blockade in human diseases: Mechanisms and future directions. Clin Immunol 2008; 126:121-136.
241. Schwarz EM, Ritchlin CT. Clinical development of anti-RANKL therapy. Arthritis Res Ther 2007; 9(Suppl 1):S7.
242. Dillon SR, Gross JA, Ansell SM et al. An APRIL to remember: Novel TNF ligands as therapeutic targets. Nat Rev Drug Discov 2006; 5:235-246.
243. Tanaka M, Suda T, Haze K et al. Fas ligand in human serum. Nat Med 1996; 2:317-322.
244. Miwa K, Hashimoto H, Yatomi T et al. Therapeutic effect of an anti-Fas ligand mAb on lethal graft-versus-host disease. Int Immunol 1999; 11:925-931.
245. Holler N, Kataoka T, Bodmer JL et al. Development of improved soluble inhibitors of FasL and CD40L based on oligomerized receptors. J Immunol Methods 2000; 237:159-173.
246. Watermann I, Gerspach J, Lehne M et al. Activation of CD95L fusion protein prodrugs by tumor-associated proteases. Cell Death Differ 2006; 14:765-774.
247. Farley SM, Purdy DE, Ryabinina OP et al. Fas ligand-induced proinflammatory transcriptional responses in reconstructed human epidermis. Recruitment of the epidermal growth factor receptor and activation of MAP kinases. J Biol Chem 2008; 283:919-928.
248. Yu KY, Kwon B, Ni J et al. A newly identified member of tumor necrosis factor receptor superfamily (TR6) suppresses LIGHT-mediated apoptosis. J Biol Chem 1999; 274:13733-13736.
249. Migone TS, Zhang J, Luo X et al. TL1A Is a TNF-like ligand for DR3 and TR6/DcR3 and functions as a T-cell costimulator. Immunity 2002; 16:479-492.
250. Wroblewski VJ, McCloud C, Davis K et al. Pharmacokinetics, metabolic stability and subcutaneous bioavailability of a genetically engineered analog of DcR3, FLINT [DcR3(R218Q)], in cynomolgus monkeys and mice. Drug Metab Dispos 2003; 31:502-507.
251. Wortinger MA, Foley JW, Larocque P et al. Fas ligand-induced murine pulmonary inflammation is reduced by a stable decoy receptor 3 analogue. Immunology 2003; 110:225-233.
252. Holler N, Tardivel A, Kovacsovics-Bankowski M et al. Two adjacent trimeric Fas ligands are required for Fas signaling and formation of a death-inducing signaling complex. Mol Cell Biol 2003; 23:1428-1440.
253. Schmidt M, Lugering N, Pauels HG et al. IL-10 induces apoptosis in human monocytes involving the CD95 receptor/ligand pathway. Eur J Immunol 2000; 30:1769-1777.
254. Schmidt M, Lugering N, Lugering A et al. Role of the CD95/CD95 ligand system in glucocorticoid-induced monocyte apoptosis. J Immunol 2001; 166:1344-1351.
255. Suda T, Hashimoto H, Tanaka M et al. Membrane Fas ligand kills human peripheral blood T-lymphocytes and soluble Fas ligand blocks the killing. J Exp Med 1997; 186:2045-2050.

256. Xiao S, Jodo S, Sung SS et al. A novel signaling mechanism for soluble CD95 ligand. Synergy with anti-CD95 monoclonal antibodies for apoptosis and NF-kappaB nuclear translocation. J Biol Chem 2002; 277:50907-50913.

257. Ogasawara J, Watanabe-Fukunaga R, Adachi M et al. Lethal effect of the anti-Fas antibody in mice. Nature 1993; 364:806-809.

258. Nishimura Y, Hirabayashi Y, Matsuzaki Y et al. In vivo analysis of Fas antigen-mediated apoptosis: effects of agonistic anti-mouse Fas mAb on thymus, spleen and liver. Int Immunol 1997; 9:307-316.

259. Nishimura-Morita Y, Nose M, Inoue T et al. Amelioration of systemic autoimmune disease by the stimulation of apoptosis-promoting receptor Fas with anti-Fas mAb. Int Immunol 1997; 9:1793-1799.

260. Ogawa Y, Kuwahara H, Kimura T et al. Therapeutic effect of anti-Fas antibody on a collagen induced arthritis model. J Rheumatol 2001; 28:950-955.

261. Ichikawa K, Yoshida-Kato H, Ohtsuki M et al. A novel murine anti-human Fas mAb which mitigates lymphadenopathy without hepatotoxicity. Int Immunol 2000; 12:555-562.

262. Nakayama J, Ogawa Y, Yoshigae Y et al. A humanized anti-human Fas antibody, R-125224, induces apoptosis in type I activated lymphocytes but not in type II cells. Int Immunol 2006; 18:113-124.

263. Hiramoto K, Inui M, Kamei T et al. mHFE7A, a newly identified monoclonal antibody to Fas, induces apoptosis in human melanoma cells in vitro and delays the growth of melanoma xenotransplants. Oncol Rep 2006; 15:409-415.

264. Kuwahara H, Tani Y, Ogawa Y et al. Therapeutic effect of novel anti-human Fas antibody HFE7a on graft-versus-host disease model. Clin Immunol 2001; 99:340-346.

265. Samel D, Muller D, Gerspach J et al. Generation of a FasL-based proapoptotic fusion protein devoid of systemic toxicity due to cell-surface antigen-restricted Activation. J Biol Chem 2003; 278:32077-32082.

266. Bremer E, ten Cate B, Samplonius DF et al. Superior activity of fusion protein scfvrit:sfasl over cotreatment with rituximab and Fas agonists. Cancer Res 2008; 68:597-604.

267. Bremer E, ten Cate B, Samplonius DF et al. CD7-restricted activation of Fas-mediated apoptosis: a novel therapeutic approach for acute T-cell leukemia. Blood 2006; 107:2863-2870.

268. Scanlan MJ, Raj BK, Calvo B et al. Molecular cloning of fibroblast activation protein alpha, a member of the serine protease family selectively expressed in stromal fibroblasts of epithelial cancers. Proc Natl Acad Sci USA 1994; 91:5657-5661.

269. Garin-Chesa P, Old LJ, Rettig WJ. Cell surface glycoprotein of reactive stromal fibroblasts as a potential antibody target in human epithelial cancers. Proc Natl Acad Sci USA 1990; 87:7235-7239.

270. Assohou-Luty C, Gerspach J, Siegmund D et al. A CD40-CD95L fusion protein interferes with CD40L-induced prosurvival signaling and allows membrane CD40L-restricted activation of CD95. J Mol Med 2006; 84:785-797.

271. Jung G, Grosse-Hovest L, Krammer PH et al. Target cell-restricted triggering of the CD95 (APO-1/Fas) death receptor with bispecific antibody fragments. Cancer Res 2001; 61:1846-1848.

272. Herrmann T, Grosse-Hovest L, Otz T et al. Construction of optimized bispecific antibodies for selective activation of the death receptor CD95. Cancer Res 2008; 68:1221-1227.

273. Gerspach J, Muller D, Munkel S et al. Restoration of membrane TNF-like activity by cell surface targeting and matrix metalloproteinase-mediated processing of a TNF prodrug. Cell Death Differ 2006; 13:273-284.

274. Wajant H, Moosmayer D, Wuest T et al. Differential activation of TRAIL-R1 and -2 by soluble and membrane TRAIL allows selective surface antigen-directed activation of TRAIL-R2 by a soluble TRAIL derivative. Oncogene 2001; 20:4101-4106.

275. Bremer E, Kuijlen J, Samplonius D et al. Target cell-restricted and -enhanced apoptosis induction by a scFv:sTRAIL fusion protein with specificity for the pancarcinoma-associated antigen EGP2. Int J Cancer 2004; 20; 109:281-290.

276. Bremer E, Samplonius DF, van Genne L et al. Simultaneous inhibition of epidermal growth factor receptor (EGFR) signaling and enhanced activation of tumor necrosis factor-related apoptosis-inducing ligand (TRAIL) receptor-mediated apoptosis induction by an scFv:sTRAIL fusion protein with specificity for human EGFR. J Biol Chem 2005; 280:10025-10033.

277. Bremer E, Samplonius DF, Peipp M et al. Target cell-restricted apoptosis induction of acute leukemic T-cells by a recombinant tumor necrosis factor-related apoptosis-inducing ligand fusion protein with specificity for human CD7. Cancer Res 2005; 65:3380-3388.

278. Stieglmaier J, Bremer E, Kellner C et al. Selective induction of apoptosis in leukemic B-lymphoid cells by a CD19-specific TRAIL fusion protein. Cancer Immunol Immunother 2008; 57:233-246.

279. Simon AK, Gallimore A, Jones E et al. Fas ligand breaks tolerance to self-antigens and induces tumor immunity mediated by antibodies. Cancer Cell 2002; 2:315-322.

280. Miwa K, Asano M, Horai R et al. Caspase 1-independent IL-1[beta] release and inflammation induced by the apoptosis inducer Fas ligand. Nat Med 1998; 4:1287-1292.

281. Behrens CK, Igney FH, Arnold B et al. CD95 ligand-expressing tumors are rejected in anti-tumor TCR transgenic perforin knockout mice. J Immunol 2001; 166:3240-3247.
282. Kang SM, Braat D, Schneider DB et al. A noncleavable mutant of Fas ligand does not prevent neutrophilic destruction of islet transplants. Transplantation 2000; 69:1813-1817.
283. Allison J, Georgiou HM, Strasser A et al. Transgenic expression of CD95 ligand on islet beta cells induces a granulocytic infiltration but does not confer immune privilege upon islet allografts. Proc Natl Acad Sci USA 1997; 94:3943-3947.
284. Petrovsky N, Silva D, Socha L et al. The role of Fas ligand in beta cell destruction in autoimmune diabetes of NOD mice. Ann N Y Acad Sci 2002; 958:204-208.
285. Silva DG, Petrovsky N, Socha L et al. Mechanisms of accelerated immune-mediated diabetes resulting from islet beta cell expression of a Fas ligand transgene. J Immunol 2003; 170:4996-5002.
286. Lau HT, Yu M, Fontana A et al. Prevention of islet allograft rejection with engineered myoblasts expressing FasL in mice. Science 1996; 273:109-112.
287. Yolcu ES, Askenasy N, Singh NP et al. Cell membrane modification for rapid display of proteins as a novel means of immunomodulation: FasL-decorated cells prevent islet graft rejection. Immunity 2002; 17:795-808.
288. Korbutt GS, Elliott JF, Rajotte RV. Cotransplantation of allogeneic islets with allogeneic testicular cell aggregates allows long-term graft survival without systemic immunosuppression. Diabetes 1997; 46:317-322.
289. Zhang H, Yang Y, Horton JL et al. Amelioration of collagen-induced arthritis by CD95 (Apo-1/Fas)-ligand gene transfer. J Clin Invest 1997; 100:1951-1957.
290. Kim SH, Kim S, Oligino TJ et al. Effective treatment of established mouse collagen-induced arthritis by systemic administration of dendritic cells genetically modified to express FasL. Mol Ther 2002; 6:584-590.
291. Guery L, Batteux F, Bessis N et al. Expression of Fas ligand improves the effect of IL-4 in collagen-induced arthritis. Eur J Immunol 2000; 30:308-315.
292. Fleck M, Zhang HG, Kern ER et al. Treatment of chronic sialadenitis in a murine model of Sjogren's syndrome by local FasL gene transfer. Arthritis Rheum 2001; 44:964-973.
293. Morelli AE, Larregina AT, Smith-Arica J et al. Neuronal and glial cell type-specific promoters within adenovirus recombinants restrict the expression of the apoptosis-inducing molecule Fas ligand to predetermined brain cell types and abolish peripheral liver toxicity. J Gen Virol 1999; 80:571-583.
294. Ambar BB, Frei K, Malipiero U et al. Treatment of experimental glioma by administration of adenoviral vectors expressing Fas ligand. Hum Gene Ther 1999; 10:1641-1648.
295. Aoki K, Akyurek LM, San H et al. Restricted expression of an adenoviral vector encoding Fas ligand (CD95L) enhances safety for cancer gene therapy. Mol Ther 2000; 1:555-565.
296. Hyer ML, Voelkel-Johnson C, Rubinchik S et al. Intracellular Fas ligand expression causes Fas-mediated apoptosis in human prostate cancer cells resistant to monoclonal antibody-induced apoptosis. Mol Ther 2000; 2:348-358.
297. Rubinchik S, Ding R, Qiu AJ et al. Adenoviral vector which delivers FasL-GFP fusion protein regulated by the tet-inducible expression system. Gene Ther 2000; 7:875-885.
298. Rubinchik S, Wang D, Yu H et al. A complex adenovirus vector that delivers FASL-GFP with combined prostate-specific and tetracycline-regulated expression. Mol Ther 2001; 4:416-426.
299. Sipo I, Hurtado PA, Wang X et al. An improved Tet-On regulatable FasL-adenovirus vector system for lung cancer therapy. J Mol Med 2006; 84:215-225.

CHAPTER 6

OX40 (CD134) and OX40L

Michael J. Gough and Andrew D. Weinberg*

Abstract

The interaction between OX40 and OX40L plays an important role in antigen-specific T-cell expansion and survival. While OX40 is expressed predominantly on T-lymphocytes early after antigen activation, OX40L is expressed on activated antigen presenting cells and endothelial cells within acute inflammatory environments. We discuss here how ligation of OX40 by OX40L leads to enhanced T-cell survival, along with local inflammatory responses that appear critical for both effective T-cell mediated responses and chronic immune pathologies. We describe how interventions that block or mimic the OX40-OX40L interaction can be applied to treat autoimmune diseases or enhance anti-tumor immune responses. The clinically relevant properties of these agents emphasize the importance of this particular TNFSF-TNFSF in health and disease.

Expression of OX40 and OX40L

The TNF family member OX40 was initially identified as a 50 kDa protein expressed on activated CD4 T-cell blasts, recognized by the OX40 antibody (thus the receptor was termed OX40).[1] Addition of the OX40 antibody to activated T-cells enhanced the T-cell proliferation late in the response.[1] Subsequent cloning of the cDNA encoding OX40 identified significant similarities to CD40 and nerve growth factor receptor,[2] placing OX40 as an early member of the now large TNF receptor superfamily (TNFRSF). Baum et al developed a murine cDNA library to clone the murine ligand for OX40 (OX40L).[3] The murine OX40L protein showed close homology and genetic linkage to the previously identified human protein gp34, which was elevated in T-cells following HTLV infection. Human gp34 was then shown to be the ligand for human OX40 and both human and mouse OX40L had similar functional properties in costimulating proliferation of CD4 T-cells.[4]

The initial description identified activated rat CD4 T-cells as expressing OX40 exclusively.[1] al-Shamkhani et al confirmed that the original anti-rat OX40 antibody and OX40L-Ig recognized the same protein and generated a new antibody to recombinant mouse OX40 that similarly identified OX40 expression on activated CD4 and CD8 T-cells in mice.[5] OX40 is not immediately induced on T-cells following T-cell receptor ligation, but is first detected 12-24 hours following stimulation and downregulated 48-96 later.[6] This in vitro data correlates well with in vivo functional responses, since OX40 agonistic antibodies must be administered within 24-48 hours of antigen administration to enhance T-cell proliferation.[7] The regulation of OX40 expression in T-cells has not been fully elucidated, but a combination of genetic and phenotypic studies has provided valuable information regarding the induction of OX40 expression in T-cells. Early papers demonstrated that like OX40L, OX40 is upregulated by HTLV tax expression in T-cells.[4,8] The OX40 promoter region was cloned by Pankow et al and tax-dependent promoter activity was localized

*Corresponding Author: Andrew D. Weinberg—Robert W. Franz Cancer Center, Earle A. Chiles Research Institute, Providence Portland Medical Center, Portland, OR 97213, USA. Email: andrew.weinberg@providence.org

Therapeutic Targets of the TNF Superfamily, edited by Iqbal S. Grewal.
©2009 Landes Bioscience and Springer Science+Business Media.

to a region containing predicted NF-κB binding sites.[9] These NF-κB sites bind p65 and c-rel after tax expression, resembling a CD28-responsive enhancer region of the CD40L gene.[10] Similar CD28-responsive elements were first identified in the IL-2 promoter and have been functionally identified within the promoter regions of CD40L[11] and CD95L.[12] Using fibroblasts or activated B cells as antigen presenting cells, it was demonstrated that OX40 could be induced in the absence of CD28 stimulation.[6,13] However, titration of T-cell receptor stimulation using plate-bound anti-CD3 antibodies demonstrated dependence on CD28 signals for OX40 expression with low dose T-cell receptor stimulation and CD28 independence for OX40 expression was observed at higher doses of T-cell receptor signals.[14] Interestingly, OX40 expression can also be upregulated by administration of TNFα,[15] which can also activate NF-κB signal transduction. These data suggest that this integration of T-cell receptor and CD28 signaling occurs via activation of NF-κB and can act through NF-κB sites within the OX40 promoter. The majority of T-cell responses in vivo, which do not involve large numbers of transgenic T-cells or high doses of antigen, will most likely require additional costimulatory signals for effective upregulation of OX40. Thus, the relative levels of OX40 expressed on T-cells can be greatly influenced by the local environment via contact with mature antigen presenting cells expressing CD80 or CD86, or via a milieu rich in TNFα or similar cytokines.

Expression of OX40L is also tightly controlled. The initial cloning of OX40L used a T-cell lymphoma cDNA library [4] and human OX40L was first identified as a HTLV tax-regulated gene in lymphoma cell lines.[4] A cloned murine OX40-Ig fusion protein identified binding activity on activated murine B-cells in vitro and in vivo[16] and a critical role for the B cell-T-cell OX40-OX40L interaction in antibody responses.[17] An antibody to cloned rat OX40L confirmed expression of OX40L on activated T-cells, B-cells and dendritic cells.[18] This antibody blocked OX40-OX40L interactions and inhibited the costimulatory activity of dendritic cells on activated T-cells,[18] emphasizing the importance of OX40-OX40L interactions on endogenous T-cell responses. OX40L has been identified on freshly isolated human natural killer (NK) cells[19] and expression is upregulated by ligation of the NK receptors.[20] The NK expression of OX40L is functional as it has been shown to costimulate autologous CD4 T-cell proliferation and increase IFNγ production.[20] Low-level expression of OX40L has also been found on activated murine CD4 and CD8 T-cells,[4] however the majority of reports have studied OX40L expression and function on activated antigen-presenting cells. OX40L was identified on endothelial cells through a search for molecules mediating adhesion between leukemia T-cell lines and endothelial cells.[21] Expression cloning identified the adhesion ligand-receptor pair as OX40 on the T-cells and OX40L on endothelial cell lines.[21] There is strong association between expression of OX40L on endothelial cells and inflammation at the site in vivo.[22] Interestingly, OX40L expression appeared to be restricted to the basal rather than the lumenal surfaces of the endothelial structures and the authors suggest that the interaction is thus not likely to be involved in the first rolling step of extravasation.[22] Microglia, as well as endothelial cells, within the inflammatory site of actively induced models of experimental allergic encephalomyelitis, were shown to express OX40L.[23,24] Microglial cells isolated from the CNS of mice with EAE drove antigen-specific proliferation of myelin-reactive T-cells that was significantly inhibited by blocking the OX40-OX40L interaction.[23] In summary, OX40L expression is found primarily at sites of inflammation. Thus, T-cells activated through the T-cell receptor that express OX40 are most likely to receive costimulation by activated antigen presenting cells, endothelia or NK cells once within the site of inflammation. This geographic restriction adds a layer of specificity to costimulation via OX40 that is analogous to situations of immunological 'danger' in vivo.[25]

Biologic Function of OX40-OX40L Interactions

TNFSF receptors and ligands show relatively consistent structural motifs, with the TNFSF ligands forming a homotrimer as membrane-bound proteins, which are often released as soluble trimeric proteins following proteolytic cleavage.[26-28] OX40L is one of the more divergent members of the TNF family, while OX40 is structurally relatively similar to the other family members.[29] The stoichiometry of interaction between OX40 and OX40L trimers was initially determined to be 3:1,[30] suggesting that three OX40 molecules bind one trimeric OX40L complex, similar to other TNF family members. This hypothesis is supported by data showing that soluble monomeric OX40 binds trimeric OX40L with low affinity and dissociates rapidly.[29,30] The crystal structure of OX40 binding to OX40L was recently solved and showed that, within the trimer-trimer interaction, each OX40 molecule bound individually to one OX40L molecule.[29]

Most TNFR family members, including OX40, signal through the TNF receptor associated factor (TRAF) family of adaptor molecules.[31] TRAF molecules consist of a highly conserved C-terminal domain, which elicits trimer assembly and receptor interaction and the less-conserved N-terminal domain that is critical for downstream signal transduction.[32] OX40 signal transduction has been linked to T-cell function in vivo through TRAF2 and TRAF5,[33,34] along with TRAF1, TRAF3 and TRAF5 in vitro.[35-37] TRAF3 can function as a negative regulator of signal transduction following OX40 ligation,[35-37] though OX40 displayed the lowest TRAF3 binding capacity of all TNFRs tested thus far.[35] Using a dominant negative TRAF2 transgenic mouse bred to a TCR-transgenic mouse strain, TRAF2 was shown to be required for the enhancement in CD4 T-cell expansion and survival elicited by the OX40 agonist antibody in vivo.[33] In the absence of TRAF5, OX40 ligation resulted in an enhanced Th2 phenotype in vitro and in vivo.[34] OX40 ligation has been shown to enhance both Th1 and Th2-type responses.[38] Since the choice between Th1 and Th2 differentiation by CD4 T-cells is determined in part by the antigen dose and strongly by the cytokine environment, it is possible that environmental factors influence the TRAF molecules interacting with OX40 following initial TCR ligation.

The crystal structure of the TRAF molecules indicates that like OX40 and OX40L, the TRAF molecules form a trimer, arranged such that each TRAF monomer binds to an OX40 monomer.[39,40] The downstream consequences of OX40 ligation are NF-κB,[36] PI-3K[41] and protein kinase B (also known as Akt) activation.[41,42] Akt is activated by a number of signal transduction pathways, including TCR ligation and IL-2 signal transduction, each via PI3-kinase[43] and can enhance T-cell proliferation and survival.[43] OX40 ligation in wild-type cells results in enhanced activation of Akt, and OX40 deficient T-cells that constitutively express active Akt have restored survival,[42] presumably through sustained expression of the anti-apoptotic molecule Bcl-xL.[43] In vitro stimulated CD4 T-cells express Bcl2 and Bcl-xL over the critical day 4-8 time period following antigen stimulation, while the expression of these genes is not sustained over this time period in OX40$^{-/-}$ cells.[44] This OX40-sustained Bcl-xL expression is similarly critical for survival of in vitro-activated CD8 T-cells.[45]

Downstream of these proximal signaling events, many changes occur in T-cells following OX40 ligation. Gene expression studies have identified a number of candidate genes that are regulated by OX40 ligation in vitro and in vivo. Ligation of OX40 has been shown to upregulate CD25, CD127 (IL-7Rα), CD212 (IL12Rβ2), IL15Rα and IFNγ mRNA in CD4 T-cells in vivo[33,46] and simultaneously to downregulate mRNA for CD152 (CTLA-4), IL-4 and Mad4.[33] Mad4 is of interest, since this protein can heterodimerize with Max, competing with Myc and thus inhibiting proliferation.[47] Decreased levels of Mad4 would thus indicate enhanced proliferative capacity following OX40 ligation. The combined effect of enhanced cytokine receptors and decreased CD152 suggests OX40 ligation shifts T-cells towards a more permissive proliferative and survival phenotype.

These data fit nicely with the observed cellular effect of T-cell-specific OX40 ligation. As described earlier, initial studies identified that antibody ligation of OX40 enhanced CD4 T-cell proliferation.[1] Administration of OX40 agonists in vivo to mice treated with soluble antigen in the absence of adjuvant resulted in an enhanced expansion of the CD4 T-cells, along with increased survival and the formation of long-term memory populations.[7,48-50] Recently OX40 ligation has also been shown to enhance expansion and survival of antigen-stimulated CD8 T-cells in vivo.[45,51-53] Moreover, OX40 ligation of CD4 T-cells indirectly enhances CD8 expansion and survival through CD4 'help'.[51,54-56] OX40 ligation does not appear to direct differentiation to either Th1 or Th2 phenotypes exclusively, since separate models demonstrate that each differentiation pathway can be

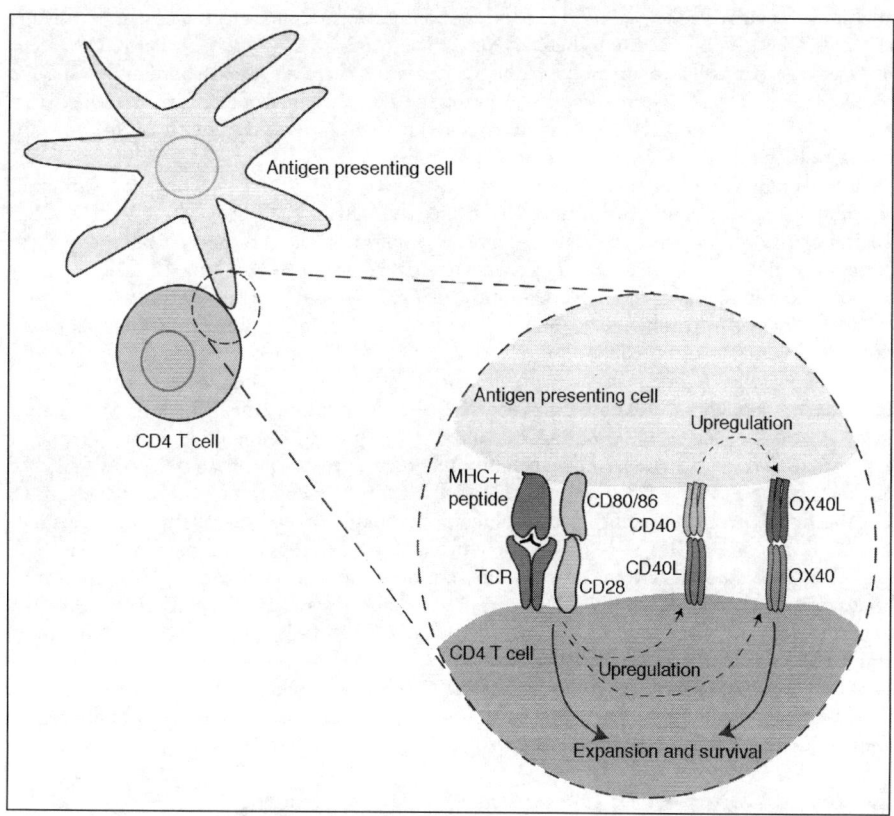

Figure 1. Specific recognition of a peptide-MHC complex on an antigen-presenting cell by the T-cell receptor combines with CD28 costimulation to upregulate first CD40L and then OX40 on the T cell. Ligation of CD40 on the antigen-presenting cell leads to expression of OX40L and costimulation of the T-cell. This reciprocal interaction will be further enhanced by environmental cytokines, such as TNFα.

enhanced by OX40 costimulation.[38,57-61] OX40 agonists have potent biologic function in OX40L sufficient hosts, suggesting that the availability of OX40L is limiting in vivo. This point is of critical importance in later discussions concerning therapeutic use of OX40 agonists and antagonists in cancer and autoimmune diseases, respectively.

Investigators have demonstrated, using in vivo vaccination models, that survival of antigen-specific OX40[-/-] CD4 T-cells is significantly impaired compared to wild-type CD4 T-cells.[62] This effect is particularly noticeable when the antigen challenge is provided along with adjuvant or as part of an immunogenic viral challenge.[62,63] In models where mice are immunized with antigen containing no adjuvant, CD4 T-cell survival is extremely poor even with functional OX40 expression,[7,64] suggesting a deficit in OX40L expression. In agreement with this analysis, administration of agonistic OX40 antibodies significantly enhances the CD4 T-cell response to soluble antigen[7] and importantly this effect is increased when given in conjunction with a strong adjuvant, such as LPS.[7,48] Adjuvants can increase expression of both OX40L on antigen-presenting cells[18,65] and OX40 on the T-cells. T-cells can also respond to several other costimulatory molecules, thus, T-cell proliferation is less dependent on the presence of functional OX40 on T-cells, particularly in the presence of strong adjuvants. Interestingly, this redundancy is particularly noticeable in CD8 compared to CD4 T-cells. For example, in response to the highly immunogenic LCMV and influenza virus challenge, the CD8 T-cell response is normal and fully functional,[63,66,67] while the CD4 T-cell response is diminished.[63,67] Nevertheless, even in those models where CD8 T-cells display full expansion and functional pathogen clearance, there is evidence of diminished CD8 recall responses and long-term survival.[55] This may be a consequence of defective CD4-mediated help to CD8 T-cells, or a lack of the necessary cytokine environment generated by OX40-OX40L interaction, to support T-cell differentiation into memory cells.

Interestingly, OX40 has been shown to provide a signal to OX40L-expressing cells. Ohshima et al demonstrated that human dendritic cells, activated through CD40 ligation, expressed OX40L.[65] Cross-linking OX40L with antibodies significantly increased the activated phenotype of these antigen presenting cells, as evidenced by production of the cytokines IL-12 and IL-1β and expression of the costimulatory molecules CD80 and CD86.[65] Activated B-cells also express OX40L and engagement via OX40 enhances immunoglobulin production in the presence of CD40 stimulation or cytokines.[68,69] Epithelial cells transfected with OX40L increased expression of c-jun and c-fos mRNA following crosslinking with agonist OX40.[70] In vascular endothelial cell lines that constitutively express OX40L, provision of OX40 also elevated c-jun mRNA[70] and resulted in an increase in CCL5 secretion.[71] Thus, OX40 and OX40L provide bi-directional signals between antigen-presenting cells and T-cells. Such bi-directional signaling has been described for other members of the TNF receptor family.[72] CD137-CD137L interactions produce similar effects to OX40-OX40L in costimulating T-cell proliferation, though the main target appears to be CD8 T-cells. Provision of CD137 has been shown to activate macrophages expressing CD137L.[73] CD30L is expressed on activated T-cells and neutrophils and cross-linking CD30L using antibodies or recombinant CD30-Ig also results in activation.[74] Similarly, CD95L has been shown to costimulate proliferation of CD8 T-cells.[75,76] Finally, CD40L-deficient T-cells are deficient in antigen-specific expansion in wild-type hosts[77] and are unable to provide proper help to normal B-cells.[78] These data from a collection of TNFSF/TNFRSF members suggest that the observed OX40-OX40L bi-directional signaling is most likely a real class-specific effect and a biologically relevant event.

Expression and Role of OX40 and OX40L in Disease

Immunohistochemistry and flow cytometry have identified OX40-expressing cells within sites of inflammation in vivo. These OX40-expressing cells are associated with the transient inflammation seen in response to vaccination or pathogen challenge, but also at sites of chronic inflammation in various disease states.[79-83] For example, Matsumura et al demonstrated that OX40 was expressed on T-cells in all psoriatic skin sites tested, but not in nonlesional skin from the same individual.[79] Importantly, a range of experiments have demonstrated that OX40 expression was found particularly on the recently activated autoantigen-specific T-cells at the inflammatory site,[80,83-86] which is in agreement with in vitro and in vivo experiments demonstrating that expression of OX40 only occurs following T-cell receptor engagement. Thus adoptive transfer of myelin basic protein-specific T-cells into animals caused experimental autoimmune encephalomyelitis, accompanied by enhanced expression of OX40 on antigen-specific T-cells at the site of inflammation and not on nonspecific host T-cells, or autoantigen-specific T-cells found at other sites.[87]

Immunohistochemistry of specimens from growing tumors of various histological types in patients has revealed the presence of OX40 on CD4 T-cells.[88-92] In two such instances, the presence of OX40 on CD4 T-cells was associated with prolonged patient survival.[90,92] T regulatory cells, defined as CD4+CD25+ cells expressing FoxP3, can also express OX40 in mice.[93-95] These cells are known to accumulate at the tumor site and their presence is mainly associated with poor prognosis,[96-98] though there is a conflicting report.[99] In our experience in studying murine tumors, a large number of the OX40-expressing cells that infiltrate tumor sites are CD4+CD25+FoxP3+ cells. Human T regulatory cells can have a different phenotype to murine T regulatory cells and OX40 has currently not been reported on human T regulatory cells. Thus, it is unclear in human immunohistochemical tumor studies whether expression of OX40 represents an accumulation of T regulatory cells or a distinct population of antigen-responsive activated effector CD4 T-cells,

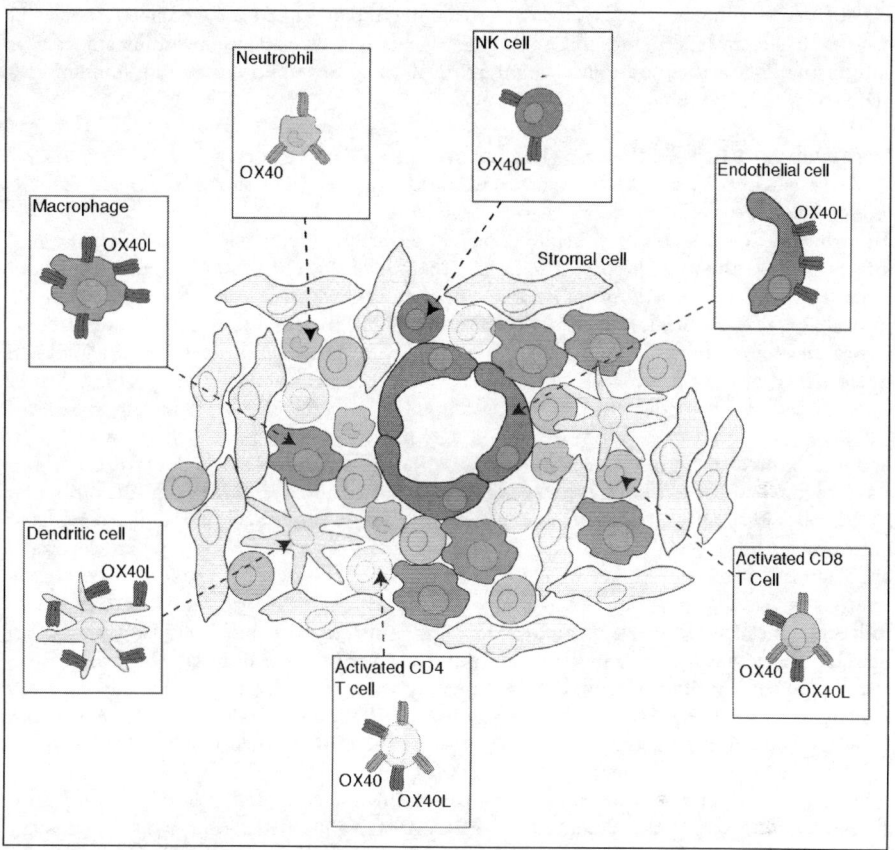

Figure 2. Within inflamed tissue sites, multiple cells provide OX40L for infiltrating T-cells. In this representation of a perivscular cuff, endothelial cells may express OX40L on their basolateral surface to infiltrating T-cells. Activated macrophages and tissue dendritic cells can also express OX40L in inflammatory sites. In addition, NK cells can upregulate OX40L following recognition of their target cells. T-cells recognizing specific antigen on stromal cells or cross-presented on dendritic cells and macrophages will upregulate OX40 and thus receive local costimulation. Neutrophils can also express OX40 and ligation by OX40L improves their survival. Thus, an inflammatory site has multiple opportunities for OX40-OX40L interaction that will sustain the local inflammatory response and these opportunities are not available at non-inflammatory tissue sites.

or both. This is relevant since it may help us to understand the consequences of OX40-directed therapies in vivo, since while agonistic antibodies to OX40 enhance the expansion and survival of CD4 and CD8 T-cells in vitro and in vivo,[7,45,48-53] they also block the inhibitory action of T regulatory cells in vitro.[94,100,101]

Importantly, while OX40 is commonly detectable on T-cells in both sites of chronic inflammation[79-86] and tumors,[88-92] cells expressing OX40L are only found at sites of inflammation[22,23,82] and not on cells invading tumors or on tumor cells themselves. Thus, the immune balance at the tumor site does not lead to a functional OX40-OX40L interaction despite the presence of OX40-expressing T-cells. These data establish a powerful rationale for intervention in the OX40-OX40L interaction for immunological therapy. In circumstances where chronic inflammation causes disease, such as rheumatoid arthritis, psoriasis or multiple sclerosis, there is combined expression of OX40 and

OX40L and this interaction plays a role in sustaining the unwanted autoimmune response. In contrast, in circumstances of insufficient 'danger signals' such as vaccination without adjuvant or chronic tumor growth, insufficient ligation of OX40 could be a limiting factor for immune-mediated destruction of tumor cells.

Intervention in OX40-OX40L Interaction for Therapy

As described earlier, in models of acute viral infection the absence or blockade of OX40-OX40L interactions allows pathogen clearance to proceed while secondary inflammation is reduced.[102,103] Though reduction in secondary inflammation may be desired in preclinical models of acute viral infection, these data provide some insight into the role of OX40-OX40L in both chronic and acute autoimmune disorders. Administration of depleting OX40 antibodies to animals exhibiting clinical signs of experimental allergic encephalomyelitis ameliorated disease by depleting the antigen-specific cells at the autoimmune site.[84] Administration of an agent that blocks OX40-OX40L interaction also reduced the severity and duration of experimental allergic encephalomyelitis in vivo.[23] In the non-obese diabetic model of autoimmune diabetes, OX40 was identified on both CD4 and CD8 T-cells along with OX40L on dendritic cells in the pancreatic-draining lymph nodes at the prediabetic 11-13 week time-point.[104] Administration of blocking OX40L antibodies at this time-point significantly reduced the incidence of diabetes. Blocking OX40L antibodies also significantly reduced intestinal inflammation in a dextran sulphate sodium-induced model of inflammatory bowel disease [105] and blocked development of disease in an adoptive transfer model of inflammatory colitis.[106] In rheumatoid arthritis patients, OX40 was detectable on T-cells in the synovial fluid and synovium and OX40L was present on cells within the synovium.[107] In mouse collagen-induced models of rheumatoid arthritis, administration of blocking OX40L antibodies significantly reduced the inflammation and thus the severity of the disease.[107] In each of these models, reducing inflammation within the target organ, for example through anti-inflammatory drug treatments, has also been shown to provide therapeutic benefit in animal models and humans. These data provide strong supportive evidence that in addition to their role in CD4 and CD8 T-cell survival and effector function, OX40-OX40L interaction may be important in sustaining a chronic site of immune reactivity both in pathogenic infection and in autoimmune pathogenesis.[23,84,102,103,105,107] Notably, blockade of the OX40-OX40L interaction may have significant advantages over systemic anti-inflammatory drug treatments: OX40 and OX40L expression is highly restricted to the inflammatory site and therefore blockade of this pathway is not predicted to have systemic immunosuppressive side effects that are seen with conventional treatments, such as corticosteroids. Such a blockade could however, interfere with developing immune responses, such as concurrent infections.

We and others have hypothesized that observations made in chronic inflammatory models could have powerful implications for cancer therapy. The tumor site is characterized by a mixed inflammatory status. Pro-inflammatory cytokines such as TNFα are commonly present, as are a range of inflammatory chemokines.[108-110] Reports have also shown anti-inflammatory cytokines such as TGFβ and IL-10[109,110] and the chemokines that encourage infiltration of T-regulatory cells rather than effector T-cells have been identified at the tumor site.[96,111] As discussed earlier, there is usually limited expression of OX40L, which based on the autoimmune literature would predict that the tumor site would be unable to sustain a long-term immune response, despite the presence of T-cells expressing OX40. Therefore, we infused OX40 agonists into tumor-bearing hosts and observed enhanced tumor immunity, leading to increased survival of animals challenged with many tumor types.[112-114] This survival benefit was dependent on both CD4 and CD8 T-cells.[113,114] It is important to note that while agonistic OX40 antibodies were effective when administered systemically, expression of OX40L within the tumor site alone is able to enhance effective anti-tumor immune responses.[115] Andarini et al demonstrated that intratumoral administration of an adenoviral vector expressing OX40L enhanced survival of treated mice.[115] These were striking results because using adenoviral-mediated gene therapy only a small proportion of the tumor cell mass will productively express the ligand. The anti-tumor response in this model was

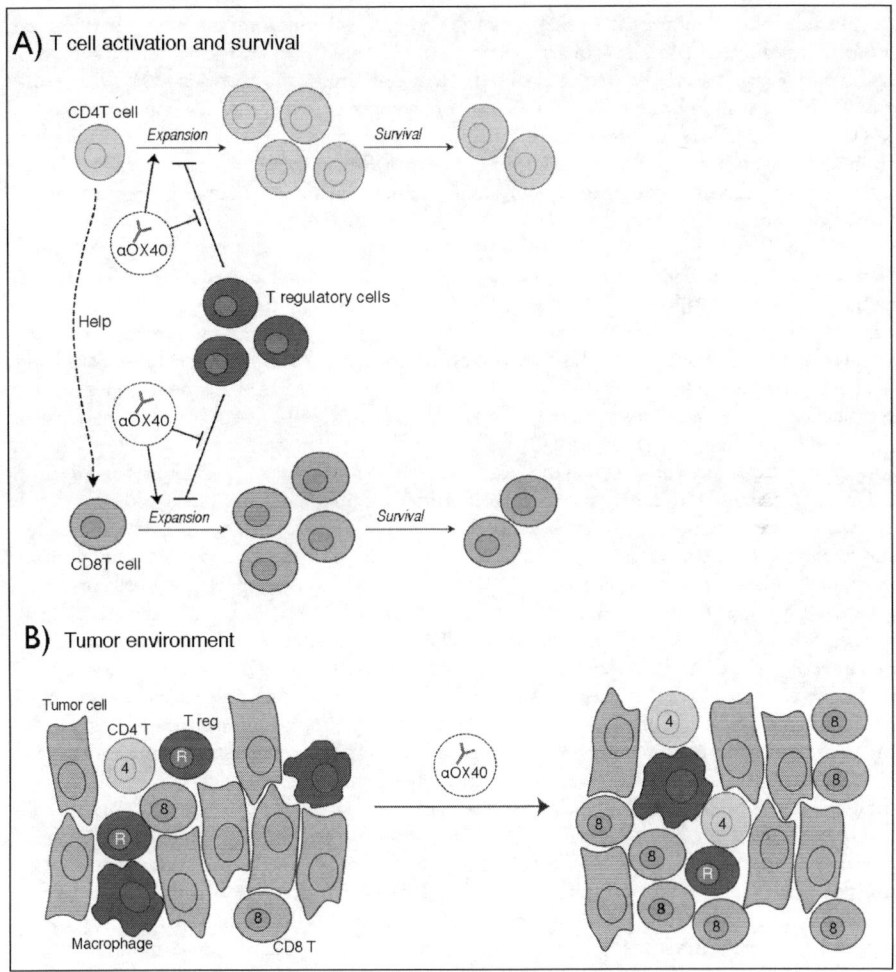

Figure 3. A) During antigen-specific activation, administration of agonistic antibodies to OX40 enhances the expansion and long-term survival of both CD4 and CD8 T-cells. In addition, these activated CD4 T-cells provide help to CD8 T-cells that further supports their activation and long-term survival. T regulatory cells can inhibit antigen-specific expansion of CD4 and CD8 T-cells, but this inhibition can be blocked by administration of agonistic antibodies to OX40. B) The environment of the growing tumor includes a mix of macrophages, anergic CD8 T-cells and T regulatory cells. Administration of agonistic antibodies to OX40 has been shown to inhibit T regulatory cells and overcome CD8 T-cell anergy, thus may dramatically alter the intratumoral environment.

also dependent on both CD4 and CD8 T-cells and generated increased T-cell infiltrates within the tumor. Current dogma concludes that the majority of tumor antigen-specific priming occurs within the lymph node draining the site of the tumor, where naïve T-cells can find simultaneous antigen presentation, costimulation, CD4 T-cell help and antigen presenting cell licensing. In such a scenario, OX40L expression exclusively at the tumor site would not be expected to enhance priming of draining lymph node cells, but could stimulate the effector cells which most likely up-regulate OX40 upon interaction with their target antigen at the tumor site. Thus, it is interesting to observe that adenoviral delivery of OX40L to tumors, while increasing survival of treated animals, was not able to cure any animals of their tumors.[115] The lack of long-term tumor-free survival was probably not due to the low level of gene expression achievable by in vivo gene therapy, since others have shown that stable, ex vivo-transduced tumor cells uniformly expressing OX40L provide only a small delay in tumor growth.[116] This is in direct contrast to delivery of agonistic antibodies to OX40, which provide a potent systemic tumor survival effect.[112-114] It is possible that systemic antibody delivery is more effective because it can ligate OX40 at multiple locations, including the tumor site and the tumor draining lymph nodes. Immunotherapies that ignore either location may be significantly less effective.

We hypothesize that OX40-OX40L interactions enhance immune responses in two ways. First, OX40 ligation significantly enhances the expansion, survival and effector differentiation of antigen-specific T-cells. This effect is likely to occur within the tumor draining lymph node, where provision of agonistic OX40 antibodies can overcome a lack of an immunological danger signal that results in inadequate OX40L to achieve tumor antigen priming. In acute viral challenge models or vaccination models with sufficient adjuvant activity, the OX40L expression is probably sufficient to provide OX40 costimulation. The second role of OX40-OX40L interactions occurs at the site of inflammation. Where both OX40 and OX40L are expressed, the ligation of OX40 on antigen-specific T-cells can enhance the local release of pro-inflammatory cytokines and ligation of OX40 on T-regulatory cells may reduce their inhibitory effects. In addition, ligation of OX40L on local antigen-presenting cells can enhance their maturation to full antigen presenting function and further increase the release of cytokines such as IL-12. With continued presence of antigen, the combination of pro-inflammatory cytokines and mature antigen presenting cells permits a prolonged site-specific inflammation that is critical for immune pathology. In chronic models, interruption of OX40-OX40L interactions at the site of inflammation is sufficient to reduce inflammation and thus disease severity, even where long-lived antigen-specific cells persist.

However, there is another mechanism by which agonistic OX40 antibodies may exact their effect, particularly in tumor models. Lathrop et al demonstrated that adoptive transfer of CD4 T-cells specific for a peptide expressed on all MHC class II-expressing cells, resulted initially in T-cell expansion, which was followed by development of an anergic phenotype.[117] In vivo administration of agonistic OX40 antibodies resulted in the reversal of anergy and activation of T-cells that proved fatal to the host.[117] Defective T-cell activation has commonly been reported in tumor models and can be reversed by strong ex vivo stimulation or provision of costimulation in vivo. It is not clear from these models whether the OX40 agonist antibodies directly reverses anergy, or whether OX40 acts indirectly by its effects on T regulatory cells,[94,100,101] which can maintain a state of T-cell anergy in vivo.[118,119] Nevertheless, overcoming anergic or tolerance in tumor-specific T-cells is likely to contribute strongly to the efficacy of OX40-mediated immunotherapy in patients with cancer.

These data provide a compelling rationale for clinical development of OX40 agonist antibodies for cancer therapy. Our laboratory has prepared a GMP clinical grade murine anti-human OX40 agonist antibody that has been FDA-approved for a phase I clinical trial. When injected into non-human primates, this agent demonstrated no acute toxicity, but did show immune enhancement as ascertained by increased T-and B-cell responses and transient enlargement of gut-associated lymph nodes and splenomegaly.[120] The OX40 agonist is currently being tested in a phase I clinical trial in cancer patients.

Conclusion

OX40 is a TNFSF receptor expressed early after T-cell receptor engagement on CD4 and CD8 T-cells while it's cognate ligand (OX40L) is expressed mainly on activated antigen presenting cells present at sites of inflammation in vivo. Effective antigen-specific CD4 and CD8 T-cell expansion and survival can be dependent on ligation of OX40, though the dependence on OX40 is most evident in CD4 T-cells. Co-expression of this receptor-ligand pair is found mainly at sites of acute and chronic inflammation in vivo and interventions that block the OX40-OX40L interaction reduce the pathologic effect of chronic inflammation in vivo. Conversely, a deficiency of OX40L within tumor sites results in inadequate anti-tumor immunity that can be enhanced significantly by in vivo administration of OX40 agonists. These data provide a strong rationale for therapeutic use of OX40 agonists in cancer patients and such a clinical trial is ongoing.

References

1. Paterson DJ, Jefferies WA, Green JR et al. Antigens of activated rat T lymphocytes including a molecule of 50,000 Mr detected only on CD4 positive T blasts. Mol Immunol 1987; 24(12):1281-1290.
2. Mallett S, Fossum S, Barclay AN. Characterization of the MRC OX40 antigen of activated CD4 positive T lymphocytes—a molecule related to nerve growth factor receptor. EMBO J 1990; 9(4):1063-1068.
3. Baum PR, Gayle RB, 3rd, Ramsdell F et al. Molecular characterization of murine and human OX40/OX40 ligand systems: identification of a human OX40 ligand as the HTLV-1-regulated protein gp.34 EMBO J 1994; 13(17):3992-4001.
4. Baum PR, Gayle RBd, Ramsdell F et al. Identification of OX40 ligand and preliminary characterization of its activities on OX40 receptor. Circ Shock 1994; 44(1):30-34.
5. al-Shamkhani A, Birkeland ML, Puklavec M et al. OX40 is differentially expressed on activated rat and mouse T-cells and is the sole receptor for the OX40 ligand. Eur J Immunol 1996; 26(8):1695-1699.
6. Gramaglia I, Weinberg AD, Lemon M et al. Ox-40 ligand: a potent costimulatory molecule for sustaining primary CD4 T-cell responses. J Immunol 1998; 161(12):6510-6517.
7. Evans DE, Prell RA, Thalhofer CJ et al. Engagement of OX40 enhances antigen-specific CD4(+) T-cell mobilization/memory development and humoral immunity: comparison of alphaOX-40 with alphaCTLA-4. J Immunol 15 2001; 167(12):6804-6811.
8. Higashimura N, Takasawa N, Tanaka Y et al. Induction of OX40, a receptor of gp,34 on T-cells by trans-acting transcriptional activator, Tax, of human T-cell leukemia virus type I. Jpn J Cancer Res 1996; 87(3):227-231.
9. Pankow R, Durkop H, Latza U et al. The HTLV-I tax protein transcriptionally modulates OX40 antigen expression. J Immunol 2000; 165(1):263-270.
10. Schubert LA, Cron RQ, Cleary AM et al. A T-cell-specific enhancer of the human CD40 ligand gene. J Biol Chem 2002; 277(9):7386-7395.
11. Parra E, Mustelin T, Dohlsten M et al. Identification of a CD28 response element in the CD40 ligand promoter. J Immunol 2001; 166(4):2437-2443.
12. Crist SA, Griffith TS, Ratliff TL. Structure/function analysis of the murine CD95L promoter reveals the identification of a novel transcriptional repressor and functional CD28 response element. J Biol Chem 2003; 278(38):35950-35958.
13. Akiba H, Oshima H, Takeda K et al. CD28-independent costimulation of T-cells by OX40 ligand and CD70 on activated B-cells. J Immunol 1999; 162(12):7058-7066.
14. Toennies HM, Green AM, Arch RH. Expression of CD30 and Ox40 on T lymphocyte subsets is controlled by distinct regulatory mechanisms. J Leukoc Biol 2004; 75(2):350-357.
15. Horai R, Nakajima A, Habiro K et al. TNF-alpha is crucial for the development of autoimmune arthritis in IL-1 receptor antagonist-deficient mice. J Clin Invest 2004; 114(11):1603-1611.
16. Calderhead DM, Buhlmann JE, van den Eertwegh AJ et al. Cloning of mouse Ox:40 a T-cell activation marker that may mediate T-B-cell interactions. J Immunol 1993; 151(10):5261-5271.
17. Stuber E, Strober W. The T-cell-B-cell interaction via OX40-OX40L is necessary for the T-cell-dependent humoral immune response. J Exp Med 1996; 183(3):979-989.
18. Satake Y, Akiba H, Takeda K et al. Characterization of rat OX40 ligand by monoclonal antibody. Biochem Biophys Res Commun 2000; 270(3):1041-1048.
19. Kashii Y, Giorda R, Herberman RB et al. Constitutive expression and role of the TNF family ligands in apoptotic killing of tumor cells by human NK cells. J Immunol 1999; 163(10):5358-5366.
20. Zingoni A, Sornasse T, Cocks BG et al. Cross-talk between activated human NK cells and CD4+ T-cells via OX40-OX40 ligand interactions. J Immunol 2004; 173(6):3716-3724.
21. Imura A, Hori T, Imada K et al. The human OX40/gp34 system directly mediates adhesion of activated T-cells to vascular endothelial cells. J Exp Med 1996; 183(5):2185-2195.
22. Matsumura Y, Imura A, Hori T et al. Localization of OX40/gp34 in inflammatory skin diseases: a clue to elucidate the interaction between activated T-cells and endothelial cells in infiltration. Arch Dermatol Res 1997; 289(11):653-656.
23. Weinberg AD, Wegmann KW, Funatake C et al. Blocking OX-40/OX-40 ligand interaction in vitro and in vivo leads to decreased T-cell function and amelioration of experimental allergic encephalomyelitis. J Immunol 1999; 162(3):1818-1826.
24. Nohara C, Akiba H, Nakajima A et al. Amelioration of experimental autoimmune encephalomyelitis with anti-OX40 ligand monoclonal antibody: a critical role for OX40 ligand in migration, but not development, of pathogenic T-cells. J Immunol 2001; 166(3):2108-2115.
25. Matzinger P. Tolerance, danger and the extended family. Ann Rev Immunol 1994; 12:991-1045.

26. Armitage RJ. Tumor necrosis factor receptor superfamily members and their ligands. Curr Opin Immunol 1994; 6(3):407-413.
27. Zhang G. Tumor necrosis factor family ligand-receptor binding. Curr Opin Struct Biol 2004; 14(2):154-160.
28. Bodmer JL, Schneider P, Tschopp J. The molecular architecture of the TNF superfamily. Trends Biochem Sci 2002; 27(1):19-26.
29. Compaan DM, Hymowitz SG. The crystal structure of the costimulatory OX40-OX40L complex. Structure 2006; 14(8):1321-1330.
30. Al-Shamkhani A, Mallett S, Brown MH et al. Affinity and kinetics of the interaction between soluble trimeric OX40 ligand, a member of the tumor necrosis factor superfamily and its receptor OX40 on activated T-cells. J Biol Chem 1997; 272(8):5275-5282.
31. Wajant H, Henkler F, Scheurich P. The TNF-receptor-associated factor family: scaffold molecules for cytokine. Cell Signal 2001; 13(6):389-400.
32. Chung JY, Park YC, Ye H et al. All TRAFs are not created equal: common and distinct molecular mechanisms of TRAF-mediated signal transduction. J Cell Sci 2002; 115(Pt 4):679-688.
33. Prell RA, Evans DE, Thalhofer C et al. OX40-mediated memory T-cell generation is TNF receptor-associated factor 2 dependent. J Immunol 2003; 171(11):5997-6005.
34. So T, Salek-Ardakani S, Nakano H et al. TNF receptor-associated factor 5 limits the induction of Th2 immune responses. J Immunol 2004; 172(7):4292-4297.
35. Hauer J, Puschner S, Ramakrishnan P et al. TNF receptor (TNFR)-associated factor (TRAF) 3 serves as an inhibitor of TRAF2/5-mediated activation of the noncanonical NF-kappaB pathway by TRAF-binding TNFRs. Proc Natl Acad Sci USA 2005; 102(8):2874-2879.
36. Kawamata S, Hori T, Imura A et al. Activation of OX40 signal transduction pathways leads to tumor necrosis factor receptor-associated factor (TRAF) 2- and TRAF5-mediated NF-kappaB activation. J Biol Chem 1998; 273(10):5808-5814.
37. Arch RH, Thompson CB. 4-1BB and Ox40 are members of a tumor necrosis factor (TNF)-nerve growth factor receptor subfamily that bind TNF receptor-associated factors and activate nuclear factor kappaB. Mol Cell Biol 1998; 18(1):558-565.
38. Rogers PR, Croft M. CD28, Ox-40, LFA-1 and CD4 modulation of Th1/Th2 differentiation is directly dependent on the dose of antigen. J Immunol 2000; 164(6):2955-2963.
39. Park YC, Burkitt V, Villa AR et al. Structural basis for self-association and receptor recognition of human TRAF2. Nature 1999; 398(6727):533-538.
40. McWhirter SM, Pullen SS, Holton JM et al. Crystallographic analysis of CD40 recognition and signaling by human TRAF2. Proc Natl Acad Sci USA 1999; 96(15):8408-8413.
41. Mestas J, Crampton SP, Hori T et al. Endothelial cell costimulation through OX40 augments and prolongs T-cell cytokine synthesis by stabilization of cytokine mRNA. Int Immunol 2005; 17(6):737-747.
42. Song J, Salek-Ardakani S, Rogers PR et al. The costimulation-regulated duration of PKB activation controls T-cell longevity. Nat Immunol 2004; 5(2):150-158.
43. Jones RG, Parsons M, Bonnard M et al. Protein kinase B regulates T lymphocyte survival, nuclear factor kappaB activation and Bcl-X(L) levels in vivo. J Exp Med 2000; 191(10):1721-1734.
44. Rogers PR, Song J, Gramaglia I et al. OX40 promotes Bcl-xL and Bcl-2 expression and is essential for long-term survival of CD4 T-cells. Immunity 2001; 15(3):445-455.
45. Song A, Tang X, Harms KM, Croft M. OX40 and Bcl-xL Promote the Persistence of CD8 T-cells to Recall Tumor-Associated Antigen. J Immunol 2005; 175(6):3534-3541.
46. Huddleston CA, Weinberg AD, Parker DC. OX40 (CD134) engagement drives differentiation of CD4+ T-cells to effector cells. Eur J Immunol 2006; 36(5):1093-1103.
47. Hurlin PJ, Queva C, Koskinen PJ et al. Mad3 and Mad:4 novel Max-interacting transcriptional repressors that suppress c-myc dependent transformation and are expressed during neural and epidermal differentiation. EMBO J 1996; 15(8):2030.
48. Maxwell JR, Weinberg A, Prell RA et al. Danger and OX40 receptor signaling synergize to enhance memory T-cell survival by inhibiting peripheral deletion. J Immunol 2000; 164(1):107-112.
49. Gramaglia I, Jember A, Pippig SD et al. The OX40 costimulatory receptor determines the development of CD4 memory by regulating primary clonal expansion. J Immunol 2000; 165(6):3043-3050.
50. Weatherill AR, Maxwell JR, Takahashi C et al. OX40 ligation enhances cell cycle turnover of Ag-activated CD4 T-cells in vivo. Cell Immunol 2001; 209(1):63-75.
51. Ruby CE, Redmond WL, Haley D et al. Anti-OX40 stimulation in vivo enhances CD8(+) memory T-cell survival and significantly increases recall responses. Eur J Immunol 2007; 37(1):157-166.
52. Lee SW, Park Y, Song A et al. Functional dichotomy between OX40 and 4-1BB in modulating effector CD8 T-cell responses. J Immunol 2006; 177(7):4464-4472.
53. Fujita T, Ukyo N, Hori T et al. Functional characterization of OX40 expressed on human CD8+ T-cells. Immunol Lett 2006; 106(1):27-33.

54. Serghides L, Bukczynski J, Wen T et al. Evaluation of OX40 ligand as a costimulator of human antiviral memory CD8 T-cell responses: comparison with B7.1 and 4-1BBL. J Immunol 2005; 175(10):6368-6377.

55. Hendriks J, Xiao Y, Rossen JW et al. During viral infection of the respiratory tract, CD27, 4-1BB and OX40 collectively determine formation of CD8+ memory T-cells and their capacity for secondary expansion. J Immunol 2005; 175(3):1665-1676.

56. Chen AI, McAdam AJ, Buhlmann JE et al. Ox40-ligand has a critical costimulatory role in dendritic cell:T-cell interactions. Immunity 1999; 11(6):689-698.

57. Akiba H, Miyahira Y, Atsuta M et al. Critical contribution of OX40 ligand to T-helper cell type 2 differentiation in experimental leishmaniasis. J Exp Med 2000; 191(2):375-380.

58. Flynn S, Toellner KM, Raykundalia C et al. CD4 T-cell cytokine differentiation: the B-cell activation molecule, OX40 ligand, instructs CD4 T-cells to express interleukin 4 and upregulates expression of the chemokine receptor, Blr-1. J Exp Med 1998; 188(2):297-304.

59. Ohshima Y, Yang LP, Uchiyama T et al. OX40 costimulation enhances interleukin-4 (IL-4) expression at priming and promotes the differentiation of naive human CD4(+) T-cells into high IL-4-producing effectors. Blood 1998; 92(9):3338-3345.

60. Linton PJ, Bautista B, Biederman E et al. Costimulation via OX40L expressed by B-cells is sufficient to determine the extent of primary CD4 cell expansion and Th2 cytokine secretion in vivo. J Exp Med 2003; 197(7):875-883.

61. Murata K, Ishii N, Takano H et al. Impairment of antigen-presenting cell function in mice lacking expression of OX40 ligand. J Exp Med. 2000; 191(2):365-374.

62. Gramaglia I, Jember A, Pippig SD et al. The OX40 costimulatory receptor determines the development of CD4 memory by regulating primary clonal expansion. J Immunol 2000; 165(6):3043-3050.

63. Kopf M, Ruedl C, Schmitz N et al. OX40-deficient mice are defective in Th cell proliferation but are competent in generating B-cell and CTL Responses after virus infection. Immunity 1999; 11(6):699-708.

64. Croft M, Duncan DD, Swain SL. Response of naive antigen-specific CD4+ T-cells in vitro: characteristics and antigen-presenting cell requirements. J Exp Med 1992; 176(5):1431-1437.

65. Ohshima Y, Tanaka Y, Tozawa H et al. Expression and function of OX40 ligand on human dendritic cells. J Immunol 1997; 159(8):3838-3848.

66. Pippig SD, Pena-Rossi C, Long J et al. Robust B-cell immunity but impaired T-cell proliferation in the absence of CD134 (OX40). J Immunol 1999; 163(12):6520-6529.

67. Dawicki W, Bertram EM, Sharpe AH, Watts TH. 4-1BB and OX40 act independently to facilitate robust CD8 and CD4 recall responses. J Immunol 2004; 173(10):5944-5951.

68. Stuber E, Neurath M, Calderhead D et al. Cross-linking of OX40 ligand, a member of the TNF/NGF cytokine family, induces proliferation and differentiation in murine splenic B-cells. Immunity 1995; 2(5):507-521.

69. Morimoto S, Kanno Y, Tanaka Y et al. CD134L engagement enhances human B cell Ig production: CD154/CD40, CD70/CD27 and CD134/CD134L interactions coordinately regulate T-cell-dependent B-cell responses. J Immunol 2000; 164(8):4097-4104.

70. Matsumura Y, Hori T, Kawamata S et al. Intracellular signaling of gp,34 the OX40 ligand: induction of c-jun and c-fos mRNA expression through gp34 upon binding of its receptor, OX40. J Immunol 1999; 163(6):3007-3011.

71. Kotani A, Hori T, Matsumura Y et al. Signaling of gp34, (OX40 ligand) induces vascular endothelial cells to produce a CC chemokine RANTES/CCL5. Immunol Lett 2002; 84(1):1-7.

72. Eissner G, Kolch W, Scheurich P. Ligands working as receptors: reverse signaling by members of the TNF superfamily enhance the plasticity of the immune system. Cytokine Growth Factor Rev 2004; 15(5):353-366.

73. Langstein J, Michel J, Fritsche J et al. CD137 (ILA/4-1BB), a member of the TNF receptor family, induces monocyte activation via bidirectional signaling. J Immunol 1998; 160(5):2488-2494.

74. Wiley SR, Goodwin RG, Smith CA. Reverse signaling via CD30 ligand. J Immunol 1996; 157(8):3635-3639.

75. Suzuki I, Martin S, Boursalian et al. Fas ligand costimulates the in vivo proliferation of CD8+ T-cells. J Immunol 2000; 165(10):5537-5543.

76. Sun M, Ames KT, Suzuki I et al. The cytoplasmic domain of Fas ligand costimulates TCR signals. J Immunol 2006; 177(3):1481-1491.

77. Grewal IS, Xu J, Flavell RA. Impairment of antigen-specific T-cell priming in mice lacking CD40 ligand. Nature 1995; 378(6557):617-620.

78. van Essen D, Kikutani H, Gray D. CD40 ligand-transduced costimulation of T-cells in the development of helper function. Nature 1995; 378(6557):620-623.

79. Matsumura Y, Hori T, Nishigori C et al. Expression of CD134 and CD134 ligand in lesional and nonlesional psoriatic skin. Arch Dermatol Res 2003; 294(12):563-566.

80. Weinberg AD, Wallin JJ, Jones RE et al. Target organ-specific up-regulation of the MRC OX-40 marker and selective production of Th1 lymphokine mRNA by encephalitogenic T-helper cells isolated from the spinal cord of rats with experimental autoimmune enciphalomyelitis. Journal of Immunology 1994; 152:4712-4721.
81. Souza HS, Elia CC, Spencer J et al. Expression of lymphocyte-endothelial receptor-ligand pairs, alpha-4beta7/MAdCAM-1 and OX40/OX40 ligand in the colon and jejunum of patients with inflammatory bowel disease. Gut 1999; 45(6):856-863.
82. Aten J, Roos A, Claessen N et al. Strong and selective glomerular localization of CD134 ligand and TNF receptor-1 in proliferative lupus nephritis. J Am Soc Nephrol 2000; 11(8):1426-1438.
83. Endres R, Luz A, Schulze H et al. Listeriosis in p47(phox–/–) and TRp55–/– mice: protection despite absence of ROI and susceptibility despite presence of RNI. Immunity 1997; 7(3):419-432.
84. Weinberg AD. Antibodies to OX-40 (CD134) can identify and eliminate autoreactive T-cells: implications for human autoimmune disease. Mol Med Today 1998; 4(2):76-83.
85. Weinberg AD, Bourdette DN, Sullivan TJ et al. Selective depletion of myelin-reactive T-cells with the anti-OX-40 antibody ameliorates autoimmune encephalomyelitis. Nat Med 1996; 2(2):183-189.
86. Weinberg AD, Lemon M, Jones AJ et al. OX-40 antibody enhances for autoantigen specific V beta 8.2+ T-cells within the spinal cord of Lewis rats with autoimmune encephalomyelitis. J Neurosci Res 1996; 43(1):42-49.
87. Weinberg AD, Wallin JJ, Jones RE et al. Target organ-specific up-regulation of the MRC OX-40 marker and selective production of Th1 lymphokine mRNA by encephalitogenic T-helper cells isolated from the spinal cord of rats with experimental autoimmune encephalomyelitis. J Immunol 1994; 152(9):4712-4721.
88. Vetto JT, Lum S, Morris A et al. Presence of the T-cell activation marker OX-40 on tumor infiltrating lymphocytes and draining lymph node cells from patients with melanoma and head and neck cancers. Am J Surg 1997; 174(3):258-265.
89. Durkop H, Latza U, Himmelreich P et al. Expression of the human OX40 (hOX40) antigen in normal and neoplastic tissues. Br J Haematol 1995; 91(4):927-931.
90. Ladanyi A, Somlai B, Gilde K et al. T-cell activation marker expression on tumor-infiltrating lymphocytes as prognostic factor in cutaneous malignant melanoma. Clin Cancer Res 2004; 10(2):521-530.
91. Ramstad T, Lawnicki L, Vetto J et al. Immunohistochemical analysis of primary breast tumors and tumor-draining lymph nodes by means of the T-cell costimulatory molecule OX-40. Am J Surg 2000; 179(5):400-406.
92. Petty JK, He K, Corless CL et al. Survival in human colorectal cancer correlates with expression of the T-cell costimulatory molecule OX-40 (CD134). Am J Surg 2002; 183(5):512-518.
93. Mottonen M, Heikkinen J, Mustonen L et al. CD4+ CD25+ T-cells with the phenotypic and functional characteristics of regulatory T-cells are enriched in the synovial fluid of patients with rheumatoid arthritis. Clin Exp Immunol 2005; 140(2):360-367.
94. Valzasina B, Guiducci C, Dislich H et al. Triggering of OX40 (CD134) on CD4(+)CD25+ T-cells blocks their inhibitory activity: a novel regulatory role for OX40 and its comparison with GITR. Blood 2005; 105(7):2845-2851.
95. Nolte-'t Hoen EN, Wagenaar-Hilbers JP, Boot EP et al. Identification of a CD4+CD25+ T-cell subset committed in vivo to suppress antigen-specific T-cell responses without additional stimulation. Eur J Immunol 2004; 34(11):3016-3027.
96. Curiel TJ, Coukos G, Zou L et al. Specific recruitment of regulatory T-cells in ovarian carcinoma fosters immune privilege and predicts reduced survival. Nat Med 2004; 10(9):942-949.
97. Sato E, Olson SH, Ahn J et al. Intraepithelial CD8+ tumor-infiltrating lymphocytes and a high CD8+/regulatory T-cell ratio are associated with favorable prognosis in ovarian cancer. Proc Natl Acad Sci USA 2005; 102(51):18538-18543.
98. Wolf D, Wolf AM, Rumpold H et al. The expression of the regulatory T-cell-specific forkhead box transcription factor FoxP3 is associated with poor prognosis in ovarian cancer. Clin Cancer Res 2005; 11(23):8326-8331.
99. Badoual C, Hans S, Rodriguez J et al. Prognostic value of tumor-infiltrating CD4+ T-cell subpopulations in head and neck cancers. Clin Cancer Res 2006; 12(2):465-472.
100. Takeda I, Ine S, Killeen N et al. Distinct roles for the OX40-OX40 ligand interaction in regulatory and nonregulatory T-cells. J Immunol 2004; 172(6):3580-3589.
101. Ito T, Wang YH, Duramad O et al. OX40 ligand shuts down IL-10-producing regulatory T-cells. Proc Natl Acad Sci USA 2006; 103(35):13138-13143.
102. Humphreys IR, Walzl G, Edwards L et al. A critical role for OX40 in T-cell-mediated immunopathology during lung viral infection. J Exp Med 2003; 198(8):1237-1242.

103. Humphreys IR, Edwards L, Walzl G et al. OX40 ligation on activated T-cells enhances the control of Cryptococcus neoformans and reduces pulmonary eosinophilia. J Immunol 2003; 170(12):6125-6132.
104. Pakala SV, Bansal-Pakala P, Halteman BS et al. Prevention of diabetes in NOD mice at a late stage by targeting OX40/OX40 ligand interactions. Eur J Immunol 2004; 34(11):3039-3046.
105. Obermeier F, Schwarz H, Dunger N et al. OX40/OX40L interaction induces the expression of CXCR5 and contributes to chronic colitis induced by dextran sulfate sodium in mice. Eur J Immunol 2003; 33(12):3265-3274.
106. Malmstrom V, Shipton D, Singh B et al. Cd134l expression on dendritic cells in the mesenteric lymph nodes drives colitis in T-cell-restored scid mice. J Immunol 2001; 166(11):6972-6981.
107. Yoshioka T, Nakajima A, Akiba H et al. Contribution of OX40/OX40 ligand interaction to the pathogenesis of rheumatoid arthritis. Eur J Immunol 2000; 30(10):2815-2823.
108. Kulbe H, Thompson R, Wilson JL et al. The inflammatory cytokine tumor necrosis factor-alpha generates an autocrine tumor-promoting network in epithelial ovarian cancer cells. Cancer Res 2007; 67(2):585-592.
109. de Visser KE, Eichten A, Coussens LM. Paradoxical roles of the immune system during cancer development. Nat Rev Cancer 2006; 6(1):24-37.
110. Coussens LM, Werb Z. Inflammation and cancer. Nature 2002; 420(6917):860-867.
111. Gough M, Crittenden M, Thanarajasingam U et al. Gene therapy to manipulate effector T-cell trafficking to tumors for immunotherapy. J Immunol 2005; 174(9):5766-5773.
112. Morris A, Vetto JT, Ramstad T et al. Induction of anti-mammary cancer immunity by engaging the OX-40 receptor in vivo. Breast Cancer Res Treat 2001; 67(1):71-80.
113. Kjaergaard J, Peng L, Cohen PA et al. Augmentation versus inhibition: effects of conjunctional OX-40 receptor monoclonal antibody and IL-2 treatment on adoptive immunotherapy of advanced tumor. J Immunol 2001; 167(11):6669-6677.
114. Weinberg AD, Rivera MM, Prell R et al. Engagement of the OX-40 receptor in vivo enhances antitumor immunity. J Immunol 2000; 164(4):2160-2169.
115. Andarini S, Kikuchi T, Nukiwa M et al. Adenovirus vector-mediated in vivo gene transfer of OX40 ligand to tumor cells enhances antitumor immunity of tumor-bearing hosts. Cancer Res 2004; 64(9):3281-3287.
116. Gri G, Gallo E, Di Carlo E et al. OX40 ligand-transduced tumor cell vaccine synergizes with GM-CSF and requires CD40-Apc signaling to boost the host T-cell antitumor response. J Immunol 2003; 170(1):99-106.
117. Lathrop SK, Huddleston CA, Dullforce PA et al. A signal through OX40 (CD134) allows anergic, autoreactive T-cells to acquire effector cell functions. J Immunol 2004; 172:6735-6743.
118. Kuniyasu Y, Takahashi T, Itoh M et al. Naturally anergic and suppressive CD25(+)CD4(+) T-cells as a functionally and phenotypically distinct immunoregulatory T-cell subpopulation. Int Immunol 2000; 12(8):1145-1155.
119. Sakaguchi S, Sakaguchi N, Shimizu J et al. Immunologic tolerance maintained by CD25+ CD4+ regulatory T-cells: their common role in controlling autoimmunity, tumor immunity and transplantation tolerance. Immunol Rev 2001; 182:18-32.
120. Weinberg AD, Thalhofer C, Morris N et al. Anti-OX40 (CD134) administration to nonhuman primates: immunostimulatory effects and toxicokinetic study. J Immunother 2006; 29(6):575-585.

CHAPTER 7

Targeting CD70 for Human Therapeutic Use

Tamar E. Boursalian, Julie A. McEarchern, Che-Leung Law
and Iqbal S. Grewal*

Abstract

Expression of CD70, a member of the tumor necrosis factor superfamily, is restricted to activated T- and B-lymphocytes and mature dendritic cells. Binding of CD70 to its receptor, CD27, is important in priming, effector functions, differentiation and memory formation of T-cells as well as plasma and memory B-cell generation. Antibody blockade of CD70-CD27 interaction inhibits the onset of experimental autoimmune encephalomyelits and cardiac allograft rejection in mice. CD70 has been also detected on hematological tumors and on carcinomas. The highly restricted expression pattern of CD70 in normal tissues and its widespread expression in various malignancies as well as its potential role in autoimmune and inflammatory conditions makes it an attractive target for antibody-based therapeutics. This chapter provides an overview of the physiological role of CD70-CD27 interactions and discusses various approaches to target this pathway for therapeutic use in cancers and autoimmunity.

Introduction

Interactions between members of the tumor necrosis factor (TNF) and the tumor necrosis factor receptor (TNFR) superfamily of ligands/receptors control multiple cellular pathways, including lymphocyte proliferation, differentiation and cell death.[1,2] While these receptors and ligands are expressed on both normal and malignant cell types, the majority of these molecules are expressed on cells of hematopoietic origin involved in the immune system.[3] They are known to play important roles in multiple cellular processes, from the development of the immune system to the regulation of both normal and pathogenic immune responses. Their effects are seen in both innate and adaptive immune responses, including defense against pathogens, inflammatory responses, autoimmunity and tumorigenesis.[1,4] The importance of TNF and TNFR superfamily members in vivo is evident in the increased risk of malignancies and development of autoimmunity observed in mice and humans carrying mutations that affect these ligands/receptors.[5-7] Thus, approaches for targeting many of these receptors are increasingly being investigated and developed for use in clinical settings.

CD70, also known as CD27L, is a member of the TNF superfamily, a family of molecules made up of over 20 proteins, some membrane-bound and others secreted.[3] The primary amino acid sequence of CD70 predicts that, like other TNF family members, it is a type II transmembrane glycoprotein.[8,9] It shares sequence homology to other TNF family members in its extracellular region, suggesting close structural similarity between it and other TNF superfamily members, which

*Corresponding Author: Iqbal S. Grewal—Vice President of Preclinical Therapeutics, Seattle Genetics, Inc. 21823 30th Drive SE, Bothell, Washington 98021. Email: igrewal@seagen.com

Therapeutic Targets of the TNF Superfamily, edited by Iqbal S. Grewal.
©2009 Landes Bioscience and Springer Science + Business Media.

include TNFα, the lymphotoxins, CD30L, CD40L, FasL, OX40L, 4-1BBL, receptor activator of NF-κB ligand (RANKL), a proliferation-inducing ligand (APRIL), B lymphocyte stimulator (BLyS), nerve growth factor (NGF) and TNF-related apoptosis-inducing ligand (TRAIL). CD70 is predominantly expressed on activated T- and B-lymphocytes and plays an important role in lymphocyte effector function. Human CD70 is comprised of 193 amino acids with an apparent molecular mass of 50 kDa. It is made up of an extracellular binding domain, a transmembrane segment and two potential N-linked glycosylation sites.[8,9] Because of its structural homology to TNFα, CD70 is predicted to exist as a homotrimer.[8,10] Only a membrane-bound form of CD70 has been observed, with no recognizable motifs for cleavage from the cell surface reported to date.

CD70 is known to bind to a unique receptor, CD27. This ligand-receptor pair is cross-reactive between human and mouse.[11] CD27 is a member of the TNFR superfamily, whose members are type I membrane proteins characterized by the presence of a cysteine-rich domain in the extracellular portion of the receptor.[3] CD27 is a type I transmembrane glycoprotein of about 55 kDa. It is expressed as a homodimer on the cell surface with a disulfide bridge that links two monomer chains.[12,13] The existence of CD27 as a homodimer suggests that interaction of CD70 with CD27 may involve three CD27 homodimers.[10] Unlike CD70, CD27 has been shown to exist in a soluble form as well (sCD27), being cleaved from the cell surface by proteases. This soluble form of CD27 is detectable in healthy individuals, but is highly upregulated in many disease situations.[13] CD27 binds to TNF-receptor associated factor (TRAF-2) and TRAF-5 adaptor proteins through a conserved motif in its cytoplasmic tail which in turn activates Nuclear factor-kappaB (NF-κB) and the c-Jun kinase pathways.[14] Additional studies show that CD27 can activate both canonical as well as alternate NF-κB pathways through the NF-κB-inducing kinase (NIK), suggesting a role for CD27 in cell proliferation, differentiation and survival.[15] While CD27 itself contains no recognizable death domain motifs in its cytoplasmic region, a limited number of studies suggests a role for CD27 in apoptosis through the receptor-associated death domain-containing adaptor protein Siva.[16] However, despite CD27 binding to the Siva adaptor molecule, concrete evidence is lacking to support Siva involvement in CD27 signaling. Thus, as CD27 has been shown convincingly to mediate conventional survival of T-cells, to date it appears that interaction between CD70 and CD27 primarily serves to deliver signals of activation rather than apoptosis (Fig. 1).

Based on its biology, CD70 makes an attractive target for antibody-based immunotherapy for autoimmune and inflammatory indications. Additionally, with its expression on multiple hematological tumor types and carcinomas, CD70 is also a viable target in oncology.

CD70 Expression and Biology

Early histological studies reported limited expression of CD70 on B- and T-lymphocytes, mainly observed in germinal center B-cells and rare T-cells in tonsils, skin and the gut.[17] Subsequently, CD70 expression has been shown on recently activated T- and B-cells, with expression waning following the removal of antigenic stimulus.[18,19] In nonlymphoid lineages, CD70 expression is induced on mature dendritic cells (DCs) through triggering of CD40 or Toll-like receptors[20-22] and a low level of CD70 expression has been observed on thymic medullar epithelial cells.[17,23] Surface expression of CD70 on activated T- and B-cells is transient, persisting for several days and is mainly observed in primed effector lymphocytes.[17,19] For example, the majority of IFN-γ producing T-cells are CD70+ , as are B-cells producing immunoglobulin in response to T-dependent antigens.[24] This highly restricted and temporally regulated expression pattern for CD70 is carefully mediated by cellular activation signals, stimulation by antigens, costimulatory signals and cytokines, thus ensuring only transient opportunity for this ligand to exert its biological functions.[17,19]

CD27 is predominantly expressed on mature T-cells, memory B-cells, germinal center B-cells and natural killer (NK) cells.[25-27] CD27 is constitutively expressed on resting T-cells; however, a marked increase in CD27 expression is observed following T-cell activation, particularly in CD45RA+ T-cells[8,28-30] and can result in shedding of sCD27 from the cell surface.[13] CD27 expression on effector T-cells is transiently upregulated, subsequently diminishes and is highly correlated with the effector functions of the T-cells.[31] In contrast to T-cells, resting naïve B-cells

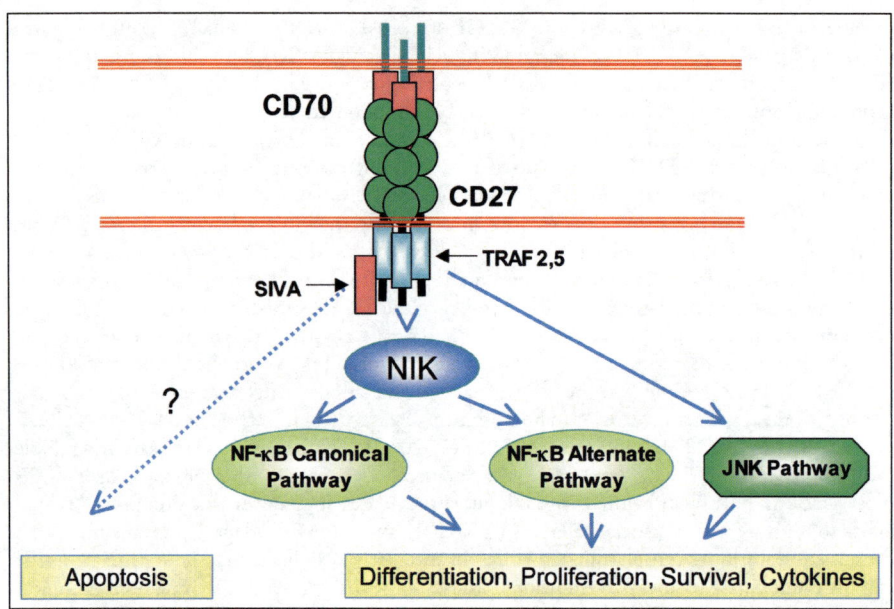

Figure 1. Signaling pathways mediated by CD70-CD27 interactions. Binding of CD70 to CD27 recruits the adaptor proteins TRAF2 and TRAF5, which activate kinases and provide a link to common signaling pathways for canonical and alternate NF-κB and JNK activation. Signals through the CD27 receptor mediate differentiation, proliferation, survival and cytokine production. Although CD27 has been shown to bind Siva and induce apoptosis, conclusive evidence for this pathway awaits further investigation (indicated by dashed arrow).

do not express CD27; however, CD27 expression can be induced by B-cell receptor triggering and is maintained over a long period of time.[32,33] Memory B-cells uniformly express CD27.[34] Neither CD27 nor CD70 expression is generally observed in nonlymphoid normal, healthy tissues, including the vital organs.

Many studies have established a requirement for CD70-CD27 interactions in efficient cooperation between activated lymphocytes during the generation of an immune response. A model depicting the role of CD70 in various facets of the immune system is illustrated in Figure 2. For T-cells, one of the key biological roles of these interactions is in the efficient priming of T-cells and the subsequent promotion of their survival, leading to the formation of effector and memory T-cells. Triggering of CD27 signals, either through interaction with CD70 or ligation through agonistic anti-CD27 antibodies, has been reported to induce proliferation and cytokine secretion by both CD4 and CD8 T-cells.[19] In addition, these signals promote the development of cytotoxic T-lymphocyte (CTL) responses by CD8 T-cells,[19] increase the survival of CD27-expressing cells[35,36] and induce TNFα production by effector T-cells.[37] In B-cells, the interaction of CD70-CD27 is important in B-cell differentiation and in the generation of plasma cells.[32,38] Additionally, CD70-CD27 interactions play several roles in T-dependent antibody production by promoting B-cell activation, germinal center formation, expansion and differentiation into plasma cells[39] and by enhancing immunoglobulin secretion.[33] In NK cells, direct cross-linking of CD27 results in the enhancement of NK cell cytolytic activity, proliferation and IFNγ production.[40,41] CD27 signaling also promotes NK cell activity in conjunction with interleukin-2 (IL-2) costimulation.[39]

A role for CD70 in cellular immune responses in vivo has been demonstrated in several studies. CD70 trangenic mice exhibit an accumulation of T-cells with an effector phenotype[42] and display increased CD8 T-cell response to influenza virus as well as enhanced tumor clearance.[43] In contrast, mice deficient in CD27 have reduced T-cell numbers in their lungs and spleens following

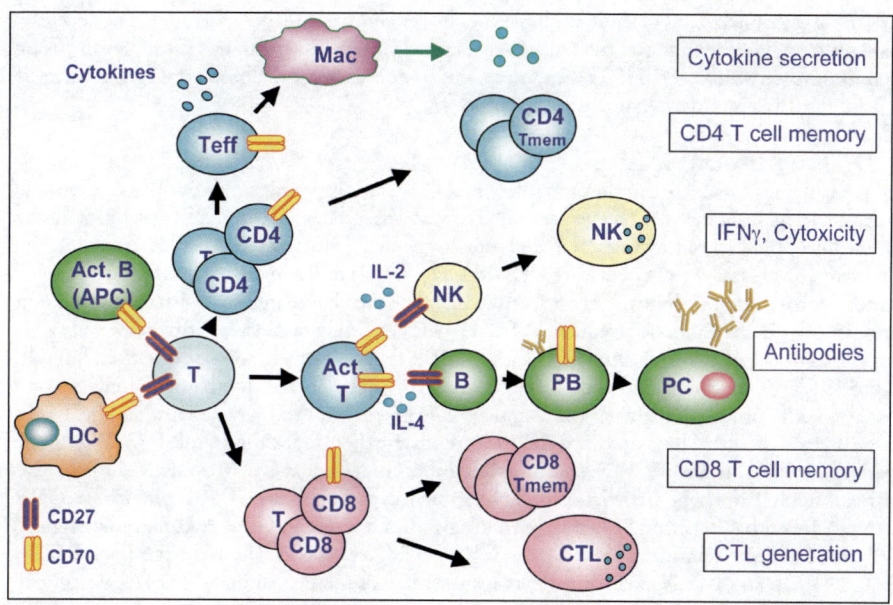

Figure 2. A model for CD70 mediated activation of lymphocytes. CD70-CD27 interactions are known to regulate multiple steps in lymphocyte activation including proliferation and generation of effector and memory T-cells, activation of NK cells and generation of plasma cells and immunoglobulin production from B cells. A model of various steps regulated by CD70-CD27 interactions are shown. DC, dendritic cell; Teff, T effector cell; PB, plasmablast; PC, plasma cell; Mac, macrophage; Act. B, Activated B cell; Act. T, activated T-cell; Tmem, T memory cell; NK, natural killer cell.

primary or secondary infection with influenza virus.[35] In vivo studies using T-cells with receptors specific for influenza but lacking CD27 expression suggest a role for CD27-CD70 interactions in the survival of T-cells in secondary and memory T-cell responses.[44] Additional in vivo studies using CD70 transfection have shown enhanced NK- as well as T-cell-dependent mechanisms of tumor clearance.[45,46] Studies with antibodies that block the interaction of CD70 and CD27 have shown efficacy in models of experimental autoimmune encephalitis (EAE)[47] and cardiac allograft rejection.[48] In the EAE model, CD70 blockade did not affect T-cell priming, immunoglobulin production or alter the balance of T-helper type 1 (T_H1) and T_H2 cells. However, it did inhibit antigen-induced TNFα production, suggesting that CD70-CD27 interaction may play a role in the enhancement of T_H1 mediated immune responses. In addition, it has been reported that CD70 expression on T-cells is enhanced by TNFα and IL-12, but is downregulated by IL-4, further supporting a role for CD70 in T_H1 responses over T_H2 responses.[19,49]

In a recent study, a novel population of CD70 expressing antigen presenting cells (APCs) was described, residing exclusively in the gut lamina propria of the mouse.[50] These cells express CD70 constitutively and are capable of presenting antigens. They were shown to mediate the expansion and differentiation of antigen-specific T-cells in the gut mucosa via CD70-dependent mechanisms. These data establish an additional role for CD70 in antigen presentation; however, these specialized tissue-specific APCs that utilize CD70 have only been observed in the mouse thus far.

In addition to delivering signals through CD27, a limited number of studies have revealed that CD70 itself possesses signaling properties. These studies report that signals delivered through CD70 activate the phosphatidylinositol-3 (PI3) kinase and MAP kinase pathways.[51,52] CD70 signals were shown to regulate cell cycle entry by primary B-cells,[51] while triggering cytotoxicity in NK, T-cell receptor (TCR) γδ+ and some TCRαβ + T-cell clones.[52] The signaling capabilities of CD70 were uncovered in these studies either under conditions where CD27 was not present, using mice whose lymphocytes constitutively express CD70 while lacking CD27,[51] or by using cells transfected with CD70.[52] As such, it remains to be seen what the biological consequence of CD70 signaling is under physiological conditions.

CD70 in Autoimmunity

Several lines of evidence implicate a role for CD70 in autoimmunity and conditions of chronic inflammation. In humans, CD70 expression has been observed on CD4 T-cells isolated from the synovium of rheumatoid arthritis (RA) and psoriatic arthritis patients.[53] Further studies also report an increased prevalence of circulating CD70+ CD4 T-cells in RA patients[54] and also in patients suffering from systemic lupus erythematosis (SLE),[55,56] when compared to healthy individuals. In the case of SLE, this increased frequency of CD70+ CD4 T-cells correlates with disease severity as measured by the SLE Disease Activity Index (SLEDAI)[55] score or with disease duration.[56] T-cells from SLE patients cocultured with B-cells elicited enhanced Ig secretion by the B-cells in comparison with normal individuals. This augmented Ig production was abrogated when the T-cells were pretreated with a blocking anti-CD70 antibody, further implicating a role for CD70 in the pathogenesis of this disease.[55] These authors and others suggest that CD70 overexpression in SLE patients results from hypomethylation of DNA sequences that flank the CD70 promotor.[55,57] DNA demethylation has been implicated in both drug-induced lupus and lupus of unknown origin.[58] Similar demethylation patterns have not been observed in RA patients. The overexpression of CD70 in CD4+ CD28- T-cells in these patients is instead attributed to an inability to downregulate CD70 expression once its expression is induced by activation of the T-cells.[54]

The role of CD70 has also been investigated in murine models of autoimmunity and inflammation. Similar to what is observed in the peripheral blood of human SLE patients, an increase in splenic CD70+ CD4 T-cells has also been observed in the lupus-prone MRL/lpr strain of mice.[59] The authors propose that this is a result of defective DNA methylation of the *Tnsf7* (CD70) gene caused by a decrease in Dnmt1 (DNA methyltransferase 1) expression, leading to upregulation of CD70 expression which correlates with age-dependent autoimmunity in these mice. In line with these observations, CD4 T-cells treated with DNA methylation inhibitors become autoreactive and will induce a lupus-like disease when adoptively transferred to syngeneic mice.[60,61]

As mentioned in the previous section, CD70 also appears to play a role in EAE, a T_H1-mediated disease, as shown by the reduction of TNF-α production following treatment with anti-CD70 antibody.[47] However, while treatment with blocking anti-CD70 was able to suppress the onset of disease, this treatment had little efficacy in established EAE. Anti-CD70 treatment was also effective at inhibiting inflammatory bowel disease (IBD) using the CD45RBhi transfer model in mice, another T_H1-mediated disease.[62] Anti-CD70 treatment resulted in either prevention or reversal of colitis as well as a reduction in key T_H1 cytokines associated with colitis. In contrast, anti-CD70 was not effective in modulation of disease in experimental *Leishmania major* infection in susceptible Balb/c mice which is predominantly a T_H2-mediated response, again supporting a role for CD70 in T_H1 over T_H2 responses.

The T_H1/T_H2 paradigm has recently been reevaluated to include a third population of T-helper cells, T_H17, named for its production of the cytokine IL-17. This subset of CD4 T-cells plays specific roles in both host defense against certain pathogens and in organ-specific autoimmunity (reviewed in ref. 63). A recent study illustrates CD70 involvement in T_H17 biology, showing that TNFα priming of monocytes generates CD70+ DCs that elicit both T_H1 and T_H17 responses.[64] Thus, this emerging area of investigation may prove to be an additional arena for CD70 targeting.

CD70 represents a promising target for antibody-directed immunotherapy given the overexpression observed in such diseases as rheumatoid and psoriatic arthritis and lupus, as well as its restricted expression pattern in normal cells. As discussed above, expression of CD70 is mostly restricted to activated lymphocytes and dendritic cells under physiological conditions and is transient in nature, waning with the removal of antigenic stimulus. Thus, in contrast to many immunosuppressive agents currently used to treat autoimmune and inflammatory conditions, targeted therapy against

CD70, whether by depletion or by blocking of CD70–CD27 interactions, is not likely to cause generalized immunosuppression, instead targeting only the activated cells of the immune system. However, a possible shortcoming of this approach presents itself in that CD70–CD27 interactions represent one of several costimulatory pathways involved in normal immune cell activation and disease, such as the CD28/CD80/CD86 pathway. Targeting only one costimulatory pathway may not be sufficient to impact disease progression. This notion is supported by the fact that anti-CD70 antibodies will only partially inhibit T-cell allogeneic responses in vitro[37] and that anti-CD70 antibody treatment does not impact EAE that is already established.[47]

CD70 in Oncology

In addition to its expression on normal lymphocytes in an ongoing immune response, CD70 expression has been documented in many different types of lymphomas and carcinomas, including tumors of neural origin.

In hematological malignancies, CD70 is expressed in tumors of both B- and T-cell origin. CD70 is expressed on malignant Hodgkin and Reed-Sternberg cells of Hodgkin lymphoma (HL).[65] CD70 is also abundantly expressed in other B-cell derived lymphomas, including non-Hodgkin lymphomas (NHL) such as diffuse large B-cell lymphoma, follicular lymphoma, B-cell lymphocytic leukemia, Burkitt's and mantle cell lymphomas,[66] as well as multiple myeloma[67] and Waldenstrom's macroglobulinemia.[68] The functional role of CD70 expression on these lymphomas and leukemias is not clear, but given the fact that CD70 expression is known to be induced on activated B-cells,[21,69] it may reflect differentiation arrest and oncogenic transformation of these cells. Alternatively, the sustained presence of CD70 on their surface may be the result of a sustained state of stimulation in tumor cells. In support of this notion, follicular NHL cells routinely undergo continuous somatic hypermutation which is a hallmark of sustained antigenic B-cell stimulation.[70,71]

Studies suggest that expression of CD70 in B-cell malignancies may play a role in immune escape as well as enhancing tumor survival and growth. In NHL, CD70+ B-cells have been reported to induce the expression of forkhead-box protein 3 (Foxp3) in tumor infiltrating CD4+ CD25- T-cells that possess immunosuppressive activity.[72] This NHL-mediated upregulation of Foxp3 can be significantly inhibited by blockade of CD70, implicating CD70 in the induction of the immune suppression. In Waldenstrom's macroglobulinemia, studies indicate that the mast cells in these patients use a CD70-dependant mechanism to upregulate CD40L and APRIL,[68] both of which (among other TNF members) have been have been reported to promote the growth of tumor cells expressing their receptors.[68,73] Thus, constitutive expression of CD70 within the tumor microenvironment or expression on the tumors themselves has the potential to promote tumor growth as well as to facilitate immune evasion.

In addition to expression of CD70, many NHLs and leukemias also express its ligand, CD27. The significance of this co-expression is not clear at this time; however, one could envision that expression of both ligand and receptor on the same tumor cell could serve to create an autocrine loop whereby the delivery of proliferative signals delivered through CD27 via its interaction with CD70 would provide growth potential to the malignant cells.[66] Indeed in studies of childhood acute lymphoblastic leukemia (ALL), upregulation of both CD70 and CD27 expression was observed in CD19+ ALL cells of the bone marrow and was shown to be important for the proliferation of the leukemic cells. Proliferation of the ALL cells in vitro was greatly reduced when the cells were treated with an anti-human CD70 antibody that blocked its interaction with CD27.[74]

With regard to nonlymphoid tumors, early studies reported CD70 expression only on undifferentiated nasopharyngeal carcinoma and embryonic carcinoma.[75] In the case of nasopharyngeal carcinoma, CD70 expression was thought to be related to Epstein-Barr virus (EBV) infection. Both nasopharyngeal carcinoma and HL are usually associated with EBV and both express CD70.[65,75] Transforming viruses like EBV and also the human T leukemia virus-1 (HTLV-1) are known to induce expression of CD70 on cells of epithelial origin, which do not normally express CD70.[75] In more recent studies, CD70 has also been detected on EBV-negative thymic carcinoma,[23] renal cell carcinoma (RCC),[76-78] glioblastoma,[79,80] astrocytoma[79,80] and ovarian cancer.[81]

The significance of CD70 expression on carcinomas is unclear. However, it may contribute to immune escape mechanisms by tumor cells. Studies investigating the potential role of CD70 expression in clear cell RCC and glioblastoma suggest that CD70 expressed on tumor cells may contribute to impaired T-cell function often observed within the tumor microenvironment, thus facilitating immune evasion by the tumor cells.[82,83] In support of this theory, expression of CD70 on glioma cells can mediate apoptosis of lymphocytes, implicating CD70 in the induction of immune suppression.[80] Similar mechanisms may come into play in the case of RCC as there are several indications that RCC is an immunological tumor: the presence of tumor infiltrating lymphocytes (TIL); response to TIL-directed therapy; response to IFNα and IL-2 therapy; and the incidence of a few known cases of complete spontaneous remission.[83] Other mediators of immunosuppression in lymphocytes are also induced by RCC, such as protaglandin E2 (PGE2).[84] Such immunomodulatory mechanisms coupled with constitutive expression of CD70 may provide a distinct advantage to RCC for immune escape as well as actively inducing immune inhibition.

In contrast to the above-mentioned in vitro studies supporting a role for CD70 in immune escape mechanisms by tumors, a limited number of in vivo studies indicate a role for CD70 in the generation of anti-tumor immunity.[85] These studies suggest that expression of CD70 on tumor cells provides an immunostimulatory effect that overrides CD70-mediated immune cell apoptosis, leading to long-lasting anti-tumor immunity. This is consistent with the fact that CD70-CD27 interactions are known to support the survival of conventional T-cells. Given the contrasting roles of immune escape versus anti-tumor immunity indicated by the above studies, clearly more investigation is warranted to determine the significance of CD70 expression on carcinomas.

In considering treatments for hematological malignancies, antibody-based immunotherapies are emerging as an important class of drugs yielding promising results in the clinic. Many monoclonal antibodies have been useful in treating B-cell-derived malignancies. Targets for these antibodies include CD20,[86] CD22,[87] CD52,[88] CD40[89] and B-cell idiotype.[90] While these targets are expressed on the surface of tumor cells, they are also expressed on the majority normal B-cells and/ or B-cell precursors and thus pose the threat that monoclonal antibodies against these molecules will also target normal B-cells. For example, rituximab, a monoclonal antibody directed against CD20 that has been successful in treating lymphomas and other indications, has been shown to deplete memory B-cells. This results in a decrease in antibody production during the course of a recall response to antigen.[91,92] The long-term consequence of the loss of memory B-cells caused by rituxan treatment is as yet unknown.

In order to mitigate the generalized immune suppression potentially caused by the targeting of pan-B-cell markers, an alternative approach is to target molecules that are transiently expressed on normal B-cells, such as activation markers. With this in mind, CD70 is an attractive target for antibody-based therapy. As discussed above, the expression pattern of CD70 is highly restricted under normal physiological conditions. It is induced upon activation of lymphocytes, expression is transient and is downregulated once antigenic stimulation subsides. While expression on normal cells is transient, CD70 is abundantly expressed on multiple tumors of hematopoietic origin, which is strong rationale for targeting this molecule using antibody-directed immunotherapy to deplete CD70-expressing tumor cells or to inhibit their growth.

In preclinical models, studies using two different mouse anti-human CD70 antibodies, LD6 (IgG2b) and Ki-24 (IgG3), have served to validate CD70 as a potential target for immunotherapy in EBV+ Burkitt's lymphoma.[93] Both antibodies exhibited efficient complement dependent cytotoxicity (CDC) activity in vitro against the EBV+ Burkitt's lymphoma cell lines, Raji and Jijoye. Moreover, these antibodies demonstrated in vivo efficacy in xenograft models of Burkitt's lymphoma in severe combined immunodeficient (SCID) mice. Additional data indicated a mechanism of action independent of inflammatory response or induction of lytic EBV, suggesting that the efficacy of the anti-CD70 antibody treatment may have stemmed at least partially from the CDC activity observed for these antibodies in vitro. Rituxan, which is effective in treating NHL, also exhibits CDC activity in vitro and is known to depend on CDC activity in vivo.[94]

The most clinically useful therapeutic antibodies are those that provide efficacy through multiple modes of action exerting cytotoxic effects on tumor cells. An example of an anti-CD70 antibody being developed for clinical use is SGN-70, a humanized anti-CD70 antibody of IgG1 isotype.[67,95] This antibody blocks binding of CD70 to CD27 and mediates Fc-dependent antibody effector functions including CDC, antibody dependent cellular cytotoxicity (ADCC) and antibody-dependent cellular phagocytosis (ADCP) of CD70+ tumor cells by macrophages. Removal of antibody-coated target cells by the reticuloendothelial system is emerging as an important component of the therapeutic activity of antibodies targeting CD20,[96,97] suggesting a role for FcγR-mediated phagocytosis in the elimination of target cells. In addition to its in vitro activities, SGN-70 treatment in vivo results in the regression of tumors and prolonged survival of mice in disseminated lymphoma and multiple myeloma xenograft models that use CD70+ tumor lines.[67,95] Additionally, in the multiple myeloma model, the prevalence of myeloma cells in the bone marrow and λ light chain levels in the sera were significantly reduced with SGN-70 treatment, both of which are measures of tumor burden.

Antibody therapies are also being considered for targeting proteins expressed on solid tumors. However, solid tumors may pose a challenge to antibody therapy by virtue of their relative impenetrability in comparison to hematoligcal malignancies, where therapeutic benefit can be achieved at low doses. Thus, alternative strategies are being pursued that build on the utility of monoclonal antibodies. Examples include radiolabeled antibodies combined with chemotherapy (which are associated with undesirable side affects) or antibody-drug conjugates (ADCs) where a cytotoxic drug is linked to the antibody, thus delivering a lethal payload within the tumor cell bearing the target. CD70 is a good candidate for this approach due to the fact that it is rapidly internalized following antibody binding,[78] ensuring the delivery of the drug inside the cell. This, combined with the fact that CD70 is constitutively expressed on multiple carcinoma types while its expression is restricted on normal tissues, makes CD70 a viable target for this type of antibody-based therapy against solid tumors. Anti-CD70 ADCs consisting of the tubulin-binding agent monomethyl auristatin F (MMAF) conjugated through either a peptide or glucuronide linker have recently been evaluated for their preclinical therapeutic utilities.[78,98,99] These ADCs have demonstrated potent, antigen-specific cytotoxic activity against CD70 expressing carcinomas in vitro and this activity was confirmed in vivo in xenograft models established with CD70+ tumor cell lines.[78,99] Most recently, another set of anti-CD70-MMAF ADCs that does not contain any enzyme-cleavable linker has also demonstrated therapeutic efficacy against CD70+ tumors in preclinical experiments.[100]

As mentioned above, there may be a relationship between CD70 expressed on inflammatory cells of the tumor microenvironment and growth and survival advantage for the tumor cells. Further investigation of this notion may support a rationale for anti-CD70 treatment regardless of CD70 expression on the tumors themselves. Upstream signals to infiltrating lymphocytes could be blocked to result in the inhibition of paracrine growth signals to the malignant cells. Thus in addition to direct targeting of CD70 on malignant cells themselves, blocking CD70-CD27 interaction may also impart therapeutic benefit by restricting growth signals and/or escape from immune surveillance.

Conclusions and Future Directions

It is now evident that CD70-CD27 interactions play a role in the activation and differentiation of different cell types in both the adaptive and innate immune systems. In particular, CD70-CD27 interactions regulate the later phases of the effector immune response. Thus, therapeutic strategies designed to perturb this interaction may provide a useful means to treat autoimmune diseases and additionally to prevent graft rejection. These strategies may include the use of anti-CD70 antibodies, development of small molecule antagonists, or recombinant soluble proteins that can block binding of CD70 to CD27. An alternative approach lies in targeting at the level of intracellular pathways of CD70-mediated signaling that include inactivation of proteins associated with the CD27 cytoplasmic tail such as TRAF2 and TRAF6. Although some of these approaches have been successful in experimental models, potential side effects must be weighed before they are applied to humans. CD70 could also be potentially exploited for beneficial roles in cancer therapy. Since it is broadly expressed on multiple tumor types of both hematological and carcinoma origin and has relative limited expression on normal tissues, the CD70 antigen offers an excellent opportunity as a tumor target for antibody-based immunotherapy. Defining the significance of CD70 expression on tumor cells remains a largely unexplored area of investigation. Although some preliminary evidence suggests an intriguing role for CD70 in immune escape mechanisms, the exact nature of CD70 involvement in this phenomenon remains to be elucidated. Further studies investigating CD70 and its relationship to immune escape may provide insights into the development of new therapeutic interventions for cancers. Since CD70–CD27 interactions regulate multiple phases of the immune response and CD70 expression is linked with malignancies, CD70 is likely to remain the subject of intense investigation, particularly in the development of beneficial therapeutic approaches.

References

1. Smith CA, Farrah T, Goodwin RG. The TNF receptor superfamily of cellular and viral proteins: activation, costimulation and death. Cell 1994; 76:959-62.
2. Gruss HJ, Dower SK. Tumor necrosis factor ligand superfamily: involvement in the pathology of malignant lymphomas. Blood 1995; 85:3378-404.
3. Aggarwal BB. Signalling pathways of the TNF superfamily: a double-edged sword. Nat Rev Immunol 2003; 3:745-56.
4. Locksley RM, Killeen N, Lenardo MJ. The TNF and TNF receptor superfamilies: integrating mammalian biology. Cell 2001; 104:487-501.
5. Renshaw BR, Fanslow WC 3rd, Armitage RJ et al. Humoral immune responses in CD40 ligand-deficient mice. J Exp Med 1994; 180:1889-900.
6. Davidson WF, Giese T, Fredrickson TN. Spontaneous development of plasmacytoid tumors in mice with defective Fas-Fas ligand interactions. J Exp Med 1998; 187:1825-38.
7. Gulino AV, Notarangelo LD. Hyper IgM syndromes. Curr Opin Rheumatol 2003; 15:422-9.
8. Goodwin RG, Alderson MR, Smith CA et al. Molecular and biological characterization of a ligand for CD27 defines a new family of cytokines with homology to tumor necrosis factor. Cell 1993; 73:447-56.
9. Bowman MR, Crimmins MA, Yetz-Aldape J et al. The cloning of CD70 and its identification as the ligand for CD27. J Immunol 1994; 152:1756-61.
10. Peitsch MC, Tschopp J. Comparative molecular modelling of the Fas-ligand and other members of the TNF family. Mol Immunol 1995; 32:761-72.
11. Bossen C, Ingold K, Tardivel A et al. Interactions of tumor necrosis factor (TNF) and TNF receptor family members in the mouse and human. J Biol Chem 2006; 281:13964-71.
12. Camerini D, Walz G, Loenen WA et al. The T-cell activation antigen CD27 is a member of the nerve growth factor/tumor necrosis factor receptor gene family. J Immunol 1991; 147:3165-9.
13. Hintzen RQ, van Lier RA, Kuijpers KC et al. Elevated levels of a soluble form of the T-cell activation antigen CD27 in cerebrospinal fluid of multiple sclerosis patients. J Neuroimmunol 1991; 35:211-7.
14. Akiba H, Nakano H, Nishinaka S et al. CD27, a member of the tumor necrosis factor receptor superfamily, activates NF-kappaB and stress-activated protein kinase/c-Jun N-terminal kinase via TRAF2, TRAF5 and NF-kappaB-inducing kinase. J Biol Chem 1998; 273:13353-8.
15. Ramakrishnan P, Wang W, Wallach D. Receptor-specific signaling for both the alternative and the canonical NF-kappaB activation pathways by NF-kappaB-inducing kinase. Immunity 2004; 21:477-89.
16. Prasad KV, Ao Z, Yoon Y et al. CD27, a member of the tumor necrosis factor receptor family, induces apoptosis and binds to Siva, a proapoptotic protein. Proc Natl Acad Sci USA 1997; 94:6346-51.
17. Hintzen RQ, Lens SM, Koopman G et al. CD70 represents the human ligand for CD27. Int Immunol 1994; 6:477-80.
18. Lens SM, de Jong R, Hooibrink B et al. Phenotype and function of human B-cells expressing CD70 (CD27 ligand). Eur J Immunol 1996; 26:2964-71.
19. Lens SM, Baars PA, Hooibrink B et al. Antigen-presenting cell-derived signals determine expression levels of CD70 on primed T-cells. Immunology 1997; 90:38-45.
20. Akiba H, Miyahira Y, Atsuta M et al. Critical contribution of OX40 ligand to T helper cell type 2 differentiation in experimental leishmaniasis. J Exp Med 2000; 191:375-80.
21. Tesselaar K, Xiao Y, Arens R et al. Expression of the murine CD27 ligand CD70 in vitro and in vivo. J Immunol 2003; 170:33-40.

22. Bullock TN, Yagita H. Induction of CD70 on dendritic cells through CD40 or TLR stimulation contributes to the development of CD8 + T-cell responses in the absence of CD4 + T-cells. J Immunol 2005; 174:710-7.
23. Hishima T, Fukayama M, Hayashi Y et al. CD70 expression in thymic carcinoma. Am J Surg Pathol 2000; 24:742-6.
24. Hintzen RQ, Lens SM, Beckmann MP et al. Characterization of the human CD27 ligand, a novel member of the TNF gene family. J Immunol 1994; 152:1762-73.
25. Hintzen RQ, de Jong R, Lens SM et al. CD27: marker and mediator of T-cell activation? Immunol Today 1994; 15:307-11.
26. Lens SM, Tesselaar K, van Oers MH et al. Control of lymphocyte function through CD27-CD70 interactions. Semin Immunol 1998; 10:491-9.
27. Borst J, Hendriks J, Xiao Y. CD27 and CD70 in T-cell and B-cell activation. Curr Opin Immunol 2005; 17:275-81.
28. de Jong R, Loenen WA, Brouwer M et al. Regulation of expression of CD27, a T-cell-specific member of a novel family of membrane receptors. J Immunol 1991; 146:2488-94.
29. Hintzen RQ, de Jong R, Lens SM et al. Regulation of CD27 expression on subsets of mature T-lymphocytes. J Immunol 1993; 151:2426-35.
30. van Lier RA, Borst J, Vroom TM et al. Tissue distribution and biochemical and functional properties of Tp55 (CD27), a novel T-cell differentiation antigen. J Immunol 1987; 139:1589-96.
31. Watts TH. TNF/TNFR family members in costimulation of T-cell responses. Annu Rev Immunol 2005; 23:23-68.
32. Jacquot S, Kobata T, Iwata S et al. CD154/CD40 and CD70/CD27 interactions have different and sequential functions in T-cell-dependent B-cell responses: enhancement of plasma cell differentiation by CD27 signaling. J Immunol 1997; 159:2652-7.
33. Kobata T, Jacquot S, Kozlowski S et al. CD27-CD70 interactions regulate B-cell activation by T-cells. Proc Natl Acad Sci USA 1995; 92:11249-53.
34. Klein U, Rajewsky K, Kuppers R. Human immunoglobulin (Ig)M + IgD + peripheral blood B-cells expressing the CD27 cell surface antigen carry somatically mutated variable region genes: CD27 as a general marker for somatically mutated (memory) B-cells. J Exp Med 1998; 188:1679-89.
35. Hendriks J, Gravestein LA, Tesselaar K et al. CD27 is required for generation and long-term maintenance of T-cell immunity. Nat Immunol 2000; 1:433-40.
36. Sugita K, Hirose T, Rothstein DM et al. CD27, a member of the nerve growth factor receptor family, is preferentially expressed on CD45RA + CD4 T-cell clones and involved in distinct immunoregulatory functions. J Immunol 1992; 149:3208-16.
37. Hintzen RQ, Lens SM, Lammers K et al. Engagement of CD27 with its ligand CD70 provides a second signal for T-cell activation. J Immunol 1995; 154:2612-23.
38. Xiao Y, Hendriks J, Langerak P et al. CD27 is acquired by primed B-cells at the centroblast stage and promotes germinal center formation. J Immunol 2004; 172:7432-41.
39. Agematsu K, Nagumo H, Oguchi Y et al. Generation of plasma cells from peripheral blood memory B-cells: synergistic effect of interleukin-10 and CD27/CD70 interaction. Blood 1998; 91:173-80.
40. Takeda K, Oshima H, Hayakawa Y et al. CD27-mediated activation of murine NK cells. J Immunol 2000; 164:1741-5.
41. Orengo AM, Cantoni C, Neglia F et al. Reciprocal expression of CD70 and of its receptor, CD27, in human long term-activated T- and natural killer (NK) cells: inverse regulation by cytokines and role in induction of cytotoxicity. Clin Exp Immunol 1997; 107:608-13.
42. Arens R, Tesselaar K, Baars PA et al. Constitutive CD27/CD70 interaction induces expansion of effector-type T-cells and results in IFNgamma-mediated B-cell depletion. Immunity 2001; 15:801-12.
43. Arens R, Schepers K, Nolte MA et al. Tumor rejection induced by CD70-mediated quantitative and qualitative effects on effector CD8 + T-cell formation. J Exp Med 2004; 199:1595-605.
44. Hendriks J, Xiao Y, Borst J. CD27 promotes survival of activated T-cells and complements CD28 in generation and establishment of the effector T-cell pool. J Exp Med 2003; 198:1369-80.
45. Nieland JD, Graus YF, Dortmans YE et al. CD40 and CD70 costimulate a potent in vivo antitumor T-cell response. J Immunother 1998; 21:225-36.
46. Kelly JM, Darcy PK, Markby JL et al. Induction of tumor-specific T-cell memory by NK cell-mediated tumor rejection. Nat Immunol 2002; 3:83-90.
47. Nakajima A, Oshima H, Nohara C et al. Involvement of CD70-CD27 interactions in the induction of experimental autoimmune encephalomyelitis. J Neuroimmunol 2000; 109:188-96.
48. Aramaki O, Shirasugi N, Akiyama Y et al. CD27/CD70, CD134/CD134 ligand and CD30/CD153 pathways are independently essential for generation of regulatory cells after intratracheal delivery of alloantigen. Transplantation 2003; 76:772-6.

49. Hartwig UF, Karlsson L, Peterson PA et al. CD40 and IL-4 regulate murine CD27L expression. J Immunol 1997; 159:6000-8.
50. Laouar A, Haridas V, Vargas D et al. CD70+ antigen-presenting cells control the proliferation and differentiation of T-cells in the intestinal mucosa. Nat Immunol 2005; 6:698-706.
51. Arens R, Nolte MA, Tesselaar K et al. Signaling through CD70 regulates B-cell activation and IgG production. J Immunol 2004; 173:3901-8.
52. Garcia P, De Heredia AB, Bellon T et al. Signalling via CD70, a member of the TNF family, regulates T-cell functions. J Leukoc Biol 2004; 76:263-70.
53. Brugnoni D, Airo P, Marino R et al. CD70 expression on T-cell subpopulations: study of normal individuals and patients with chronic immune activation. Immunol Lett 1997; 55:99-104.
54. Lee WW, Yang ZZ, Li G et al. Unchecked CD70 expression on T-cells lowers threshold for T-cell activation in rheumatoid arthritis. J Immunol 2007; 179:2609-15.
55. Oelke K, Lu Q, Richardson D et al. Overexpression of CD70 and overstimulation of IgG synthesis by lupus T-cells and T-cells treated with DNA methylation inhibitors. Arthritis Rheum 2004; 50:1850-60.
56. Han BK, White AM, Dao KH et al. Increased prevalence of activated CD70+ CD4+ T-cells in the periphery of patients with systemic lupus erythematosus. Lupus 2005; 14:598-606.
57. Lu Q, Wu A, Richardson BC. Demethylation of the same promoter sequence increases CD70 expression in lupus T-cells and T-cells treated with lupus-inducing drugs. J Immunol 2005; 174:6212-9.
58. Sawalha AH, Richardson B. DNA methylation in the pathogenesis of systemic lupus erythematosus. Current Pharmacogenomics 2005; 3:73-8.
59. Sawalha AH, Jeffries M. Defective DNA methylation and CD70 overexpression in CD4+ T-cells in MRL/lpr lupus-prone mice. Eur J Immunol 2007; 37:1407-13.
60. Quddus J, Johnson KJ, Gavalchin J et al. Treating activated CD4+ T-cells with either of two distinct DNA methyltransferase inhibitors, 5-azacytidine or procainamide, is sufficient to cause a lupus-like disease in syngeneic mice. J Clin Invest 1993; 92:38-53.
61. Yung RL, Quddus J, Chrisp CE et al. Mechanism of drug-induced lupus. I. Cloned Th2 cells modified with DNA methylation inhibitors in vitro cause autoimmunity in vivo. J Immunol 1995; 154:3025-35.
62. Manocha S, Rietdijk S, Laouar A et al. CD70 antibody therapy for the prevention and treatment of experimental inflammatory bowel disease (IBD). FASEB J 2008; 22:Abstract 859.10.
63. Korn T, Oukka M, Kuchroo V et al. Th17 cells: effector T-cells with inflammatory properties. Semin Immunol 2007; 19:362-71.
64. Iwamoto S, Iwai S, Tsujiyama K et al. TNF-alpha drives human CD14+ monocytes to differentiate into CD70+ dendritic cells evoking Th1 and Th17 responses. J Immunol 2007; 179:1449-57.
65. Gruss HJ, Kadin ME. Pathophysiology of hodgkin's disease: functional and molecular aspects. Baillieres Clin Haematol 1996; 9:417-46.
66. Lens SM, Drillenburg P, den Drijver BF et al. Aberrant expression and reverse signalling of CD70 on malignant B-cells. Br J Haematol 1999; 106:491-503.
67. McEarchern JA, Smith LM, McDonagh CF et al. Preclinical characterization of SGN-70, a humanized antibody directed against CD70. 2008; Manuscript submitted
68. Ho AW, Hatjiharissi E, Ciccarelli BT et al. CD27-CD70 interactions in the pathogenesis of Waldenstrom's Macroglobulinemia. Blood 2008;
69. Lens SM, Keehnen RM, van Oers MH et al. Identification of a novel subpopulation of germinal center B-cells characterized by expression of IgD and CD70. Eur J Immunol 1996; 26:1007-11.
70. Bahler DW, Levy R. Clonal evolution of a follicular lymphoma: evidence for antigen selection. Proc Natl Acad Sci USA 1992; 89:6770-4.
71. Bahler DW, Zelenetz AD, Chen TT et al. Antigen selection in human lymphomagenesis. Cancer Res 1992; 52:5547s-5551s.
72. Yang ZZ, Novak AJ, Ziesmer SC et al. CD70+ nonHodgkin lymphoma B-cells induce Foxp3 expression and regulatory function in intratumoral CD4+ CD25 T-cells. Blood 2007; 110:2537-44.
73. Tournilhac O, Santos DD, Xu L et al. Mast cells in Waldenstrom's macroglubulinemia support lymphoplasmacytic cell growth through CD154/CD40 signaling. Ann Oncol 2006; 17:1275-82.
74. Nilsson A, de Milito A, Mowafi F et al. Expression of CD27-CD70 on early B-cell progenitors in the bone marrow: implication for diagnosis and therapy of childhood ALL. Exp Hematol 2005; 33:1500-7.
75. Agathanggelou A, Niedobitek G, Chen R et al. Expression of immune regulatory molecules in Epstein-Barr virus-associated nasopharyngeal carcinomas with prominent lymphoid stroma. Evidence for a functional interaction between epithelial tumor cells and infiltrating lymphoid cells. Am J Pathol 1995; 147:1152-60.

76. Junker K, Hindermann W, von Eggeling F et al. CD70: a new tumor specific biomarker for renal cell carcinoma. J Urol 2005; 173:2150-3.
77. Diegmann J, Junker K, Gerstmayer B et al. Identification of CD70 as a diagnostic biomarker for clear cell renal cell carcinoma by gene expression profiling, real-time RT-PCR and immunohistochemistry. Eur J Cancer 2005; 41:1794-801.
78. Law CL, Gordon KA, Toki BE et al. Lymphocyte activation antigen CD70 expressed by renal cell carcinoma is a potential therapeutic target for anti-CD70 antibody-drug conjugates. Cancer Res 2006; 66:2328-37.
79. Held-Feindt J, Mentlein R. CD70/CD27 ligand, a member of the TNF family, is expressed in human brain tumors. Int J Cancer 2002; 98:352-6.
80. Wischhusen J, Jung G, Radovanovic I et al. Identification of CD70-mediated apoptosis of immune effector cells as a novel immune escape pathway of human glioblastoma. Cancer Res 2002; 62:2592-9.
81. Aggarwal S, He T, Fitzhugh W et al. Membrane proteomic analyses of ovarian cancer identifies the immune modulators CD70 and B7-H2 as candidate markers of cisplatin response. Proceedings of the 99th Annual Meeting for the American Association for Cancer Research 2008:Abstract 2430.
82. Chahlavi A, Rayman P, Richmond AL et al. Glioblastomas induce T-lymphocyte death by two distinct pathways involving gangliosides and CD70. Cancer Res 2005; 65:5428-38.
83. Diegmann J, Junker K, Loncarevic IF et al. Immune escape for renal cell carcinoma: CD70 mediates apoptosis in lymphocytes. Neoplasia 2006; 8:933-8.
84. Smyth GP, Stapleton PP, Barden CB et al. Renal cell carcinoma induces prostaglandin E2 and T-helper type 2 cytokine production in peripheral blood mononuclear cells. Ann Surg Oncol 2003; 10:455-62.
85. Aulwurm S, Wischhusen J, Friese M et al. Immune stimulatory effects of CD70 override CD70-mediated immune cell apoptosis in rodent glioma models and confer long-lasting antiglioma immunity in vivo. Int J Cancer 2006; 118:1728-35.
86. McLaughlin P, Grillo-Lopez AJ, Link BK et al. Rituximab chimeric anti-CD20 monoclonal antibody therapy for relapsed indolent lymphoma: half of patients respond to a four-dose treatment program. J Clin Oncol 1998; 16:2825-33.
87. Leonard JP, Link BK. Immunotherapy of non-Hodgkin's lymphoma with hLL2 (epratuzumab, an anti-CD22 monoclonal antibody) and Hu1D10 (apolizumab). Semin Oncol 2002; 29:81-6.
88. Lundin J, Kimby E, Bjorkholm M et al. Phase II trial of subcutaneous anti-CD52 monoclonal antibody alemtuzumab (Campath-1H) as first-line treatment for patients with B-cell chronic lymphocytic leukemia (B-CLL). Blood 2002; 100:768-73.
89. Law CL, Grewal IS. Therapeutic interventions targeting CD40L (CD154) and CD40: The opportunities and challenges. In: Grewal IS, ed. Therapeutic Targets of the TNF Superfamily. Austin: Landes Bioscience, 2008;8-36.
90. Miller RA, Maloney DG, Warnke R et al. Treatment of B-cell lymphoma with monoclonal anti-idiotype antibody. N Engl J Med 1982; 306:517-22.
91. Nishio M, Endo T, Fujimoto K et al. Persistent panhypogammaglobulinemia with selected loss of memory B-cells and impaired isotype expression after rituximab therapy for posttransplant EBV-associated auto-immune hemolytic anemia. Eur J Haematol 2005; 75:527-9.
92. van der Kolk LE, Baars JW, Prins MH et al. Rituximab treatment results in impaired secondary humoral immune responsiveness. Blood 2002; 100:2257-9.
93. Israel BF, Gulley M, Elmore S et al. Anti-CD70 antibodies: a potential treatment for EBV+ CD70-expressing lymphomas. Mol Cancer Ther 2005; 4:2037-44.
94. Di Gaetano N, Cittera E, Nota R et al. Complement activation determines the therapeutic activity of rituximab in vivo. J Immunol 2003; 171:1581-7.
95. McEarchern JA, Oflazoglu E, Francisco L et al. Engineered anti-CD70 antibody with multiple effector functions exhibits in vitro and in vivo antitumor activities. Blood 2007; 109:1185-92.
96. Uchida J, Hamaguchi Y, Oliver JA et al. The innate mononuclear phagocyte network depletes B-lymphocytes through Fc receptor-dependent mechanisms during anti-CD20 antibody immunotherapy. J Exp Med 2004; 199:1659-69.
97. Gong Q, Ou Q, Ye S et al. Importance of cellular microenvironment and circulatory dynamics in B-cell immunotherapy. J Immunol 2005; 174:817-26.
98. Jeffrey SC, Andreyka JB, Bernhardt SX et al. Development and properties of beta-glucuronide linkers for monoclonal antibody-drug conjugates. Bioconjug Chem 2006; 17:831-40.
99. Doronina SO, Mendelsohn BA, Bovee TD et al. Enhanced activity of monomethylauristatin F through monoclonal antibody delivery: effects of linker technology on efficacy and toxicity. Bioconjug Chem 2006; 17:114-24.
100. Oflazoglu E, Stone IJ, Wood CG et al. Potent anticarcinoma activity of the humanized anti-CD70 antibody h1F6 conjugated to the tubulin inhibitor auristatin via an uncleavable linker. Clin Cancer Res 2008; In Press.

CHAPTER 8

4-1BB as a Therapeutic Target for Human Disease

Seung-Woo Lee and Michael Croft*

Abstract

4-1BB (CD137) is being thought of as an attractive target for immunotherapy of many human immune diseases based on encouraging results with 4-1BB agonistic antibody treatment in mouse models of cancer, autoimmune disease, asthma and additionally as a means to improve vaccination. In this review, we will summarize the results of basic research on 4-1BB and 4-1BB immunotherapy of disease and provide some potential mechanistic insights into the many stimulatory and regulatory functions of 4-1BB.

Introduction to Basic Research

4-1BB (CD137, ILA, TNFRSF9), a member of the tumor-necrosis factor receptor (TNFR) superfamily, was originally identified as an inducible costimulatory molecule on activated T-cells.[1-4] The ligand of 4-1BB (4-1BBL, TNFSF9), a member of the TNF super-family, was later found expressed on activated antigen-presenting cells (APC) such as B-cells, macrophages and dendritic cells (DC).[3,5-7] Based on these expression characteristics and early functional data, it was thought that 4-1BBL expressed on activated APC binds to 4-1BB that is induced on T-cells, generating positive signals inside T-cells to help them function and to augment various aspects of immunity. Many in vitro studies have supported this concept showing that ligation of 4-1BB by either agonistic antibody, a soluble 4-1BBL molecule, or 4-1BBL-expressed on fibroblast cells can costimulate both CD4 and CD8 T-cells, leading to enhanced proliferation and cytokine secretion.[9-11] In line with this positive regulation of T-cells, similar to other members of the TNFR family, the ligation of 4-1BB can recruit TNFR-associated factor (TRAF) adaptor molecules,[12-14] and activate pro-inflammatory signaling pathways involving phosphatidylinositol-3-kinase (PI3K), protein kinase B (PKB, also known as Akt) and nuclear factor κB (NF-κB) pathways, as well as up-regulate expression of anti-apoptotic Bcl-2 family molecules that aid in survival.[15,16]

4-1BB$^{-/-}$ and 4-1BBL$^{-/-}$ mice show no obvious defects in the development of lymphocytes and lymphoid organs.[17,18] The in vivo role of 4-1BB and 4-1BBL in T-cell immunity has largely been addressed in 4-1BBL$^{-/-}$ mice in various infectious model systems such as monitoring response to Listeria,[19] LCMV,[20] and influenza virus.[21,22] Overall, 4-1BBL$^{-/-}$ mice were observed to generate decreased CD8 T-cell responses, although some variations in the deficiency were seen between models, ranging from moderate to pronounced, with the deficiency tending to manifest late after infection. On the other hand, 4-1BBL$^{-/-}$ mice have been observed to generate normal CD4 T-cell responses to viruses, prompting the suggestion that 4-1BB/4-1BBL preferentially influences CD8 T-cell responses. Arguing against this strict dichotomy are the in vitro results demonstrating costimulation of CD4 cells,[8,9] and adoptive transfer experiments with CD4 T-cells showing

*Corresponding Authors: Michael Croft—Molecular Immunology, La Jolla Institute for Allergy and Immunology, 9420 Athena Circle, La Jolla, California 92037, USA. Email: mick@liai.org

Therapeutic Targets of the TNF Superfamily, edited by Iqbal S. Grewal.
©2009 Landes Bioscience and Springer Science+Business Media.

normal expansion to protein Ag in LPS in 4-1BBL[-/-] mice, but defects in the late primary phase and in secondary responses.[23]

In contrast to these results, other data suggest the biology of 4-1BB is much more complicated than positively regulating the interactions between T-cells and APC. A number of studies that will be described in more detail below have shown apparent negative effects of agonistic antibodies to 4-1BB when administered in vivo, particularly in autoimmune situations and other inflammatory responses where these reagents surprisingly suppressed T-cell responsiveness and inflammation. Furthermore, splenocytes from 4-1BB[-/-] mice displayed hyper-, not hypo-, proliferation to mitogens[17] and adoptive transfer experiments with antigen-specific T-cells that could not express 4-1BB clearly showed enhanced rather than suppressed initial CD4 and CD8 T-cell responses in vivo.[24,25] These results have promoted the idea that in the physiological setting, 4-1BB can play both a negative regulatory role in immunity in addition to its apparent positive role. Here, we will review some of the more recent literature on 4-1BB and discuss the implications of these findings with regard to potential targeting of 4-1BB and 4-1BBL for therapy of immune disease.

Expression of 4-1BB and 4-1BBL

The duration of 4-1BB expression on activated CD4 and CD8 T-cells is variable depending on experimental conditions. It can be seen several hours after T-cell activation and peak within 2 days,[4] but can be long-lasting in some cases and be expressed for as long as a 7 day period following antigen challenge.[25] Exceptions to inducible expression of 4-1BB on T-cell subsets are now recognized, with CD4+CD25+ regulatory T-cells (Treg)[26-28] and natural killer T-cells (NKT), including invariant Vα14 NKT (Lee, S.-W. and Croft, M. unpublished results), showing constitutive expression of 4-1BB without further stimulation. Some T-lymphoma cell lines express 4-1BBL[6] but so far there are no reports of 4-1BBL being expressed on primary T-cells.

Although originally thought to be exclusive to T-cells, recent studies have shown that the expression of 4-1BB in vivo is very promiscuous. Natural killer (NK) cells express 4-1BB whose ligation can induce proliferation and secretion of IFN-γ.[29,30] Some NK-cells express 4-1BB constitutively and others might up-regulate it after stimulation. It is interesting that some myeloid lineage cells, such as DC,[6,31,32] granulocytes[33] and mast cells,[34] also express 4-1BB. DC express both 4-1BB and 4-1BBL upon activation. So far it has been reported that follicular DC,[31] spleen DC,[6,32] and GM-CSF-induced bone marrow (BM) DC[32] express 4-1BB and 4-1BBL. It is not clear why DC express both molecules, possibly at the same time, but the cross-linking of 4-1BB or 4-1BBL on these cells can induce cytokines such as IL-12 and IL-6.[6,31,35] 4-1BB and 4-1BBL can also be expressed on BM-derived mast cells after stimulation through the high-affinity receptor for IgE (FcεRI).[34] Both 4-1BB[-/-] and 4-1BBL[-/-] mast cells have defects in cellular function such as degranulation and cytokine production upon FcεRI stimulation, suggesting that 4-1BB/4-1BBL interactions can costimulate mast cells perhaps analogous to the action on T-cells. Collectively, the expression profiles of 4-1BB and 4-1BBL on various subsets of immune cells raise the interesting notion that both molecules might control innate and adaptive immunity by bridging multiple cell-to-cell interactions.

Therapeutic Effects of Targeting 4-1BB or 4-1BBL

Cancer Immunology

Following the initial observation that the ligation of 4-1BB with agonistic antibody augmented the activity of T-cells, 4-1BB has been thought of as an attractive target for many diseases in which augmentation of the numbers and reactivity of antigen-specific T-cells might be desirable. In particular, the efficacy of targeting 4-1BB has been investigated in many murine tumor models (Table 1). Ligation of 4-1BB by either agonistic antibody treatment in vivo, or by transfecting tumor cells directly with 4-1BBL, can lead to expansion of tumor-reactive T-cells and suppression of tumor growth and in some cases regression of established tumors.[36-38] Moreover, anti-4-1BB has also been found effective for regression of poorly immunogenic tumors, such as C3 and

Table 1. Immunotherapy of tumors in mice through targeting 4-1BB

Method	Tumor Type	Immune Cells Involved	Ref.
Agonist 4-1BB-specific antibody	Sarcoma, mastocytoma	CD8 and CD4	36
Tumor transfected with 4-1BBL	Sarcoma, mastocytoma	CD8	37
Tumor transfected with 4-1BBL	Lymphoma	CD8	38
Agonist 4-1BB-specific antibody	Fibrosarcoma	CD8	62
Agonist 4-1BB-specific antibody	Lung carcinoma,	CD8	39
Tumor transfection with Fv of 4-1BB-specific antibody	melanoma Melanoma	CD4 and NK	41
Agonist 4-1BB-specific antibody with adenovirus expressing IL-12	Colon carcinoma	CD8 and NK	43
Agonist 4-1BB-specific antibody with dendritic cell vaccine	Fibrosarcoma	CD8, NK, CD4	42
Adenovirus expressing Ig-4-1BBL	Hepatic colon carcinoma	CD8	44

melanoma, when given in combination with peptide immunization.[39] Similarly, anti-4-1BB was also shown to be capable of breaking tolerance of CD4 T-cells in more experimental settings and reversing poor T-cell responsiveness that is characteristic of growing old.[40] These results suggest that the strong costimulatory signal imparted by agonistic antibody can transform the immune status of T-cells from being inert (i.e., where ignorance and tolerance are operative) into being active. The majority of tumor studies have shown that antigen-specific CD8 cells are crucial for tumor immunotherapy mediated by anti-4-1BB, with the assumption that the T-cell is the direct recipient of 4-1BB signals. However, roles for CD4 and NK-cells in these processes have been highlighted,[41-43] implying multiple targets of action. Furthermore, another approach was recently developed for systemic delivery of 4-1BBL through recombinant adenovirus, which could be easily translated into immunotherapy of human cancer with human 4-1BBL.[44]

Viral Immunology

Based partially on results showing that 4-1BBL[-/-] mice generate reduced CD8 T-cell responses against certain viruses, 4-1BB stimulation has also been exploited for boosting anti-viral immunity. 4-1BB agonistic antibody was shown to enhance the numbers and reactivity of viral antigen-specific CD8 cells following intranasal infection with influenza and interestingly, it was shown to result in strongly enhanced CD8 cell responses to subdominant peptide epitopes of influenza that might also be useful for protection.[45] More recently, several groups have additionally used anti-4-1BB to boost immune responses following vaccination. Codelivery of an agonistic antibody with DNA[46] or recombinant adenovirus[47] vaccination strategies augmented T-cell immunity to human immunodeficiency virus (HIV) and hepatitis C virus (HCV) proteins, respectively. Another protocol used a recombinant poxvirus encoding 4-1BBL and viral antigen to enhance anti-viral immunity.[48] Although more studies are needed to evaluate 4-1BB as a realistic target for augmenting the efficacy of anti-viral vaccination, these studies do suggest that 4-1BB may be a promising candidate as an adjuvant for developing vaccines against human viruses.

Autoimmunity

Another avenue of immunotherapy that has recently emerged as a potential application of targeting 4-1BB is in autoimmune disease. The most logical route to therapy of these diseases, based on the idea that 4-1BB binding to 4-1BBL augments T-cell and APC activity, would be to suppress these interactions using blocking reagents to 4-1BBL. This has been examined in some animal models but with largely unimpressive results. Treatment with anti-4-1BBL blocking antibody reduced the development of collagen-induced arthritis (CIA) only moderately with no evident suppressive action against established CIA.[49] Furthermore, anti-4-1BBL could not inhibit the induction of experimental allergic conjunctivitis (EAC).[50]

In contrast to these results, it was very surprising when the group of Fu and colleagues found that the same agonistic 4-1BB antibody used to promote anti-tumor immunity also resulted in ameliorating both the incidence and severity of experimental autoimmune encephalomyelitis (EAE), a mouse model of multiple sclerosis (MS). Interestingly, anti-4-1BB also inhibited the relapse that occurs in EAE that is characteristic of the human disease.[51] Since this result was published, many other studies have followed and also injected anti-4-1BB into various autoimmune disease models with the majority of data demonstrating strong inhibition of the development and progression of these diseases (Table 2).

Agonistic 4-1BB antibody successfully ameliorated acute and established lupus-like symptoms in MRL/lpr[52] and NZB × NZW F1[53] mouse strains that develop spontaneous disease resembling human systemic lupus erythematosus (SLE). In both animal strains, 4-1BB targeting reduced autoantibody production and renal disease, which suggests that anti-4-1BB ultimately inhibited pathogenic B-cell responses. In MRL/lpr mice, anti-4-1BB depleted B-cells in the periphery through an unclear mechanism involving apoptosis and IFN-γ.[52] In contrast, B-cell loss was not seen in the NZB × NZW F1 strain, however, germinal center (GC) formation, which is central to the development of functional class-switched B-cells, was abolished.[53] Correlating with these studies, a recent report also showed that anti-4-1BB inhibited GC formation apparently by diminishing FDC networks in B-cell follicles.[54]

Agonistic 4-1BB antibody also inhibited the development of CIA in DBA/1 mice which is a common animal model reminiscent of human rheumatoid arthritis.[49] Similar to the EAE study, anti-4-1BB suppressed antigen (collagen)-specific CD4 T-cell responses. In this case, it was proposed that IFN-γ secretion was also involved in the suppressive activity along with indoleamine-2,3-dioxygenase (IDO), an enzyme that regulates tryptophan metabolism.[55] The source of these molecules was not clear but anti-4-1BB treatment resulted in expansion of a novel population of cells expressing CD8 and CD11c that were proposed to directly or indirectly mediate the suppression.[49] More recently, anti-4-1BB immunotherapy was also applied to Type-I diabetes that arises spontaneously in non-obese diabetic (NOD) mice. 4-1BB is a candidate gene thought to be involved in autoimmune diabetes and was mapped in the Idd (insulin dependent diabetes) loci known to be associated with susceptibility to this disease.[56] Similar to the other autoimmune studies, anti-4-1BB treatment in NOD mice strongly prevented diabetes.[28] Although the mechanism of action was again not clear, of note antibody treatment significantly increased the numbers of CD4+CD25+FOXP-3+ regulatory T-cells (Treg), which may aid in dampening the action of pathogenic T-cells.

Inflammation and Transplantation

Anti-4-1BB treatment has also been used in other disease scenarios in mice, such as in models of allergic asthma[57,58] and chronic graft-versus-host disease (cGVHD).[59] Quite remarkably, this antibody was again shown to prevent the development of the symptoms associated with these immune reactions and also reversed established disease. Anti-4-1BB in these cases was described to down-regulate the activity of CD4 T-cells, although suggested mechanisms of action varied between the reports. In the asthma model, CD4 T-cells from 4-1BB antibody-treated mice did not proliferate when restimulated with antigen in vitro, but did proliferate to IL-2, leading to the suggestion that targeting 4-1BB induced an anergic state in CD4 T-cells.[57] In contrast, in the cGVHD model, it was suggested that the antibody accelerated activation-induced cell death (AICD) of donor CD4 T-cells, whose expansion and survival was critical for inducing disease.[59] Furthermore, the therapeutic effect of anti-4-1BB in the asthma model was partly dependent on CD8 T-cells and IFN-γ but in the cGVHD model CD8 cells and IFN-γ had no apparent roles.

Thus, although a common theme has been that anti-4-1BB suppresses immune disease, the mechanism by which it has done so has not been clear in many cases and might have involved both similar and dissimilar processes depending on the target disease.

Table 2. Amelioration of autoimmune disease in mice through agonistic 4-1BB antibody therapy

Disease Model	Effect on B Cell Number	Effect on Ig Response	Effect on T-Cell Response*	Effect of IFN-γ Neutralization**	Reference
Lupus in NZB x NZW F1	↔	↓↓ (IgG)	ND	ND	53
Inflammatory bowl disease in Balb/c	ND	ND	CD4 ↓, CD8 ↑ CD4+CD25+Treg ↑	ND	61
Lupus in MRL/lpr	↓↓↓	↓↓ (IgG)	CD4 ↓↓, CD8 ↑	Blocking of pathogenic B-cell depletion	52
Experimental allergic conjunctivitis in Balb/c	↑	↓↓ (IgE)	CD4# ↑, CD8 ↑↑	No effect#	50
Rheumatoid arthritis in DBA	ND	↓↓ (IgG)	CD4# ↓↓↓, CD8 ↑↑	Reversed antibody effect	49
Hg-autoimmunity in A.SW	↓↓↓	↓↓↓ (IgE, IgG)	CD4 ↑↑, CD8 ↑↑	Partial blocking of B-cell loss	63
Experimental autoimmune encephalomyelitis in C57BL/6	ND	ND	CD4# ↓↓↓	ND	51
Autoimmune diabetes in NOD	ND	ND	CD4+CD25+ Treg ↑	ND	28

*Represents effect on total T-cells in spleen except #indicating antigen-specific recall responses.
**IFN-γ was neutralized by anti-IFN-γ treatment except ##indicating IFN-γ−/− mice.
ND, not done.
Note, in all cases, disease symptoms and pathology were strongly suppressed by anti-4-1BB.

Possible Mechanisms of Action of 4-1BB Agonistic Antibodies

A challenging feature of agonistic 4-1BB antibody-mediated therapy, particularly if this type of reagent is to be considered for the clinic, is how it modulates immune responses in completely contrasting disease situations. The same agonistic antibody operates positively to augment immunity against tumors and infectious pathogens, while it functions negatively to suppress immunity and reduce pathology in autoimmune diseases and inflammatory situations. One of the reasons might be the promiscuous expression of 4-1BB on many kinds of immune cells that have specific and perhaps opposing roles in various patho-physiological circumstances. As discussed earlier 4-1BB is expressed on T-cells including Treg and NKT, as well as NK-cells, DC, granulocytes and mast cells, leading to one hypothesis that the cellular target of anti-4-1BB dictates whether its action becomes stimulatory or suppressive. Whether this is truly a factor is not clear, as the expression of 4-1BB in most disease situations has not been characterized.

A positive role of anti-4-1BB in vivo is perhaps straightforward in that the antibody most likely directly stimulates T-cells, NK-cells, or mast cells, leading to augmented activities of these cell types that could participate in anti-tumor or anti-viral activity (Fig. 1). The majority of in vitro data clearly support this especially in T-cells, showing biochemical changes in pro-inflammatory intracellular signaling pathways after 4-1BB stimulation.[3,4] On the other hand, a regulatory role, or resultant suppressive activity, of anti-4-1BB is likely quite complicated. For example, it has been suggested that the negative effects of administering anti-4-1BB could be due to promoting apoptosis of CD4 cells[59] or inducing a state of unresponsiveness or anergy in CD4 cells.[57] Alternatively, 4-1BB antibody treatment has been proposed to directly induce regulatory cells in the CD8 lineage. In one study, such regulatory CD8 cells were suggested to suppress other T-cells through TGF-β in an IFN-γ dependent manner.[60] Whereas in another study, a population of CD8 cells expressing CD11c were found to expand after targeting 4-1BB. Through secretion of IFN-γ these CD8 cells directly or indirectly were reported to regulate IDO production, a powerful suppressor of T-cell proliferation, from macrophages and/or DC.[49] Interestingly in these settings, it can still be argued that the action of anti-4-1BB was again positive and stimulatory, even though the ultimate outcome was negative and suppressive for the immune response. In terms of augmenting CD8

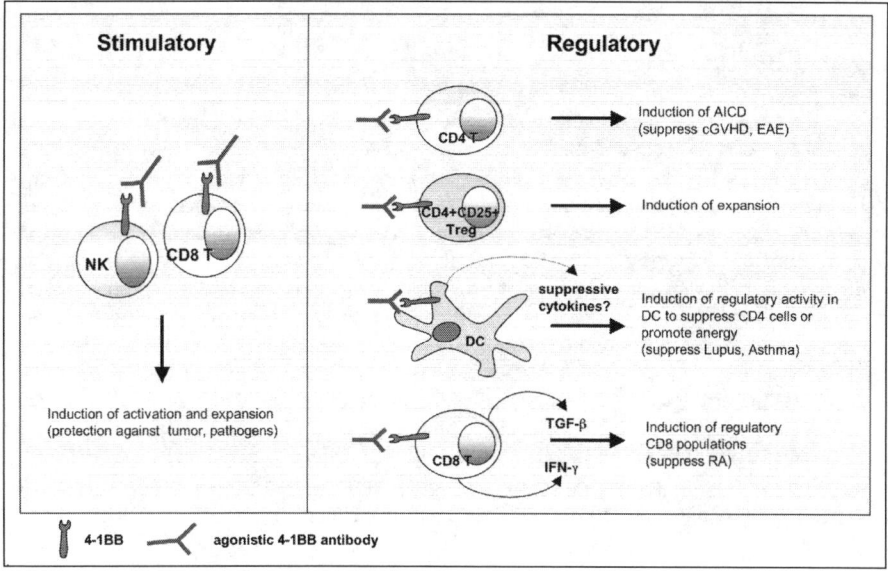

Figure 1. Possible mechanisms underlying the dual function of anti-41BB in augmenting or suppressing immunity.

activity associated with anti-tumor immunity or anti-viral responses, as opposed to augmenting CD8 regulatory activity, the issue then becomes whether the CD8 cells in each individual situation were really different. The CD8 populations that were characterized to be regulatory appeared to represent alternate subsets of cells, since one population expressed CD11c and did not produce TGF-β, whereas the other did not express CD11c but did produce TGF-β. Despite these apparent differences, both populations exerted suppressive activity that was dependent on IFN-γ, a feature that was shared with CD8 cells elicited by anti-4-1BB that protected against tumor growth and viral replication. Further studies will be required to understand whether 4-1BB signaling can differentially induce alternate subsets of T-cells and if so what will dictate whether they become regulatory or nonregulatory.

Possibly related to the latter point, but relevant to potential effects on CD4 cells as opposed to CD8 cells, is the finding that 4-1BB is also constitutively expressed on CD4+CD25+Treg cells. In one report, agonistic 4-1BB antibody had no effect on expansion of these Treg cells but it did neutralize their suppressive function.[27] In contrast, 4-1BB ligation by 4-1BBL was shown to expand Treg cell numbers in vitro and in vivo without a loss in their suppressive activity.[26] Furthermore, anti-4-1BB enhanced the number of CD4+CD25+ Treg in NOD mice[28] and in mice undergoing colitis,[61] situations in which the antibody suppressed these diseases. These data then also raise the possibility that 4-1BB stimulation may preferentially modulate the number and/or function of several types of Treg and the nature of these regulatory populations could vary in specific disease situations.

Another possible target of anti-4-1BB was highlighted in the lupus studies with NZB × NZW F1 mice. Here, anti-4-1BB mediated suppression of disease was abolished after adoptive transfer of autoantigen-primed CD4 T-cells or bone marrow derived DC.[53] This suggested that the regulatory function of the agonistic antibody might have been transmitted in this case through DC. It is certainly plausible that 4-1BB antibodies target DC directly as many activated DC can express 4-1BB and DC are known to be capable of both stimulatory or suppressive activity, e.g., through production of pro-inflammatory cytokines such as IL-6 and IL-12, or secreting inhibitory cytokines such as IL-10 and TGF-β. As before, more studies are needed to test the hypothesis that signals to DC from 4-1BB can impact immune disease and explain some of the dramatic effects of anti-4-1BB therapy.

Concluding Remarks

Based on very promising results from many different disease models, 4-1BB agonistic antibody immunotherapy is indeed a candidate for clinical modulation of human diseases. One important issue will be potential side effects. For example, anti-4-1BB treatment dramatically reduces pathogenic T- and B-cell responses in many autoimmune disease situations (Table 2), however, it seems to globally influence nonpathogenic immune responses. The repeated injection of anti-4-1BB in naïve mice leads to development of severe immunological anomalies, including splenomegaly, lymphadenopathy, hepatomegaly, multi-focal hepatitis and anemia.[64] These adverse effects are again apparently dependent on activation of CD8 T-cells and involve production of several cytokines such as IFN-γ, TNF and Type I IFN. More studies will then be needed to determine any unwanted immunopathological consequences of administering anti-4-1BB in disease models, as well as to understand any dosage effects of the antibody in terms of pro- or anti-inflammatory activities. It does not need to be stressed that testing in preclinical animal models of disease and in nonhuman primates is essential before contemplating human clinical trials. Recent approaches with systemic delivery of soluble 4-1BBL by recombinant viruses is an alternative to the use of anti-4-1BB, although at present there is no information on whether 4-1BBL will replicate the therapeutic activity of the antibody or lead to similar side effects.

References

1. Kwon BS, Weissman SM. cDNA sequences of two inducible T-cell genes. Proc Natl Acad Sci USA 1989; 86:1963.
2. Schwarz H, Blanco FJ, von Kempis J et al. ILA, a member of the human nerve growth factor/tumor necrosis factor receptor family, regulates T-lymphocyte proliferation and survival. Blood 1996; 87:2839-2845.
3. Watts TH. TNF/TNFR family members in costimulation of T-cell responses. Annu Rev Immunol 2005; 23:23.
4. Croft M. Costimulatory members of the TNFR family: keys to effective T-cell immunity? Nat Rev Immunol 2003; 3:609.
5. Goodwin RG, Din WS, Davis-Smith T et al. Molecular cloning of a ligand for the inducible T-cell gene 4-1BB: a member of an emerging family of cytokines with homology to tumor necrosis factor. Eur J Immunol 1993; 23:2631.
6. Futagawa T, Akiba H, Kodama T et al. Expression and function of 4-1BB and 4-1BB ligand on murine dendritic cells. Int Immunol 2002; 14:275.
7. Schwarz H. Biological activities of reverse signal transduction through CD137 ligand. J Leukoc Biol 2004; 77:281.
8. Gramaglia I, Cooper D, Miner KT et al. Costimulation of antigen-specific CD4 T-cells by 4-1BB ligand. Eur J Immunol 2000; 30:392.
9. Cannons JL, Lau P, Ghumman B et al. 4-1BB ligand induces cell division, sustains survival and enhances effector function of CD4 and CD8 T-cells with similar efficacy. J Immunol 2001; 167:1313.
10. Shuford WW, Klussman K, Tritchler DD et al. 4-1BB costimulatory signals preferentially induce CD8+ T-cell proliferation and lead to the amplification in vivo of cytotoxic T-cell responses. J Exp Med 1997; 186:47.
11. Bukczynski J, Wen T, Wang C et al. Enhancement of HIV-specific CD8 T-cell responses by dual co-stimulation with CD80 and CD137L. J Immunol 2005; 175:6378.
12. Arch RH, Thompson CB. 4-1BB and Ox40 are members of a tumor necrosis factor (TNF)-nerve growth factor receptor subfamily that bind TNF receptor-associated factors and activate nuclear factor kappaB. Mol Cell Biol 1998; 18:558.
13. Jang IK, Lee ZH, Kim YJ et al. Human 4-1BB (CD137) signals are mediated by TRAF2 and activate nuclear factor-kappa B. Biochem Biophys Res Commun 1998; 242:613.
14. Ma BY, Mikolajczak SA, Danesh A et al. The expression and the regulatory role of OX40 and 4-1BB heterodimer in activated human T-cells. Blood 2005; 106:2002.
15. Starck L, Scholz C, Dorken B et al. Costimulation by CD137/4-1BB inhibits T-cell apoptosis and induces Bcl-xL and c-FLIP(short) via phosphatidylinositol 3-kinase and AKT/protein kinase B. Eur J Immunol 2005; 35:1257.
16. Lee HW, Park SJ, Choi BK et al. 4-1BB promotes the survival of CD8+ T-lymphocytes by increasing expression of Bcl-xL and Bfl-1. J Immunol 2002; 169:4882.
17. Kwon BS, Hurtado JC, Lee ZH et al. Immune responses in 4-1BB (CD137)-deficient mice. J Immunol 2002; 168:5483.
18. DeBenedette MA, Wen T, Bachmann MF et al. Analysis of 4-1BB ligand (4-1BBL)-deficient mice and of mice lacking both 4-1BBL and CD28 reveals a role for 4-1BBL in skin allograft rejection and in the cytotoxic T-cell response to influenza virus. J Immunol 1999; 163:4833.
19. Shedlock DJ, Whitmire JK, Tan J et al. Role of CD4 T-cell help and costimulation in CD8 T-cell responses during Listeria monocytogenes infection. J Immunol 2003; 170:2053.
20. Tan JT, Whitmire JK, Ahmed R et al. 4-1BB ligand, a member of the TNF family, is important for the generation of antiviral CD8 T-cell responses. J Immunol 1999; 163:4859.
21. Bertram EM, Lau P, Watts TH. Temporal segregation of 4-1BB versus CD28-mediated costimulation: 4-1BB ligand influences T-cell numbers late in the primary response and regulates the size of the T-cell memory response following influenza infection. J Immunol 2002; 168:3777.
22. Bertram EM, Dawicki W, Sedgmen B et al. A switch in costimulation from CD28 to 4-1BB during primary versus secondary CD8 T-cell response to influenza in vivo. J Immunol 2004; 172:981.
23. Dawicki W, Bertram EM, Sharpe AH et al. 4-1BB and OX40 act independently to facilitate robust CD8 and CD4 recall responses. J Immunol 2004; 173:5944.
24. Lee SW, Vella AT, Kwon BS et al. Enhanced CD4 T-cell responsiveness in the absence of 4-1BB. J Immunol 2005; 174:6803.
25. Lee SW, Park Y, Song A et al. Functional dichotomy between OX40 and 4-1BB in modulating effector CD8 T-cell responses. J Immunol 2006; 177:4464.
26. Zheng G, Wang B, Chen A. The 4-1BB costimulation augments the proliferation of CD4+CD25+ regulatory T-cells. J Immunol 2004; 173:2428.

27. Choi BK, Bae JS, Choi EM et al. 4-1BB-dependent inhibition of immunosuppression by activated CD4+CD25+ T-cells. J Leukoc Biol 2004; 75:785.
28. Irie J, Wu Y, Kachapati K et al. Modulating protective and pathogenic CD4+ subsets via CD137 in type 1 diabetes. Diabetes 2007; 56:186.
29. Melero I, Johnston JV, Shufford WW et al. NK1.1 cells express 4-1BB (CDw137) costimulatory molecule and are required for tumor immunity elicited by anti-4-1BB monoclonal antibodies. Cell Immunol 1998; 190:167.
30. Wilcox RA, Tamada K, Strome SE et al. Signaling through NK-cell-associated CD137 promotes both helper function for CD8+ cytolytic T-cells and responsiveness to IL-2 but not cytolytic activity. J Immunol 2002; 169:4230.
31. Lindstedt M, Johansson-Lindbom B, Borrebaeck CA. Expression of CD137 (4-1BB) on human follicular dendritic cells. Scand J Immunol 2003; 57:305.
32. Wilcox RA, Chapoval AI, Gorski KS et al. Cutting edge: Expression of functional CD137 receptor by dendritic cells. J Immunol 2002; 168:4262.
33. Lee SC, Ju SA, Pack HN et al. 4-1BB (CD137) is required for rapid clearance of Listeria monocytogenes infection. Infect Immun 2005; 73:5144.
34. Nishimoto H, Lee SW, Hong H et al. Costimulation of mast cells by 4-1BB, a member of the tumor necrosis factor receptor superfamily, with the high-affinity IgE receptor. Blood 2005; 106:4241.
35. Kim YJ, Li G, Broxmeyer HE. 4-1BB ligand stimulation enhances myeloid dendritic cell maturation from human umbilical cord blood CD34+ progenitor cells. J Hemathother Stem Cell Res 2002; 11:895.
36. Melero I, Shuford WW, Newby SA et al. Monoclonal antibodies against the 4-1BB T-cell activation molecule eradicate established tumors. Nat Med 1997; 3:682.
37. Melero I, Bach N, Hellstrom KE et al. Amplification of tumor immunity by gene transfer of the costimulatory 4-1BB ligand: synergy with the CD28 costimulatory pathway. Eur J Immunol 1998; 28:1116.
38. Guinn BA, DeBenedette MA, Watts TH et al. 4-1BBL cooperates with B7-1 and B7-2 in converting a B-cell lymphoma cell line into a long-lasting antitumor vaccine. J Immunol 1999; 162:5003.
39. Wilcox RA, Flies DB, Zhu G et al. Provision of antigen and CD137 signaling breaks immunological ignorance, promoting regression of poorly immunogenic tumors. J Clin Invest 2002; 109:651.
40. Bansal-Pakala P, Croft M. Defective T-cell priming associated with aging can be rescued by signaling through 4-1BB (CD137). J Immunol 2002; 169:5005.
41. Ye Z, Hellstrom I, Hayden-Ledbetter M et al. Gene therapy for cancer using single-chain Fv fragments specific for 4-1BB. Nat Med 2002; 8:343.
42. Ito F, Li Q, Shreiner AB et al. Anti-CD137 monoclonal antibody administration augments the antitumor efficacy of dendritic cell-based vaccines. Cancer Res 2004; 64:8411.
43. Pan PY, Gu P, Li Q et al. Regulation of dendritic cell function by NK-cells: mechanisms underlying the synergism in the combination therapy of IL-12 and 4-1BB activation. J Immunol 2004; 172:4779.
44. Xu DP, Sauter BV, Huang TG et al. The systemic administration of Ig-4-1BB ligand in combination with IL-12 gene transfer eradicates hepatic colon carcinoma. Gene Ther 2005; 12:1526.
45. Halstead ES, Mueller YM, Altman JD et al. In vivo stimulation of CD137 broadens primary antiviral CD8+ T-cell responses. Nat Immunol 2002; 3:536.
46. Munks MW, Mourich DV, Mittler RS et al. 4-1BB and OX40 stimulation enhance CD8 and CD4 T-cell responses to a DNA prime, poxvirus boost vaccine. Immunology 2004; 112:559.
47. Arribillaga L, Sarobe P, Arina A et al. Enhancement of CD4 and CD8 immunity by anti-CD137 (4-1BB) monoclonal antibodies during hepatitis C vaccination with recombinant adenovirus. Vaccine 2005; 23:3493.
48. Harrison JM, Bertram EM, Boyle DB et al. 4-1BBL coexpression enhances HIV-specific CD8 T-cell memory in a poxvirus prime-boost vaccine. Vaccine 2006; 24:6867.
49. Seo SK, Choi JH, Kim YH et al. 4-1BB-mediated immunotherapy of rheumatoid arthritis. Nat Med 2004; 10:1088.
50. Fukushima A, Yamaguchi T, Ishida W et al. Engagement of 4-1BB inhibits the development of experimental allergic conjunctivitis in mice. J Immunol 2005; 175:4897.
51. Sun Y, Lin X, Chen HM et al. Administration of agonistic anti-4-1BB monoclonal antibody leads to the amelioration of experimental autoimmune encephalomyelitis. J Immunol 2002; 68:1457.
52. Sun Y, Chen HM, Subudhi SK et al. Costimulatory molecule-targeted antibody therapy of a spontaneous autoimmune disease. Nat Med 2002; 8:1405.
53. Foell J, Strahotin S, O'Neil SP et al. CD137 costimulatory T-cell receptor engagement reverses acute disease in lupus-prone NZB × NZW F1 mice. J Clin Invest 2003; 111:1505.
54. Sun Y, Blink SE, Chen JH et al. Regulation of follicular dendritic cell networks by activated T-cells: the role of CD137 signaling. J Immunol 2005; 175:884.
55. Mellor AL, Munn DH. IDO expression by dendritic cells:tolerance and tryptophan catabolism. Nat Rev Immunol 2004; 4:762.

56. Cannons JL, Chamberlain G, Howson J et al. Genetic and functional association of the immune signaling molecule 4-1BB (CD137/TNFRSF9) with type 1 diabetes. J Autoimmun 2005; 25:13.
57. Polte T, Foell J, Werner C et al. CD137-mediated immunotherapy for allergic asthma. J Clin Invest 2006; 116:1025.
58. Sun Y, Blink SE, Liu W et al. Inhibition of Th2-mediated allergic airway inflammatory disease by CD137 costimulation. J Immunol 2006; 177:814.
59. Kim J, Choi WS, La S et al. Stimulation with 4-1BB (CD137) inhibits chronic graft-versus-host disease by inducing activation-induced cell death of donor CD4+ T-cells. Blood 2005; 105:2206.
60. Myers L, Croft M, Kwon BS et al. Peptide-specific CD8 T regulatory cells use IFN-β to elaborate TGF-γ-based suppression. J Immunol 2005; 174:7625.
61. Lee J, Lee EN, Kim EY et al. Administration of agonistic anti-4-1BB monoclonal antibody leads to the amelioration of inflammatory bowel disease. Immunol Lett 2005; 101:210.
62. Miller RE, Jones J, Le T et al. 4-1BB-specific monoclonal antibody promotes the generation of tumor-specific immune responses by direct activation of CD8 T-cells in a CD40-dependent manner. J Immunol 2002; 169:1792.
63. Vinay DS, Kim JD, Kwon BS. Amelioration of mercury-induced autoimmunity by 4-1BB. J Immunol 2006; 177:5708.
64. Niu L, Strahotin S, Hewes B et al. Cytokine-mediated disruption of lymphocyte trafficking, hemopoiesis, and induction of lymphopenia, anemia, and thrombocytopenia in anti-CD137-treated mice. J Immunol 2007; 178:4194.

CHAPTER 9

RANK(L) as a Key Target for Controlling Bone Loss

Andreas Leibbrandt and Josef M. Penninger*

Abstract

Bone-related diseases, such as osteoporosis or rheumatoid arthritis, affect hundreds of millions of people worldwide and pose a tremendous burden to health care. By deepening our understanding of the molecular mechanisms of bone metabolism and bone turnover, it became possible over the past years to devise new and promising strategies for treating such diseases. In particular, three molecules, the receptor activator of NF-κB (RANK), its ligand RANKL and the decoy receptor of RANKL, osteoprotegerin (OPG), attracted the attention of scientists and pharmaceutical companies alike. Genetic experiments evolving around these molecules established their pivotal role as central regulators of osteoclast function. RANK-RANKL signaling not only activates a variety of downstream signaling pathways required for osteoclast development, but crosstalk with other signaling pathways also fine-tunes bone homeostasis both in normal physiology and disease. Consequently, novel drugs specifically targeting RANK-RANKL and their signaling pathways in osteoclasts are expected to revolutionize the treatment of various ailments associated with bone loss, such as arthritis, cancer metastases, or osteoporosis.

Overview

During life, bone is constantly being remodeled, involving the resorption of bone by osteoclasts and the synthesis of bone matrix by osteoblasts. Disturbing this intricate balance between resorption and synthesis of bone ultimately leads to the development of skeletal abnormalities, such as osteoporosis and osteopetrosis.[1-4] Osteoporosis is a disease characterized by a decline in bone mineral density and structural deterioration of bone tissue, leading to bone fragility and an increased susceptibility to fractures especially of the hip, spine and wrist. In the US, 10 million people are estimated to already have osteoporosis, while 34 million are predicted to be osteopenic, increasing their risk for osteoporosis. Osteoporosis becomes manifest predominantly in older people aged 50 and over, in particular women (80% of those affected by osteoporosis) and accounts for more than 1.5 million fractures annually. By contrast, osteopetrosis is a heterogeneous group of rare heritable conditions, primarily based on a defect in bone resorption by osteoclasts and is associated with an increased skeletal mass due to abnormally dense bones.[5]

The landmark discoveries of three essential factors for the control of osteoclast function and hence osteoporosis and other bone diseases, respectively, has moved bone research into a new era. These factors are the receptor activator of NF-κB (RANK),[6] its ligand RANKL,[6-9] and the decoy receptor for RANKL, osteoprotegerin (OPG).[10-12] Importantly, although various calciotropic hormones and cytokines, such as PTHrP, Vitamin D3, IL-1β, or TNF-α, have all been shown

*Corresponding Author: Josef M. Penninger—IMBA, Institute of Molecular Biotechnology of the Austrian Academy of Sciences, Dr. Bohr-Gasse 3, A-1030 Vienna, Austria.
Email: Josef.Penninger@imba.oeaw.ac.at

Therapeutic Targets of the TNF Superfamily, edited by Iqbal S. Grewal.
©2009 Landes Bioscience and Springer Science+Business Media.

to affect osteoclastogenesis at distinct stages of development,[2] only RANK(L) has proven to be absolutely required for osteoclast development in vivo as evidenced by the complete absence of osteoclasts in RANKL and RANK knockout mice, respectively.[13-15]

While binding of RANKL to its receptor RANK is crucial for osteoclast development from haematopoietic progenitor cells and activation of mature osteoclasts, binding of OPG to RANKL prevents binding to RANK and signaling and therefore inhibits bone turnover by osteoclasts. Since patients with diseases such as osteoporosis, metastases, or rheumatoid arthritis all show an increased activity of osteoclasts, it seems as if the RANKL-RANK-OPG axis is the most relevant therapeutic target for osteoclast-regulated bone diseases. Here we discuss the importance of the RANKL-RANK-OPG axis in bone metabolism and how this knowledge is translated into novel therapeutic approaches to treat diseases of the bone, such as arthritis, osteoporosis and bone metastases.

Basic Characteristics of the RANKL-RANK-OPG Axis

RANKL

RANKL (also known as osteoprotegerin ligand OPGL, osteoclast differentiation factor ODF, TNFSF11, TRANCE, CD254) was independently cloned by four groups.[6-9] Human RANKL is a member of the tumor necrosis factor (ligand) superfamily (for an overview of the TNF super-family, see http://www.gene.ucl.ac.uk/nomenclature/genefamily/tnfsf.php) and encodes a type II transmembrane glycoprotein of 317 amino acids. RANKL exists in two biologically active forms, a cellular, membrane-bound form (40-45 kDa) and a soluble form (31 kDa) derived from alternative splicing or proteolytical cleavage either by ADAM metallopeptidase domain family members or matrix metalloproteases (MMPs).[16-20] In its active form, RANKL assembles into homotrimers as evidenced by the crystal structure of the extracellular domain of murine RANKL.[21,22] RANKL is most highly expressed in skeletal and lymphoid tissues that are active in mediating the immune response, but RANKL expression can also be detected in heart, skeletal muscle, lung, stomach, placenta, thyroid gland and brain.[2,4,23]

RANK

The receptor for RANKL is RANK (receptor activator of NF-κB, also known as TNFRSF11A, OFE, ODFR, TRANCE-R, ODAR, CD265), a member of the TNF receptor superfamily (see http://www.gene.ucl.ac.uk/nomenclature/genefamily/tnfrsf.php). Human RANK cDNA encodes a type I transmembrane glycoprotein of 616 amino acids with a 29 amino acid signal peptide, an extracellular domain of 183 amino acids, a transmembrane domain of 21 amino acids and a large cytoplasmic domain of 383 amino acids. In the style of TNF receptors Fas, TNFR1, or TNFR2, it is believed that RANK preassembles into trimeric complexes on the cell surface prior to ligand binding, a prerequisite for RANKL binding and signal transmission.[24-27] RANK is ubiquitously expressed, with highest levels in skeletal muscle, thymus, liver, colon, small intestine and adrenal gland.[4,6]

OPG

OPG (also called TNFRSF11B, osteoprotegerin, OCIF, TR1, or FDRC1) is a member of the TNFR superfamily and binds to RANKL. Human OPG is synthesized as a 401 amino acid precursor protein, of which a 21 amino acid signal peptide is cleaved off to give rise to the mature peptide. Unlike other TNFR family members, OPG lacks a hydrophobic transmembrane-spanning domain and is thus secreted as a soluble protein. OPG is synthesized as a monomer (55-62 kDa) and is finally secreted as a homodimeric glycoprotein of ~110 kDa. OPG is expressed at highest levels in the lung, heart, kidney and placenta.[10-12, 28,29]

Bone Remodeling and the RANKL-RANK-OPG Axis

The first molecule identified in the RANK-RANKL-OPG axis was OPG, which was initially cloned as a potential inhibitor of osteoclastogenesis.[11,12] In line with this, transgenic mice bearing high levels of OPG in their circulation or mice treated with recombinant OPG both exhibited a marked increase in bone density and osteopetrosis, respectively.[12] Conversely, ablation of OPG in mice by targeted deletion resulted in early-onset osteoporosis.[30,31] Taken together, these landmark studies demonstrated for the first time a critical requirement for endogenous OPG in the normal development of skeletal architecture and maintenance of postnatal bone mass, respectively. Moreover, those studies implied that OPG might neutralize a TNF-related factor that would stimulate osteoclast development, thus inhibiting osteoclast maturation.

That factor was soon to be found in RANKL by expression cloning and met the expectations: RANKL specifically bound to OPG, enhanced differentiation of bone marrow cells into osteoclasts in an in vitro osteoclast coculture system which could be blocked by OPG and could activate mature osteoclasts to resorb bone both in vitro and in vivo.[8,9] Thus, RANKL plays a pivotal role in regulating osteoclast function and, indirectly, bone mass. The definite proof of the essential function of RANKL in osteoclastogenesis was delivered shortly thereafter by the generation of *Rankl*-deficient mice. In a breakthrough study, it was shown that mice with a targeted deletion of RANKL show severe osteopetrosis and defective tooth eruption resulting from a complete lack of osteoclasts.[14] These findings were complemented by showing that the receptor for RANKL, RANK, which was known from previous studies albeit in a cellular context initially not related to osteoclastogenesis (see below),[6,7] is essential for osteoclast differentiation and activation induced by RANKL.[32,33] Most importantly, *Rank* knockout mice are exact phenocopies of *Rankl*[-/-] mice, i.e., they are osteopetrotic, have a defect in tooth eruption and lack osteoclasts.[13,15] Taken together, these findings unambiguously established the pivotal role of RANKL-RANK interactions in positively regulating osteoclastogenesis, counteracted and balanced by OPG which functions as a decoy receptor for RANKL (Fig. 1).

Intriguingly, essentially all factors that inhibit or enhance bone resorption by osteoclasts also positively or negatively influence RANKL and OPG mRNA/protein levels (summarized in Table 1). Since genetic ablation experiments of those factors have shown that these factors are not essential for osteoclast development in vivo,[2] the surprising conclusion has to be drawn that the complex process of osteoclast-mediated bone remodeling converges at the RANKL-RANK-OPG axis.

Mutations in RANK and OPG have also been found in patients with bone disorders. Familial expansile osteolysis (FEO, OMIM #174810) and Paget disease of the bone (PDB, OMIM #602080) are rare autosomal dominant bone dysplasia characterized by focal areas of increased bone remodeling, but distinguished clinically by the distribution of osteolytic lesions (focal skeletal lesions mainly affect the appendicular skeleton in FEO and the axial skeleton in PDB, respectively). In four families with FEO and PDB, two heterozygous insertion mutations—a 18 base pair and a 27 base pair tandem duplication—in exon 1 of RANK have been identified. Both insertion mutations affect the signal peptide region of RANK and result in reduced expression levels and increased RANK-mediated NF-κB signaling in vitro.[34] An insertion of 15 base pairs in exon 1 of RANK—remarkably similar to the FEO mutation—was also identified as the cause of expansile skeletal hyperphosphatasia (ESH), a familial metabolic bone disease characterized by expanding hyperostotic long bones, early onset deafness, premature tooth loss and episodic hypercalcemia.[35,36] In contrast, Juvenile Paget disease (JPD, OMIM #239000) is an autosomal recessive osteopathy characterized by rapidly remodeling woven bone, osteopenia, fractures and progressive skeletal deformity which can be ascribed to several mutations in OPG, frequently affecting the ligand binding domain of OPG.[36-38]

Thus, the functions of the RANKL-RANK-OPG axis in bone remodeling, initially unraveled by different mouse models, have direct relevance to human bone diseases and opened the door for the development of new drugs targeting those molecules.

RANK(L) Signaling Pathways

Binding of RANKL to RANK results in the activation of signaling cascades that control lineage commitment and activation of osteoclasts. Here, we only provide an overview of the signaling cascades downstream of RANKL-RANK, but the reader is referred to recent reviews for further details and crosstalks with other signaling pathways, respectively.[4,39]

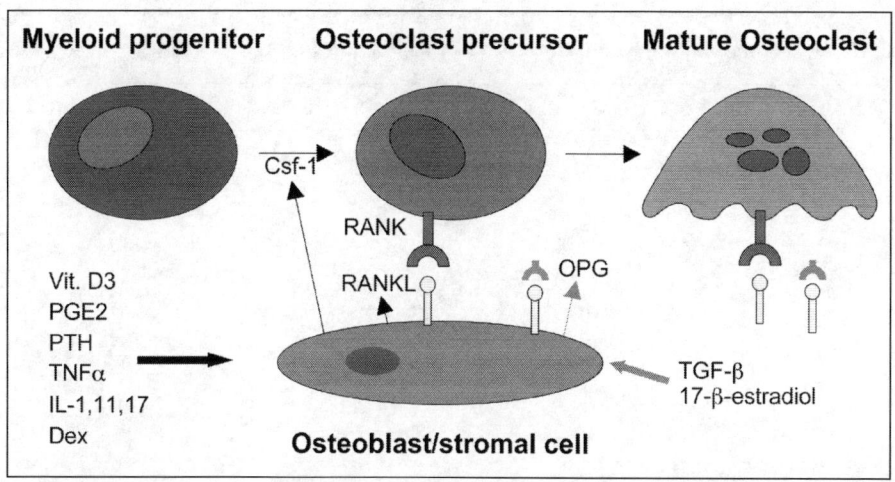

Figure 1. Regulation of osteoclastogenesis in bone tissues. Calciotropic factors such as vitamin D3, prostaglandin E2 (PGE2), cytokines, or dexamethasone (Dex) induce RANKL expression on osteoblasts. RANKL binding to RANK on osteoclastic progenitors results in the activation of signaling cascades leading to maturation and activation of osteoclasts in the presence of Csf-1. Csf-1 is a survival factor for osteoclasts, but is not essential for the commitment to osteoclast lineage, since it can be replaced by Bcl-2 overexpression. RANKL also stimulates bone resorption in mature osteoclasts via RANK. OPG is secreted from osteoblasts and acts as a decoy receptor for RANKL and inhibits osteoclastogenesis by binding to RANKL. TGF-β, which is released from bone during active bone resorption, has been suggested as a feedback mechanism upregulating OPG in osteoblasts. Importantly, estrogen (17-β-estradiol) also enhances OPG expression in osteoblasts and thus provides one explanation for the susceptibility of postmenopausal women to osteoporosis and gender bias in osteoporosis, respectively. Reduced ovarian function leads to reduced estrogen levels and thus fewer osteoblasts are stimulated to produce OPG. Lower OPG levels result in higher levels of active RANKL thereby shifting the intricate balance of bone synthesis and resorption towards the latter and osteoporosis, respectively.

In its 383-amino acid cytoplasmic domain, RANK contains binding sites for TNF receptor-associated factors (TRAFs), adaptor proteins that recruit and activate downstream signaling transducers.[40] RANK interacts with TRAFs 1, 2, 3, 5 and 6 in vitro and in cells. TRAF binding sites were shown to cluster in two distinct domains within the cytoplasmic tail of RANK, a C-terminal region (amino acids 544-616) affecting multiple TRAF binding (TRAFs 1, 2, 3, 5, 6) and a membrane-proximal (amino acids 340-421), which binds TRAF6 exclusively. These TRAF binding domains were shown to be functionally important for NF-κB and c-Jun NH2-terminal kinase (JNK) activities in response to RANK stimulation. When the membrane-proximal TRAF6 interaction domain is deleted, RANK-mediated NF-κB signaling is completely inhibited while residual JNK activation is still possible, suggesting that interactions with TRAFs are necessary for NF-κB activation but not essential for JNK pathway activation.[41-44]

The importance of TRAF6 downstream of RANK(L) has been substantiated in *Traf6* mutant mice that exhibit bone phenotypes similar to *Rankl*[-/-] and *Rank*[-/-] mice due to a partial block in osteoclastogenesis and defective activation of mature osteoclasts.[45-48] However, *Traf6*[-/-] mice still have TRAP[+] osteoclasts,[45] whereas NF-κB1/NF-κB2 double mutant mice lack TRAP[+] osteoclasts.[49,50] Thus, TRAF6 is an important transducer of RANKL-RANK signals through NF-κB for the activation of mature osteoclasts, but other TRAFs (and possibly other molecules) seem to at least partially compensate for *Traf6*-deficiency during osteoclast development.

Table 1. Factors that modulate expression of RANKL and OPG

	RANKL	OPG	References
Hormones			
Vitamin D3	↑	↑	9, 111
PTH	↑	↓	9
Estradiol		↑	112
Cytokines			
TNF-α	↑	↑	111, 113, 114
TNF-β		↑	113
IL-1α		↑	115
IL-1β	↑	↑	111, 114
IL-6*	↑	↑	116
IL-11	↑		9
IL-17	↑		104
CD40L		↑	60
Growth factors			
TGF-β	↓	↑	117
BMP-2		↑	111
LIF	↑	↑	116
IGF-I	↑	↓	118
Glucocorticoids			
Dexamethasone	↑	↓	9, 119, 120
Hydrocortisone		↓	119
Immunosuppressants			
Rapamycin	↑	↓	121
Cyclosporine A	↑	↓	121
FK-506	↑	↓	121
Others			
Prostaglandin E2	↑	↓	9, 122, 123
Calcium	↑	↑	124
LPS		↑	125

*In different studies, IL-6 did not influence OPG and RANKL levels, respectively.[114,115]

RANKL also activates the anti-apoptotic serine/threonine kinase Akt/PKB through a signaling complex involving c-Src and TRAF6.[51] c-Src and TRAF6 interact with each other and with RANK following receptor engagement and a deficiency in c-Src or addition of Src family kinase inhibitors blocks RANKL-mediated Akt/PKB activation in osteoclasts. TRAF6, in turn, enhances the kinase activity of c-Src leading to tyrosine phosphorylation of downstream signaling molecules such as c-Cbl.[51] Moreover, RANK can recruit TRAF6, Cbl family scaffolding proteins and the phospholipid kinase PI3-K in a ligand- and Src-dependent manner. RANKL mediated Akt/PKB activation is defective in *cbl-b*[-/-] dendritic cells.[52] These findings implicate Cbl family proteins as positive as well as negative modulators of TNFR superfamily signaling. Moreover, these data provided the first evidence of a cross-talk between TRAF proteins and Src family kinases. Importantly, the targeted deletion of c-Src results in an osteopetrotic phenotype in mice confirming its positioning in the RANK(L) signaling cascade inferred from biochemical studies in vitro.[53]

Recently, another molecular adapter was found to be important for RANK signaling. Grb2 associated binder 2 (Gab2) associates with RANK and mediates RANK-induced NF-κB, Akt and JNK activation. Genetic inactivation of *Gab2* in mice results in osteopetrosis and decreased bone resorption due to defective osteoclast differentiation.[54] Importantly, the contribution of

Gab2 to osteoclastogenesis is relevant not only to mice but also to humans, since siRNA-mediated inactivation of *Gab2* in human peripheral blood derived progenitor cells likewise prohibited osteoclastogenesis (Fig. 2).[54]

RANK(L) Signaling in the Immune System

Initially, RANKL was identified as a molecule which became strongly upregulated on activated T-cells shortly after stimulation,[7] while the receptor RANK was cloned from a dendritic cell (DC) cDNA library,[6] pointing towards a crucial function of RANKL-RANK signaling in T-cell—DC interactions.

It turned out that RANKL-RANK signaling from stimulated T-cells to DCs can induce cluster formation, DC survival by upregulating the anti-apoptotic molecule Bcl-x$_L$, DC-mediated T-cell proliferation, cytokine production in DCs and CD40 upregulation.[6,55-58] Interestingly, OPG can also be found on the cell surface of DCs and was furthermore shown to bind to the TNF-family molecule TRAIL, which is produced by activated T-cells to induce apoptosis of DCs.[59,60] Thus, it seems as if the balance between RANKL and TRAIL—both produced from activated T-cells—could influence DC survival and OPG might modulate that regulatory loop. However, since the binding affinity of OPG to TRAIL is rather low (~10000 times less binding to TRAIL than to RANKL),[8] it is still unclear whether OPG-TRAIL interactions have any functional relevance in vivo. Although dispensable for T-cells and DC development in vivo, as judged by the analysis of knockout mice,[13,15,61,62] the RANK-RANKL signal from the DC to the T-cell still seems to be critical for the optimum activation of T-cells. Therefore, it is tempting to speculate that controlling DC fate specifically via the RANKL-RANK-OPG axis might be useful to modulate immune responses in vivo and efficacy of DC-based antitumor vaccinations or of treating autoimmune diseases (Fig. 3).

In fact, it was recently shown that RANKL expression in the skin is also important in regulating the number of regulatory T-cells (Tregs). Tregs, in particular CD4$^+$ CD25$^+$ Tregs expressing the transcription factor Foxp3, are a functionally distinct T-cell subpopulation and function by suppressing autoaggressive T-cells. Thereby, Tregs maintain immunological self-tolerance and suppress excessive immune responses to self-antigens, such as in autoimmune diseases or allergies.[63] Despite the importance of DCs in inducing immunity to infections, it has been shown that DCs can also induce expansion of CD4$^+$ CD25$^+$ Tregs and thereby induce T-cell tolerance.[64] Given that activation of epidermal Langerhans cells (LCs; dendritic cells of the skin) by CD40L, a TNF family member closely related to RANKL, can induce severe systemic autoimmunity[65] and the aforementioned importance of RANKL signaling in T-cell-DC interactions, it was tempting to ask if RANK(L) signals might also be important for immune homeostasis in the skin. RANKL expression is evident in keratinocytes of the skin and strongly upregulated following inflammation, e.g., by UV irradiation of the skin. However, in contrast to transgenic overexpression of CD40L, RANKL overexpression in keratinocytes inhibited cutaneous contact hypersensitivity responses and concomitantly resulted in a marked increase of Tregs.[66] The RANKL receptor RANK is expressed in LCs and enhanced signaling between RANKL-overexpressing keratinocytes and RANK-expressing LCs increased their survival and rendered LCs more effective in enhancing Treg proliferation.[66] To this end, RANKL overexpression in keratinocytes could fully rescue the autoimmunity phenotype caused by CD40L overexpression in K14-RANKL/CD40L double transgenic mice.[66] Taken together, these findings provide a rationale for the long known immunosuppressive effect of ultraviolet exposure: UV irradiation upregulates RANKL in keratinocytes which in turn activate LCs through RANKL-RANK interactions. RANKL-activated LCs preferentially trigger expansion of Tregs and thus suppress immune reactions in the skin and other tissues. To genetically test this hypothesis, mice harboring a conditional allele of *Rank* have recently been generated and will be used to ablate RANK specifically in LCs (A. Leibbrandt, J. Penninger, unpublished). These findings also have several clinical implications: local induction of RANKL-RANK in the skin could be used as a new therapeutic approach for allergies as well as for systemic autoimmunity through increasing Tregs while avoiding systemic side effects.[66]

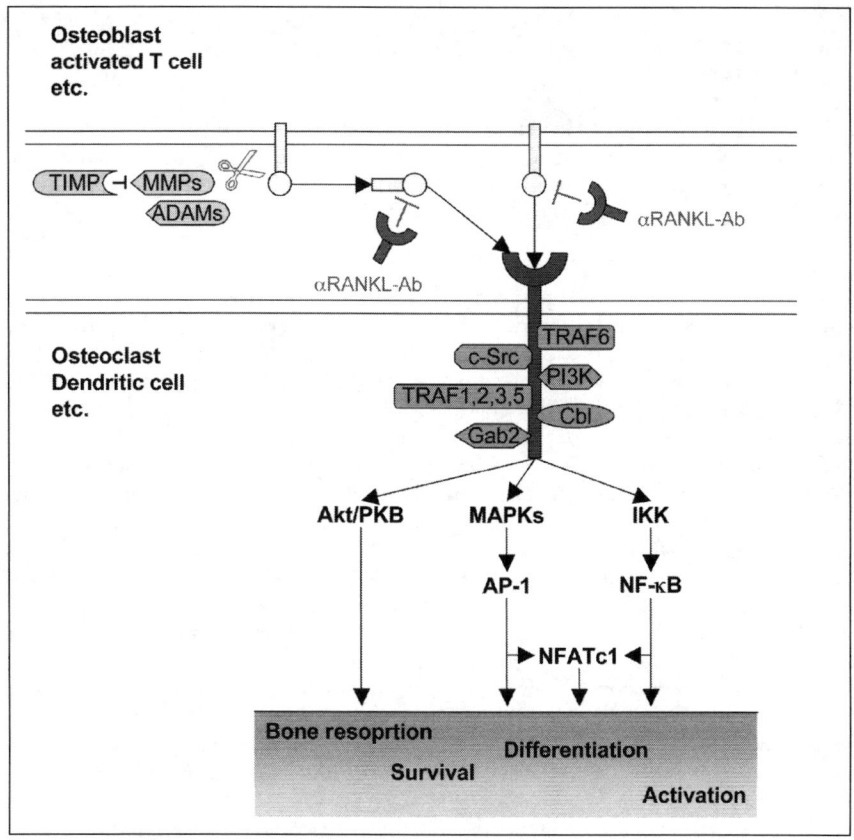

Figure 2. RANKL–RANK signaling pathways. Either membrane-bound RANKL or soluble RANKL produced by alternative splicing or cleavage by MMPs or ADAMs binds and activates the receptor RANK. RANK activation leads to the cellular context-dependent association of adaptor molecules such as TRAFs and Gab2 or Cbl proteins and consequently results in the activation and/or modulation of the NF-κB, MAPK, PI3 kinase and Calcineurin/NFATc1 pathways. In turn, activation of these pathways regulates bone resorption, activation, survival and differentiation of osteoclasts and dendritic cells. The pivotal role of RANKL in inducing osteoclastogenesis and hence bone resorption puts RANKL into the limelight as a prime drug target for bone diseases. Interference with RANKL through administration of a specific antiRANKL antibody is currently being evaluated in clinical trials and seems to be a very promising therapeutic approach to stall bone loss in osteoporosis, bone metastases, periodontitis, or RA.

As mentioned above, bone remodeling and bone loss are controlled by the RANKL-RANK-OPG axis. Moreover, RANKL is also induced in T-cells following antigen receptor engagement. Piecing these findings together, it was intriguing to ask if T-cell-derived RANKL could also regulate the development and activation of osteoclasts, i.e., would activated T-cells modulate bone turnover via RANKL? In an in vitro cell culture system of haematopoietic bone marrow precursors, activated CD4[+] T-cells induced osteoclastogenesis. Conversely, osteoclastogenesis could be blocked by addition of the physiological decoy receptor of RANKL, OPG, and was not dependent on T-cell-derived cytokines such as IL-1 or TNF-α, which could also upregulate RANKL expression in stromal cells (see Table 1).[67] Activated T-cells can also affect bone physiology in vivo, as judged by the severe osteoporotic phenotype of *Ctla4* knockout mice, in which T-cells are spontaneously

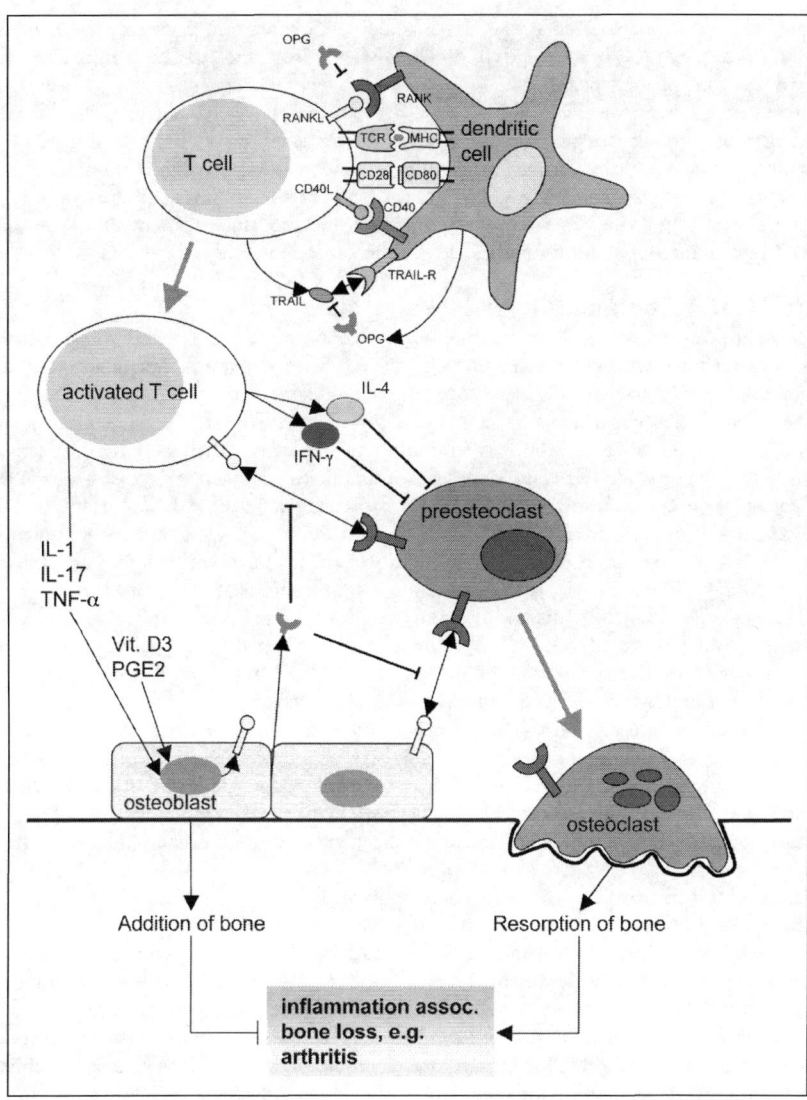

Figure 3. RANKL-RANK interactions and osteoimmunology. DCs are professional antigen-presenting cells required for T-cell-mediated immunity. DCs capture and process antigens and present them to naïve T-cells. T-cells activate DCs through CD40L and in turn receive activating and costimulatory signals through TCR:MHC and CD80:CD28 interactions. Activated T-cells express RANKL which binds to RANK on DCs and enhances activation and survival of DCs by upregulation of Bcl-xL. However, activated T-cells also express TRAIL, a TNF-family molecule which induces apoptosis of DCs to avoid excessive immune responses. OPG, which is produced by DCs and binds to RANKL and TRAIL, might negatively modulate and balance the T-cell-DC interaction, respectively. Activated T-cells produce inflammatory cytokines (IL-1, TNF-α, etc.), which together with calciotropic factors (Vitamin D3, PGE2, etc.), stimulate RANKL expression in osteoblasts (OBs). Activated T-cells and OBs induce OC differentiation from progenitors via RANKL-RANK signaling, which results in bone resorption by mature osteoclasts. OC differentiation is balanced by OPG secreted from OBs and also by cytokines IL-4 and IFN-γ produced by activated T-cells.

activated. Likewise, transferred *Ctla4*[-/-] T-cells led to a decrease in bone mineral density in lymphocyte-deficient *Rag1*[-/-] mice and continued OPG administration to *Ctla4*[-/-] mice diminished their osteoporotic phenotype.[67,68]

These results unequivocally established the pivotal role of systemically activated T-cells in resorbing bone through upregulation of RANKL, thereby stressing the importance of T-cells as crucial mediators of bone loss in vivo. The results provided a novel paradigm for immune cells as regulators of bone physiology and gave birth to the field of osteoimmunology to account for the interplay between the adaptive immune system and bone metabolism. It also gave a new perspective to certain inflammatory or autoimmune diseases, such as rheumatoid arthritis.

RANKL and Rheumatoid Arthritis

Rheumatoid arthritis (RA) is a common human autoimmune disease with 1% people affected. RA is characterized by chronic inflammation of synovial joints, progressive destruction of cartilage and bone, severe joint pain and ultimately life-long crippling.[69] Since osteoclasts are found at areas of bone erosion in RA patients,[70] it was tempting to speculate that RANKL might be a key mediator of bone erosion in RA patients. Moreover, in an adjuvant-induced arthritis model (AdA), activated T-cells (which express RANKL, Fig. 3) specific for the eliciting antigen can transfer the disease.[71] Consequently, the contribution of RANKL to RA was analyzed in an AdA model in Lewis rats. The AdA condition in rats mimics many of the clinical and pathological features of human RA, i.e., severe inflammation in the bone marrow and soft tissues surrounding joints, accompanied by extensive local bone and cartilage destruction, loss of bone mineral density and crippling,[72] and T-cells in the inflamed joints and draining lymph nodes produce many pro-inflammatory cytokines.[73] AdA rats expressed RANKL on the surface of activated T-cells isolated from synovial joints at the onset of disease.[67] Although inhibition of RANKL through OPG did not influence the severity of inflammation, OPG treatment abolished the loss of mineral bone in inflamed joints of arthritic rats in a dose-dependent manner. Bone destruction in untreated arthritic animals correlated with a dramatic increase in osteoclast numbers, which was not observed in OPG-treated rats.[67] As a consequence, OPG-treated arthritic rats exhibited minimal loss of cortical and trabecular bone, whereas untreated AdA animals developed severe bone lesions characterized by partial to complete destruction of cortical and trabecular bone and positively affected erosion of the articular cartilages. These results unequivocally demonstrated the importance of RANKL in mediating joint destruction and bone loss in AdA arthritis.

An important step in the etiology of arthritis is the alteration of cartilage structures leading to cartilage collapse in the joints. It is unclear whether cartilage destruction occurs independently of bone loss, or whether damage to the subchondral bone indirectly causes cartilage deterioration.[74] In AdA rats, partial or complete erosion of cartilage in the central and peripheral regions of joint surfaces is observed, which can be preserved in AdA rats treated with OPG. Neither cartilage erosion nor matrix degeneration in the centers of joint surfaces occurred in OPG-treated animals.[67] OPG could protect the cartilage by maintaining the underlying subchondral bone and insulating the overlying cartilage from the inflammatory cell infiltrates in the bone marrow. Since both RANKL and RANK are expressed on chondrocytes,[8,33] and *Rankl* as well as *Rank* mutant mice exhibit significant changes in the columnar alignment of chondrocytes at the growth plate,[14,15] it is possible that RANKL/RANK play a direct role in cartilage growth and cartilage homeostasis. These data provided the first evidence that inhibition of RANKL activity by OPG can also prevent cartilage destruction, a critical, irreversible step in the pathogenesis of arthritis.

Noteworthy, arthritis can also develop in the absence of activated T-cells, as shown by the K/BxN serum transfer model of spontaneous autoimmunity.[75,76] RANKL-deficient mice still develop inflammation in the K/BxN serum transfer arthritic model, but showed a dramatic reduction in bone erosion in line with the absolute requirement of RANKL in osteoclast development.[77] However, cartilage damage was still observed in both arthritic *Rankl* knockout mice and arthritic control mice, but a trend toward milder cartilage damage in the *Rankl* KO mice was noted. Thus, it appears that RANKL is not essential for cartilage destruction, but clearly plays an as yet unidentified modulatory role.[77]

In several other rodent arthritis models, such as in TNF-α- or collagen-induced arthritis,[78,79] OPG application also prevented bone erosion.[80-82] Thus, RANKL is the trigger of bone loss and crippling in all animal models of arthritis studied so far, making RANKL a prime drug candidate for therapeutic intervention in different forms of arthritis.

Importantly, RANKL expression could be detected in inflammatory cells isolated from the synovial fluid of patients with adult or juvenile RA and patients with osteoarthritis, while OPG was not detectable.[67] Thus, the correlation between RANKL expression in inflamed joints and arthritis appears to be absolute. To distinguish which cells were producing RANKL, inflammatory synovial fluids were separated into T- and nonT-cell populations. Consistent with results in rats, both synovial T- and nonT-cell populations from RA patients expressed RANKL, but not OPG. In line with this, the capacity of human T-cells expressing RANKL to directly induce osteoclastogenesis from human monocytes has been confirmed.[83] Moreover, RANKL expression is also upregulated in rheumatoid synovial fibroblasts which in turn can efficiently induce osteoclastogenesis in vitro.[84] These data confirm the findings in rodent adjuvant arthritis and suggest that RANKL signals from T-cells and synoviocytes are the principal mediators of bone destruction in human arthritis.

RANK(L), T-Cells and More

These findings also provide a molecular explanation for the observed bone loss in many other humans diseases leading to chronic systemic T-cell activation, such as adult and childhood leukemia,[85] chronic infections such as hepatitis C or HIV,[86] autoimmune disorders such as diabetes mellitus and lupus erythematosus,[87,88] allergic diseases such as asthma,[89] and lytic bone metastases in multiple cancers such as breast cancer.[90] These bone disorders can all cause irreversible crippling and thereby severely affect the quality of life of a high number of patients. For example, many patients with lupus require hip replacement surgery and essentially all children that survive leukemia experience severe bone loss and growth retardation. In addition, T-cell-derived RANKL contributes to alveolar bone resorption and tooth loss in an animal model that mimics human periodontal disease. Human peripheral blood lymphocytes from periodontitis patients were transplanted into immune-compromised NOD/SCID mice and challenged with a bacterial strain (*Actinobacillus actinomycetemcomitans*) that can cause periodontitis in humans. In response to stimulation by that microorganism, CD4+ T-cells upregulate RANKL and as a consequence induce osteoclastogenesis and bone destruction, respectively. Most importantly, inhibition of RANKL by the decoy receptor OPG significantly reduced alveolar bone resorption around the teeth.[91] Building on those results, a recent study suggests that targeting RANKL might also help to prevent periodontitis in diabetic patients which are at high risk of developing that disease.[92] Nonobese diabetic (NOD) mice—the analog of human type 1 diabetes—were orally infected with *A. actinomycetemcomitans* and it turned out that diabetic NOD mice manifested significantly higher alveolar bone loss than nondiabetic control mice. The observed bone loss was correlated with pathogen-specific proliferation and RANKL expression in local CD4+ T-cells and could be reduced to baseline levels by OPG administration.[92] Taken together, these findings suggest that specific interference with RANKL signaling pathways might be of great therapeutic value for treating inflammatory bone disorders, such as human periodontitis, or even bone loss in diabetic patients at high risk.

Since disease pathogenesis correlates with the activation of T-cells in many osteopenic disorders, the obvious question arises why the T-cells in our body, of which a certain proportion is activated at any time since they are constantly engaged in fighting off the universe of foreign antigens to which we are permanently exposed, do not cause extensive bone loss? Also, in some chronic T-cell and TNF-α-mediated diseases such as ankylosis spondylitis,[93] T-cell activation does not result in bone loss. One mechanism that counteracts RANKL-mediated bone resorption of activated T-cells seems to be the upregulation of interferon-γ (IFN-γ) in these cells. IFN-γ blocks RANKL-induced osteoclastogenesis in vitro and mice that lack IFN-γ receptor are more prone to osteoclast formation in a model of endotoxin-induced bone resorption than their wildtype littermates.[94] In line with this study, IFN-γ receptor knockout mice show also enhanced severity in the collagen-induced model of T-cell-mediated autoimmune arthritis.[95,96]

Mechanistically, IFN-γ activates the ubiquitin-proteasome pathway in osteoclasts, which results in TRAF6 degradation and therefore blocks RANK signaling. Thus, it appears that IFN-γ can prevent uncontrolled bone loss during inflammatory T-cell responses. Moreover, T-cell-derived IL-12 alone and IL-12 in synergy with IL-18 inhibits osteoclast formation in vitro,[97] and IL-4 can abrogate osteoclastogenesis through STAT6-dependent inhibition of NF-κB signaling.[98,99] Thus, multiple T-cell-derived cytokines might be able to interfere with RANK(L) signaling and therefore osteoclastogenesis and osteoclast functions. It will be interesting to determine the precise mechanism that controls the balance between T-cell-mediated bone loss and inhibition of osteoclastogenesis

A recent report suggests that a certain subset of CD4+ T helper cells, namely Th17, function as osteoclastogenic helper T-cells.[100] Th17 cells, which are derived from naïve T-cells through a mechanism distinct from Th1 and Th2 development,[101,102] produce IL-17 and are thus responsible for a variety of autoimmune inflammatory effects.[103] Since IL-17 is also a potent inducer of RANKL expression and osteoclastogenesis, respectively and found in the synovial fluid from RA patients,[104] Th17 cells seem to be the prime candidate for the osteoclastogenic Th cell subset. Indeed, Th17 cells, but not Th1, Th2, or Treg cells, could stimulate osteoclastogenesis in vitro.[100] From this study, a model emerges which implies Th17 cells as key mediators of bone destruction in RA patients by stimulating local inflammation through IL-17, expressing RANKL on themselves and inducing RANKL on osteoblast or synovial fibroblasts, thereby contributing to accelerated bone erosin. That positive Th17 effect on osteoclastogenesis is counterbalanced by Th1 and Th2 cells mainly through their production of the cytokines IFN-γ and IL-4, respectively.[100] Thus, targeting Th17 might also be a powerful approach to prevent bone destruction associated with T-cell activation in RA and other inflammatory bone diseases. Further studies will have to clarify the precise relationship and regulatory crosstalk of Th1, Th2 and Th17 subsets, respectively.

RANKL Inhibition—From Bench to Bedside

A fully human monoclonal IgG$_2$ antibody to human RANKL, denosumab (AMG 162), has been developed and is currently in late-stage clinical trials for postmenopausal osteoporosis, cancer-induced bone diseases and RA. Binding of denosumab to RANKL is selective and does not cross-react with TNF-α, TNF-β, CD40L, or TRAIL.[105] In a randomized, placebo-controlled, dose-ranging phase 2 study of 412 postmenopausal women with low bone mineral density (BMD), subcutaneous application of denosumab at 3-month or 6-month intervals over a period of 12 months resulted in a sustained decrease in bone turnover and a rapid increase in BMD.[106] In a similar study in patients with breast cancer (n = 29) or multiple myeloma (n = 25) with radiologically confirmed bone lesions, a single dose of denosumab resulted in the rapid and sustained decrease through 84 days of markers indicative for bone resorption.[107] Lastly, in an ongoing study with 227 patients with mild or moderately active RA, RANKL inhibition by denosumab also increased BMD.[108-110] In all cases, denosumab administration was well tolerated and at least as good or superior to current standard medication, but further clinical trials will be required to substantiate the indicative benefits of RANKL inhibition on suppressing bone destruction.

Conclusions

Identifying RANKL, its receptor RANK and the decoy receptor OPG as the key regulators for osteoclast development and the activation of mature osteoclasts, respectively, has opened the doors for the development of highly effective and rational drugs to treat bone loss in millions of patients. The finding that RANKL is produced by activated T-cells and that these cells in turn can directly induce osteoclastogenesis, provided a molecular explanation for the bone loss associated with diseases having immune system involvement, such as T-cell leukemias, autoimmunity, various viral infections, RA, or periodontitis. Inhibition of RANKL function e.g., via a specific antibody such as denosumab might therefore ameliorate many osteopenic conditions and prevent bone destruction and cartilage damage, e.g., in osteoporosis and arthritis, thereby dramatically enhancing the patients' quality of life.

References

1. Karsenty G, Wagner EF. Reaching a genetic and molecular understanding of skeletal development. Dev Cell 2002; 2(4):389-406.
2. Theill LE, Boyle WJ, Penninger JM. RANK-L and RANK: T-cells, bone loss and mammalian evolution. Annu Rev Immunol 2002; 20:795-823.
3. Boyle WJ, Simonet WS, Lacey DL. Osteoclast differentiation and activation. Nature 2003; 423(6937):337-342.
4. Wada T, Nakashima T, Hiroshi N et al. RANKL-RANK signaling in osteoclastogenesis and bone disease. Trends Mol Med 2006; 12(1):17-25.
5. Tolar J, Teitelbaum SL, Orchard PJ. Osteopetrosis. N Engl J Med 2004; 351(27):2839-2849.
6. Anderson DM, Maraskovsky E, Billingsley WL et al. A homologue of the TNF receptor and its ligand enhance T-cell growth and dendritic-cell function. Nature 1997; 390(6656):175-179.
7. Wong BR, Rho J, Arron J et al. TRANCE is a novel ligand of the tumor necrosis factor receptor family that activates c-Jun N-terminal kinase in T-cells. J Biol Chem 1997; 272(40):25190-25194.
8. Lacey DL, Timms E, Tan HL et al. Osteoprotegerin ligand is a cytokine that regulates osteoclast differentiation and activation. Cell 1998; 93(2):165-176.
9. Yasuda H, Shima N, Nakagawa N et al. Osteoclast differentiation factor is a ligand for osteoprotegerin/osteoclastogenesis-inhibitory factor and is identical to TRANCE/RANKL. Proc Natl Acad Sci USA 1998; 95(7):3597-3602.
10. Yasuda H, Shima N, Nakagawa N et al. Identity of osteoclastogenesis inhibitory factor (OCIF) and osteoprotegerin (OPG): a mechanism by which OPG/OCIF inhibits osteoclastogenesis in vitro. Endocrinology. 1998; 139(3):1329-1337.
11. Tsuda E, Goto M, Mochizuki S et al. Isolation of a novel cytokine from human fibroblasts that specifically inhibits osteoclastogenesis. Biochem Biophys Res Commun 1997; 234(1):137-142.
12. Simonet WS, Lacey DL, Dunstan CR et al. Osteoprotegerin: a novel secreted protein involved in the regulation of bone density. Cell 1997; 89(2):309-319.
13. Dougall WC, Glaccum M, Charrier K et al. RANK is essential for osteoclast and lymph node development. Genes Dev 1999; 13(18):2412-2424.
14. Kong YY, Yoshida H, Sarosi I et al. OPGL is a key regulator of osteoclastogenesis, lymphocyte development and lymph-node organogenesis. Nature 1999; 397(6717):315-323.
15. Li J, Sarosi I, Yan XQ et al. RANK is the intrinsic hematopoietic cell surface receptor that controls osteoclastogenesis and regulation of bone mass and calcium metabolism. Proc Natl Acad Sci USA 2000; 97(4):1566-1571.
16. Chesneau V, Becherer JD, Zheng Y et al. Catalytic properties of ADAM19. J Biol Chem 2003; 278(25):22331-22340.
17. Schlondorff J, Lum L, Blobel CP. Biochemical and pharmacological criteria define two shedding activities for TRANCE/OPGL that are distinct from the tumor necrosis factor alpha convertase. J Biol Chem 2001; 276(18):14665-14674.
18. Lum L, Wong BR, Josien R et al. Evidence for a role of a tumor necrosis factor-alpha (TNF-alpha)-converting enzyme-like protease in shedding of TRANCE, a TNF family member involved in osteoclastogenesis and dendritic cell survival. J Biol Chem 1999; 274(19):13613-13618.
19. Ikeda T, Kasai M, Utsuyama M et al. Determination of three isoforms of the receptor activator of nuclear factor-kappaB ligand and their differential expression in bone and thymus. Endocrinology 2001; 142(4):1419-1426.
20. Lynch CC, Hikosaka A, Acuff HB et al. MMP-7 promotes prostate cancer-induced osteolysis via the solubilization of RANKL. Cancer Cell 2005; 7(5):485-496.
21. Lam J, Nelson CA, Ross FP et al. Crystal structure of the TRANCE/RANKL cytokine reveals determinants of receptor-ligand specificity. J Clin Invest 2001; 108(7):971-979.
22. Ito S, Wakabayashi K, Ubukata O et al. Crystal structure of the extracellular domain of mouse RANK ligand at 2.2-A resolution. J Biol Chem 2002; 277(8):6631-6636.
23. Hofbauer LC, Khosla S, Dunstan CR et al. The roles of osteoprotegerin and osteoprotegerin ligand in the paracrine regulation of bone resorption. J Bone Miner Res 2000; 15(1):2-12.
24. Chan FK, Chun HJ, Zheng L et al. A domain in TNF receptors that mediates ligand-independent receptor assembly and signaling. Science 2000; 288(5475):2351-2354.
25. Siegel RM, Frederiksen JK, Zacharias DA et al. Fas preassociation required for apoptosis signaling and dominant inhibition by pathogenic mutations. Science 2000; 288(5475):2354-2357.
26. Chan KF, Siegel MR, Lenardo JM. Signaling by the TNF receptor superfamily and T-cell homeostasis. Immunity 2000; 13(4):419-422.
27. Locksley RM, Killeen N, Lenardo MJ. The TNF and TNF receptor superfamilies: integrating mammalian biology. Cell 2001; 104(4):487-501.

28. Tan KB, Harrop J, Reddy M et al. Characterization of a novel TNF-like ligand and recently described TNF ligand and TNF receptor superfamily genes and their constitutive and inducible expression in hematopoietic and nonhematopoietic cells. Gene 1997; 204(1-2):35-46.

29. Kwon BS, Wang S, Udagawa N et al. TR1, a new member of the tumor necrosis factor receptor superfamily, induces fibroblast proliferation and inhibits osteoclastogenesis and bone resorption. FASEB J 1998; 12(10):845-854.

30. Bucay N, Sarosi I, Dunstan CR et al. osteoprotegerin-deficient mice develop early onset osteoporosis and arterial calcification. Genes Dev 1998; 12(9):1260-1268.

31. Mizuno A, Amizuka N, Irie K et al. Severe osteoporosis in mice lacking osteoclastogenesis inhibitory factor/osteoprotegerin. Biochem Biophys Res Commun 1998; 247(3):610-615.

32. Nakagawa N, Kinosaki M, Yamaguchi K et al. RANK is the essential signaling receptor for osteoclast differentiation factor in osteoclastogenesis. Biochem Biophys Res Commun. 18 1998; 253(2):395-400.

33. Hsu H, Lacey DL, Dunstan CR et al. Tumor necrosis factor receptor family member RANK mediates osteoclast differentiation and activation induced by osteoprotegerin ligand. Proc Natl Acad Sci USA 1999; 96(7):3540-3545.

34. Hughes AE, Ralston SH, Marken J et al. Mutations in TNFRSF11A, affecting the signal peptide of RANK, cause familial expansile osteolysis. Nat Genet 2000; 24(1):45-48.

35. Whyte MP, Mills BG, Reinus WR et al. Expansile skeletal hyperphosphatasia: a new familial metabolic bone disease. J Bone Miner Res 2000; 15(12):2330-2344.

36. Whyte MP, Hughes AE. Expansile skeletal hyperphosphatasia is caused by a 15-base pair tandem duplication in TNFRSF11A encoding RANK and is allelic to familial expansile osteolysis. J Bone Miner Res 2002; 17(1):26-29.

37. Cundy T, Hegde M, Naot D et al. A mutation in the gene TNFRSF11B encoding osteoprotegerin causes an idiopathic hyperphosphatasia phenotype. Hum Mol Genet 2002; 11(18):2119-2127.

38. Chong B, Hegde M, Fawkner M et al. Idiopathic hyperphosphatasia and TNFRSF11B mutations: relationships between phenotype and genotype. J Bone Miner Res 2003; 18(12):2095-2104.

39. Takayanagi H. Mechanistic insight into osteoclast differentiation in osteoimmunology J Mol Med 2005; 83(3):170-179.

40. Inoue J, Ishida T, Tsukamoto N et al. Tumor necrosis factor receptor-associated factor (TRAF) family: adapter proteins that mediate cytokine signaling. Exp Cell Res 2000; 254(1):14-24.

41. Darnay BG, Haridas V, Ni J et al. Characterization of the intracellular domain of receptor activator of NF-kappaB (RANK). Interaction with tumor necrosis factor receptor-associated factors and activation of NF-kappab and c-Jun N-terminal kinase. J Biol Chem 1998; 273(32):20551-20555.

42. Galibert L, Tometsko ME, Anderson DM et al. The involvement of multiple tumor necrosis factor receptor (TNFR)-associated factors in the signaling mechanisms of receptor activator of NF-kappaB, a member of the TNFR superfamily. J Biol Chem 1998; 273(51):34120-34127.

43. Wong BR, Josien R, Lee SY et al. The TRAF family of signal transducers mediates NF-kappaB activation by the TRANCE receptor. J Biol Chem 1998; 273(43):28355-28359.

44. Lee ZH, Kwack K, Kim KK et al. Activation of c-Jun N-terminal kinase and activator protein 1 by receptor activator of nuclear factor kappaB. Mol Pharmacol 2000; 58(6):1536-1545.

45. Lomaga MA, Yeh WC, Sarosi I et al. TRAF6 deficiency results in osteopetrosis and defective interleukin-1, CD40 and LPS signaling. Genes Dev 1999; 13(8):1015-1024.

46. Naito A, Azuma S, Tanaka S et al. Severe osteopetrosis, defective interleukin-1 signalling and lymph node organogenesis in TRAF6-deficient mice. Genes Cells 1999; 4(6):353-362.

47. Kobayashi N, Kadono Y, Naito A et al. Segregation of TRAF6-mediated signaling pathways clarifies its role in osteoclastogenesis. EMBO J 2001; 20(6):1271-1280.

48. Kobayashi T, Walsh PT, Walsh MC et al. TRAF6 is a critical factor for dendritic cell maturation and development. Immunity 2003; 19(3):353-363.

49. Franzoso G, Carlson L, Xing L et al. Requirement for NF-kappaB in osteoclast and B-cell development. Genes Dev 1997; 11(24):3482-3496.

50. Iotsova V, Caamano J, Loy J et al. Osteopetrosis in mice lacking NF-kappaB1 and NF-kappaB2. Nat Med 1997; 3(11):1285-1289.

51. Wong BR, Besser D, Kim N et al. TRANCE, a TNF family member, activates Akt/PKB through a signaling complex involving TRAF6 and c-Src. Mol Cell 1999; 4(6):1041-1049.

52. Arron JR, Vologodskaia M, Wong BR et al. A positive regulatory role for Cbl family proteins in tumor necrosis factor-related activation-induced cytokine (trance) and CD40L-mediated Akt activation. J Biol Chem 2001; 276(32):30011-30017.

53. Soriano P, Montgomery C, Geske R et al. Targeted disruption of the c-src proto-oncogene leads to osteopetrosis in mice. Cell 1991; 64(4):693-702.

54. Wada T, Nakashima T, Oliveira-dos-Santos AJ et al. The molecular scaffold Gab2 is a crucial component of RANK signaling and osteoclastogenesis. Nat Med 2005; 11(4):394-399.

55. Wong BR, Josien R, Lee SY et al. TRANCE (tumor necrosis factor [TNF]-related activation-induced cytokine), a new TNF family member predominantly expressed in T-cells, is a dendritic cell-specific survival factor. J Exp Med 1997; 186(12):2075-2080.
56. Bachmann MF, Wong BR, Josien R et al. TRANCE, a tumor necrosis factor family member critical for CD40 ligand-independent T helper cell activation. J Exp Med 1999; 189(7):1025-1031.
57. Josien R, Wong BR, Li HL et al. TRANCE, a TNF family member, is differentially expressed on T-cell subsets and induces cytokine production in dendritic cells. J Immunol 1999; 162(5):2562-2568.
58. Josien R, Li HL, Ingulli E et al. TRANCE, a tumor necrosis factor family member, enhances the longevity and adjuvant properties of dendritic cells in vivo. J Exp Med 2000; 191(3):495-502.
59. Emery JG, McDonnell P, Burke MB et al. Osteoprotegerin is a receptor for the cytotoxic ligand TRAIL. J Biol Chem 1998; 273(23):14363-14367.
60. Yun TJ, Chaudhary PM, Shu GL et al. OPG/FDCR-1, a TNF receptor family member, is expressed in lymphoid cells and is up-regulated by ligating CD40. J Immunol 1998; 161(11):6113-6121.
61. Kong YY, Boyle WJ, Penninger JM. Osteoprotegerin ligand: a common link between osteoclastogenesis, lymph node formation and lymphocyte development. Immunol Cell Biol 1999; 77(2):188-193.
62. Kim N, Odgren PR, Kim DK et al. Diverse roles of the tumor necrosis factor family member TRANCE in skeletal physiology revealed by TRANCE deficiency and partial rescue by a lymphocyte-expressed TRANCE transgene. Proc Natl Acad Sci USA 2000; 97(20):10905-10910.
63. Sakaguchi S. Naturally arising Foxp3-expressing CD25+CD4+ regulatory T-cells in immunological tolerance to self and nonself. Nat Immunol 2005; 6(4):345-352.
64. Steinman RM, Hawiger D, Nussenzweig MC. Tolerogenic dendritic cells. Annu Rev Immunol 2003; 21:685-711.
65. Mehling A, Loser K, Varga G et al. Overexpression of CD40 ligand in murine epidermis results in chronic skin inflammation and systemic autoimmunity. J Exp Med 2001; 194(5):615-628.
66. Loser K, Mehling A, Loeser S et al. Epidermal RANKL controls regulatory T-cell numbers via activation of dendritic cells. Nat Med 2006; 12(12):1372-1379.
67. Kong YY, Feige U, Sarosi I et al. Activated T-cells regulate bone loss and joint destruction in adjuvant arthritis through osteoprotegerin ligand. Nature 1999; 402(6759):304-309.
68. Waterhouse P, Penninger JM, Timms E et al. Lymphoproliferative disorders with early lethality in mice deficient in Ctla-4. Science 1995; 270(5238):985-988.
69. Feldmann M, Brennan FM, Maini RN. Rheumatoid arthritis. Cell 1996; 85(3):307-310.
70. Takayanagi H, Oda H, Yamamoto S et al. A new mechanism of bone destruction in rheumatoid arthritis: synovial fibroblasts induce osteoclastogenesis. Biochem Biophys Res Commun 1997; 240(2):279-286.
71. Panayi GS, Lanchbury JS, Kingsley GH. The importance of the T-cell in initiating and maintaining the chronic synovitis of rheumatoid arthritis. Arthritis Rheum 1992; 35(7):729-735.
72. Bendele A, McComb J, Gould T et al. Animal models of arthritis: relevance to human disease. Toxicol Pathol 1999; 27(1):134-142.
73. Feldmann M, Brennan FM, Maini RN. Role of cytokines in rheumatoid arthritis. Annu Rev Immunol 1996; 14:397-440.
74. Muller-Ladner U, Gay RE, Gay S. Molecular biology of cartilage and bone destruction. Curr Opin Rheumatol 1998; 10(3):212-219.
75. Kouskoff V, Korganow AS, Duchatelle V et al. Organ-specific disease provoked by systemic autoimmunity. Cell 1996; 87(5):811-822.
76. Korganow AS, Ji H, Mangialaio S et al. From systemic T-cell self-reactivity to organ-specific autoimmune disease via immunoglobulins. Immunity 1999; 10(4):451-461.
77. Pettit AR, Ji H, von Stechow D et al. TRANCE/RANKL knockout mice are protected from bone erosion in a serum transfer model of arthritis. Am J Pathol 2001; 159(5):1689-1699.
78. Keffer J, Probert L, Cazlaris H et al. Transgenic mice expressing human tumour necrosis factor: a predictive genetic model of arthritis. EMBO J 1991; 10(13):4025-4031.
79. Mori H, Kitazawa R, Mizuki S et al. RANK ligand, RANK and OPG expression in type II collagen-induced arthritis mouse. Histochem Cell Biol 2002; 117(3):283-292.
80. Redlich K, Hayer S, Maier A et al. Tumor necrosis factor alpha-mediated joint destruction is inhibited by targeting osteoclasts with osteoprotegerin. Arthritis Rheum 2002; 46(3):785-792.
81. Romas E, Sims NA, Hards DK et al. Osteoprotegerin reduces osteoclast numbers and prevents bone erosion in collagen-induced arthritis. Am J Pathol 2002; 161(4):1419-1427.
82. Nakashima T, Wada T, Penninger JM. RANKL and RANK as novel therapeutic targets for arthritis. Curr Opin Rheumatol 2003; 15(3):280-287.
83. Kotake S, Udagawa N, Hakoda M et al. Activated human T-cells directly induce osteoclastogenesis from human monocytes: possible role of T-cells in bone destruction in rheumatoid arthritis patients. Arthritis Rheum 2001; 44(5):1003-1012.

84. Takayanagi H, Iizuka H, Juji T et al. Involvement of receptor activator of nuclear factor kappaB ligand/ osteoclast differentiation factor in osteoclastogenesis from synoviocytes in rheumatoid arthritis. Arthritis Rheum 2000; 43(2):259-269.
85. Oliveri MB, Mautalen CA, Rodriguez Fuchs CA et al. Vertebral compression fractures at the onset of acute lymphoblastic leukemia in a child. Henry Ford Hosp Med J 1991; 39(1):45-48.
86. Stellon AJ, Davies A, Compston J et al. Bone loss in autoimmune chronic active hepatitis on maintenance corticosteroid therapy. Gastroenterology 1985; 89(5):1078-1083.
87. Piepkorn B, Kann P, Forst T et al. Bone mineral density and bone metabolism in diabetes mellitus. Horm Metab Res 1997; 29(11):584-591.
88. Seitz M, Hunstein W. Enhanced prostanoid release from monocytes of patients with rheumatoid arthritis and active systemic lupus erythematosus. Ann Rheum Dis 1985; 44(7):438-445.
89. Ebeling PR, Erbas B, Hopper JL et al. Bone mineral density and bone turnover in asthmatics treated with long-term inhaled or oral glucocorticoids. J Bone Miner Res 1998; 13(8):1283-1289.
90. Lipton A. Future treatment of bone metastases. Clin Cancer Res 2006; 12(20 Pt 2):6305s-6308s.
91. Teng YT, Nguyen H, Gao X et al. Functional human T-cell immunity and osteoprotegerin ligand control alveolar bone destruction in periodontal infection. J Clin Invest 2000; 106(6):R59-67.
92. Mahamed DA, Marleau A, Alnaeeli M et al. G(-) anaerobes-reactive CD4+ T-cells trigger RANKL-mediated enhanced alveolar bone loss in diabetic NOD mice. Diabetes 2005; 54(5):1477-1486.
93. Brandt J, Haibel H, Cornely D et al. Successful treatment of active ankylosing spondylitis with the antitumor necrosis factor alpha monoclonal antibody infliximab. Arthritis Rheum 2000; 43(6):1346-1352.
94. Takayanagi H, Ogasawara K, Hida S et al. T-cell-mediated regulation of osteoclastogenesis by signalling cross-talk between RANKL and IFN-gamma. Nature 2000; 408(6812):600-605.
95. Vermeire K, Heremans H, Vandeputte M et al. Accelerated collagen-induced arthritis in IFN-gamma receptor-deficient mice. J Immunol 1997; 158(11):5507-5513.
96. Manoury-Schwartz B, Chiocchia G, Bessis N et al. High susceptibility to collagen-induced arthritis in mice lacking IFN-gamma receptors. J Immunol 1997; 158(11):5501-5506.
97. Horwood NJ, Elliott J, Martin TJ et al. IL-12 alone and in synergy with IL-18 inhibits osteoclast formation in vitro. J Immunol 2001; 166(8):4915-4921.
98. Abu-Amer Y. IL-4 abrogates osteoclastogenesis through STAT6-dependent inhibition of NF-kappaB. J Clin Invest 2001; 107(11):1375-1385.
99. Bendixen AC, Shevde NK, Dienger KM et al. IL-4 inhibits osteoclast formation through a direct action on osteoclast precursors via peroxisome proliferator-activated receptor gamma 1. Proc Natl Acad Sci USA 2001; 98(5):2443-2448.
100. Sato K, Suematsu A, Okamoto K et al. Th17 functions as an osteoclastogenic helper T-cell subset that links T-cell activation and bone destruction. J Exp Med 2006; 203(12):2673-2682.
101. Harrington LE, Hatton RD, Mangan PR et al. Interleukin 17-producing CD4+ effector T-cells develop via a lineage distinct from the T helper type 1 and 2 lineages. Nat Immunol 2005; 6(11):1123-1132.
102. Park H, Li Z, Yang XO et al. A distinct lineage of CD4 T-cells regulates tissue inflammation by producing interleukin 17. Nat Immunol 2005; 6(11):1133-1141.
103. Dong C. Diversification of T-helper-cell lineages: finding the family root of IL-17-producing cells. Nat Rev Immunol. 2006; 6(4):329-333.
104. Kotake S, Udagawa N, Takahashi N et al. IL-17 in synovial fluids from patients with rheumatoid arthritis is a potent stimulator of osteoclastogenesis. J Clin Invest 1999; 103(9):1345-1352.
105. Dougall WC, Chaisson M. The RANK/RANKL/OPG triad in cancer-induced bone diseases. Cancer Metastasis Rev 2006.
106. McClung MR, Lewiecki EM, Cohen SB et al. Denosumab in postmenopausal women with low bone mineral density. N Engl J Med 2006 ;354(8):821-831.
107. Body JJ, Facon T, Coleman RE et al. A study of the biological receptor activator of nuclear factor-kappaB ligand inhibitor, denosumab, in patients with multiple myeloma or bone metastases from breast cancer. Clin Cancer Res 2006; 12(4):1221-1228.
108. Lane NE, Iannini M, Atkins C et al. RANKL Inhibition with Denosumab Decreases Markers of Bone and Cartilage Turnover in Patients with Rheumatoid Arthritis. Arthritis Rheum 2006; 54(9 (Supplement)):S225-226.
109. Dore R, Hurd E, Palmer W et al. Denosumab Increases Bone Mineral Density in Patients With Rheumatoid Arthritis. Arthritis Rheum. 2006; 54(9 (Supplement)):S240.
110. Cohen SB, Valen P, Ritchlin C et al. RANKL Inhibition with Denosumab Reduces Progression of Bone Erosions in Patients with Rheumatoid Arthritis: Month 6 MRI Results. Arthritis Rheum 2006; 54(9 (Supplement)):S831-832.
111. Hofbauer LC, Dunstan CR, Spelsberg TC et al. Osteoprotegerin production by human osteoblast lineage cells is stimulated by vitamin D, bone morphogenetic protein-2 and cytokines. Biochem Biophys Res Commun 1998; 250(3):776-781.

112. Hofbauer LC, Khosla S, Dunstan CR et al. Estrogen stimulates gene expression and protein production of osteoprotegerin in human osteoblastic cells. Endocrinology 1999; 140(9):4367-4370.
113. Brandstrom H, Jonsson KB, Vidal O et al. Tumor necrosis factor-alpha and -beta upregulate the levels of osteoprotegerin mRNA in human osteosarcoma MG-63 cells. Biochem Biophys Res Commun 1998; 248(3):454-457.
114. Hofbauer LC, Lacey DL, Dunstan CR et al. Interleukin-1beta and tumor necrosis factor-alpha, but not interleukin-6, stimulate osteoprotegerin ligand gene expression in human osteoblastic cells. Bone 1999; 25(3):255-259.
115. Vidal ON, Sjogren K, Eriksson BI et al. Osteoprotegerin mRNA is increased by interleukin-1 alpha in the human osteosarcoma cell line MG-63 and in human osteoblast-like cells. Biochem Biophys Res Commun 1998; 248(3):696-700.
116. Palmqvist P, Persson E, Conaway HH et al. IL-6, leukemia inhibitory factor and oncostatin M stimulate bone resorption and regulate the expression of receptor activator of NF-kappa B ligand, osteoprotegerin and receptor activator of NF-kappa B in mouse calvariae. J Immunol 2002; 169(6):3353-3362.
117. Takai H, Kanematsu M, Yano K et al. Transforming growth factor-beta stimulates the production of osteoprotegerin/osteoclastogenesis inhibitory factor by bone marrow stromal cells. J Biol Chem 1998; 273(42):27091-27096.
118. Rubin J, Ackert-Bicknell CL, Zhu L et al. IGF-I regulates osteoprotegerin (OPG) and receptor activator of nuclear factor-kappaB ligand in vitro and OPG in vivo. J Clin Endocrinol Metab 2002; 87(9):4273-4279.
119. Vidal NO, Brandstrom H, Jonsson KB et al. Osteoprotegerin mRNA is expressed in primary human osteoblast-like cells: down-regulation by glucocorticoids. J Endocrinol 1998; 159(1):191-195.
120. Hofbauer LC, Gori F, Riggs BL et al. Stimulation of osteoprotegerin ligand and inhibition of osteoprotegerin production by glucocorticoids in human osteoblastic lineage cells: potential paracrine mechanisms of glucocorticoid-induced osteoporosis. Endocrinology 1999; 140(10):4382-4389.
121. Hofbauer LC, Shui C, Riggs BL et al. Effects of immunosuppressants on receptor activator of NF-kappaB ligand and osteoprotegerin production by human osteoblastic and coronary artery smooth muscle cells. Biochem Biophys Res Commun 2001; 280(1):334-339.
122. Brandstrom H, Jonsson KB, Ohlsson C et al. Regulation of osteoprotegerin mRNA levels by prostaglandin E2 in human bone marrow stroma cells. Biochem Biophys Res Commun 1998; 247(2):338-341.
123. Murakami T, Yamamoto M, Ono K et al. Transforming growth factor-beta1 increases mRNA levels of osteoclastogenesis inhibitory factor in osteoblastic/stromal cells and inhibits the survival of murine osteoclast-like cells. Biochem Biophys Res Commun 1998; 252(3):747-752.
124. Takami M, Takahashi N, Udagawa N et al. Intracellular calcium and protein kinase C mediate expression of receptor activator of nuclear factor-kappaB ligand and osteoprotegerin in osteoblasts. Endocrinology 2000; 141(12):4711-4719.
125. Nagasawa T, Kobayashi H, Kiji M et al. LPS-stimulated human gingival fibroblasts inhibit the differentiation of monocytes into osteoclasts through the production of osteoprotegerin. Clin Exp Immunol 2002; 130(2):338-344.

CHAPTER 10

Targeting the LIGHT-HVEM Pathway

Carl F. Ware*

Abstract

Tumor necrosis factor (TNF)-related cytokines function as key communication systems between cells of the immune system and mediate inflammation and tissue destruction. LIGHT (TNFSF14) is a key component of the communication system that controls the responses of T-Cells. LIGHT activates two cell surface receptors, the Herpesvirus Entry Mediator (HVEM) and the Lymphotoxin-β Receptor and is inhibited by soluble decoy receptor-3. The LIGHT-HVEM pathway is an important cosignaling pathway for T-Cells, whereas LIGHT-LTβR modifies the functions of dendritic cells and stromal cells by creating tissue microenvironments, which promote immune responses. HVEM also binds an Ig superfamily member, B and T lymphocyte attenuator (BTLA) that inhibits T-Cell activation. Thus, HVEM serves as a molecular switch between stimulatory and inhibitory signaling. Studies in humans and experimental animal models reveal that LIGHT contributes to inflammation and pathogenesis in mucosal, hepatic, joint and vascular tissues. LIGHT is accessible to biologic-based therapeutics, which can be used to target this molecule during inflammation-driven diseases.

Introduction

Signals mediated through tumor necrosis factor (TNF)-related cytokines and their receptors modulate immune and inflammatory responses,[1] thus blockade of signaling may suppress symptoms associated with inflammatory and immune mediated diseases. This concept was validated by the clinical impact of TNF inhibitors (Remicade™, an anti-TNF antibody and Enbrel™, a decoy receptor-Ig fusion protein) in patients with autoimmune diseases, such as rheumatoid arthritis, psoriasis and inflammatory bowel syndrome.[2] However, successful responses were limited to a subset of the patients and in other autoimmune diseases TNF inhibitors failed to alleviate symptoms. These clinical results and support from experimental animal models, indicate that other members of the TNF superfamily may be operative in immune mechanisms underlying pathogenic processes.

Several members of the TNF superfamily are involved in regulating T-Cell homeostasis by orchestrating the balance of proliferation and elimination of antigen-activated T lymphocytes. The genes encoding TNF-related cytokines modulating T-Cell homeostasis are clustered in four regions of the genome paralogous with the major histocompatibility complex (MHC)(Fig. 1).[3] The TNF gene is located on chromosome 6p21 within the MHC in a closely linked tripartite locus with genes for Lymphotoxin (LT)α and LTβ sandwiched between class I and II antigen presenting molecules. The conservation of the TNF related MHC paralogs is reflected in their exon-intron organization, transcriptional orientation and functional activity. The cellular receptors that bind these ligands belong to a corresponding superfamily (TNFR superfamily) defined by an extracellular ligand binding region comprised of several cysteine-rich domains (CRD). The receptors that bind these TNF related ligands are genetically linked in two clusters: *TNFR-1*,

*Carl F. Ware—Division of Molecular Immunology, La Jolla Institute for Allergy and Immunology 9420 Athena Circle, La Jolla, California 92037, USA. Email: cware@liai.org

Therapeutic Targets of the TNF Superfamily, edited by Iqbal S. Grewal.

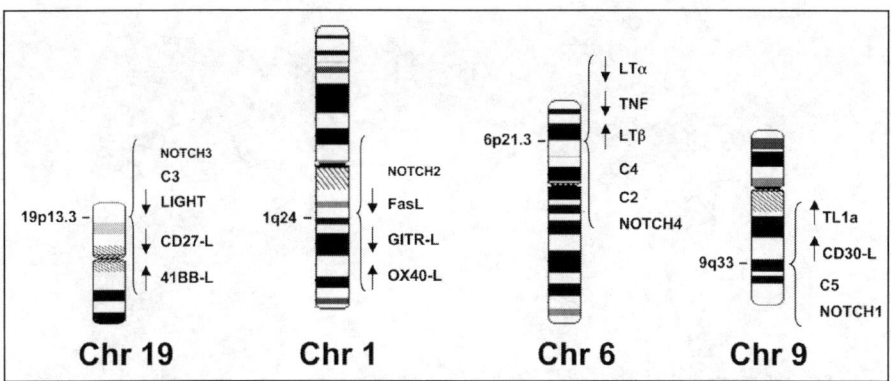

Figure 1. Organization of the TNF superfamily genes within the MHC paralogous regions present on chromosomes 1, 9, 6 and 19. Arrows indicate gene transcriptional orientation and solid blocks represent exons. *LIGHT* is 7.78kb from *C3* and ~79kb from *CD27L*. CD27L is ~235 kb from *4-1BBL*. *FasL* is separated from *GITRL* by 374kb, while *GITRL* and *OX40L* are 134k apart. *TNF* is 2.9 kb from *LTβ* and 1.3kb from *LTα*.

LTβR, CD27 reside on Chr12p13 and the others, *41BB, GITR, Ox40, TNFR-2, DR3* and herpesvirus entry mediator (*HVEM*) on Chr 1p36 (*Fas* is an exception and resides on Chr10q24). The paralogous TNFR superfamily members such CD27, 41BB and OX40 (see for example[4,5]), either function as costimulatory molecules enhancing T-lymphocyte activation and survival, or else they induce elimination of activated T-Cells, e.g., TNFR1 and Fas. Receptor signaling is mediated through two distinct types of cytoplasmic modules: the death domain module (TNFR1, Fas and DR3), which activate caspases and the TRAF binding motif, which activates cell survival

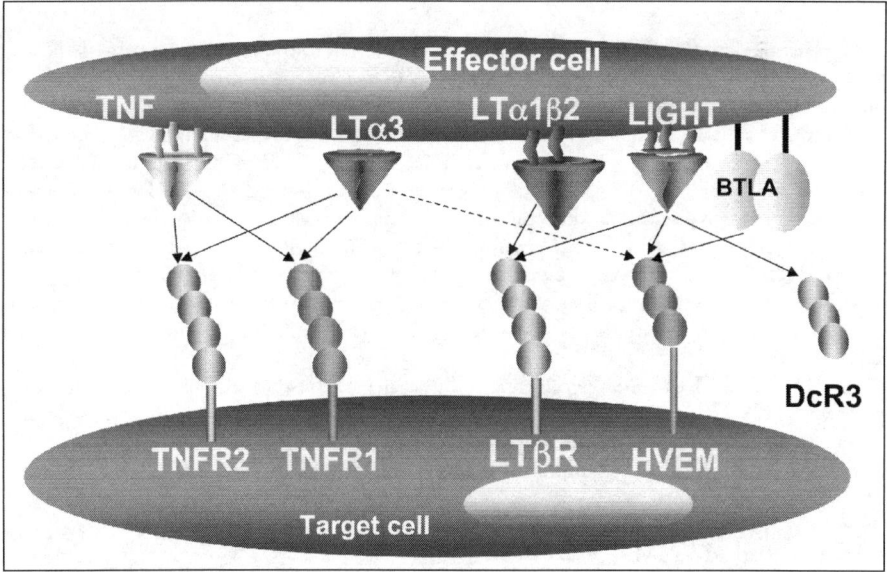

Figure 2. The Members of the immediate TNF/LT family. Arrows indicate binding interactions. Each ligand receptor interaction defines a system and these shared systems create a signaling circuit.

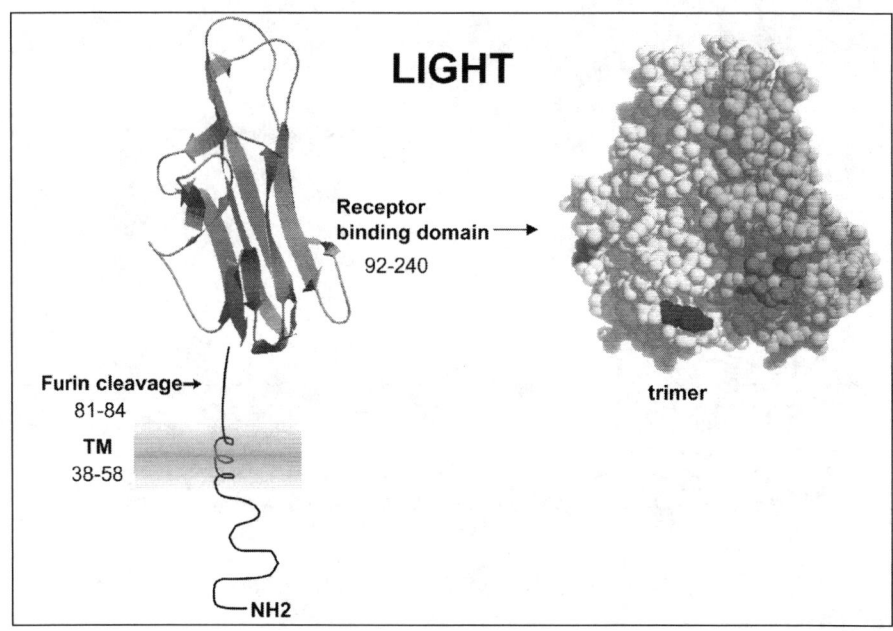

Figure 3. Molecular model of LIGHT. The theoretical LIGHT model was generated by SwissModel and encompasses amino acids Ser103 to Val240 and based on the templates for LTα and TNF (2TUN.pdb and 1TNR.pdb).[11] The domain structure of LIGHT is depicted on the left and the assembled trimeric form of the TNF homology domain is shown in space filling mode. Each subunit is shown in a different color with atoms colored red and blue have been identified as contact residues for LTβR and HVEM binding.

genes controlled by NFκB. The evolutionary conservation of the TNF-related ligands dedicated to T-Cell homeostasis and linkage to antigen recognition molecules mirrors their importance in fine-tuning antigen recognition and immune tolerance.

A broader functional link between several members of the TNF superfamily is revealed in shared ligand-receptor binding interactions. TNF, LTαβ and LIGHT overlap in binding to several cognate receptors (Fig. 2). This group, often referred to as the immediate TNF family, is viewed as an integrated signaling circuit that controls T-Cell homeostasis and a variety of other immune processes.[6] The TNF-TNFR-1 system is an important sentinel signaling system that orchestrates inflammation induced by innate recognition systems as well as by T-Cells. The LTαβ-LTβR system controls lymphoid tissue development and structure, but is also involved in regulating cellular immune processes by differentiation of stromal cells, which create microenvironments that promote cellular interactions.[7-9]

LIGHT (TNFSF14, homologous to *L*ymphotoxins exhibits inducible expression and competes with HSV glycoprotein D for *H*VEM, a receptor expressed by T-lymphocytes) displays a unique receptor binding profile that imparts its physiological functions. LIGHT has emerged as a key factor controlling T-Cell immune responses and thus is a candidate to target in different immune-mediated diseases.

LIGHT and HVEM

LIGHT follows the canonical paradigm of a TNF superfamily member configured as a type II transmembrane protein containing a C-terminal TNF homology domain that folds into a β-sheet sandwich, which assembles into a functional homotrimer[10,11] (Fig. 3). LIGHT engages two specific cellular receptors, the LTβR and HVEM. These TNFR are type I membrane glycoproteins that

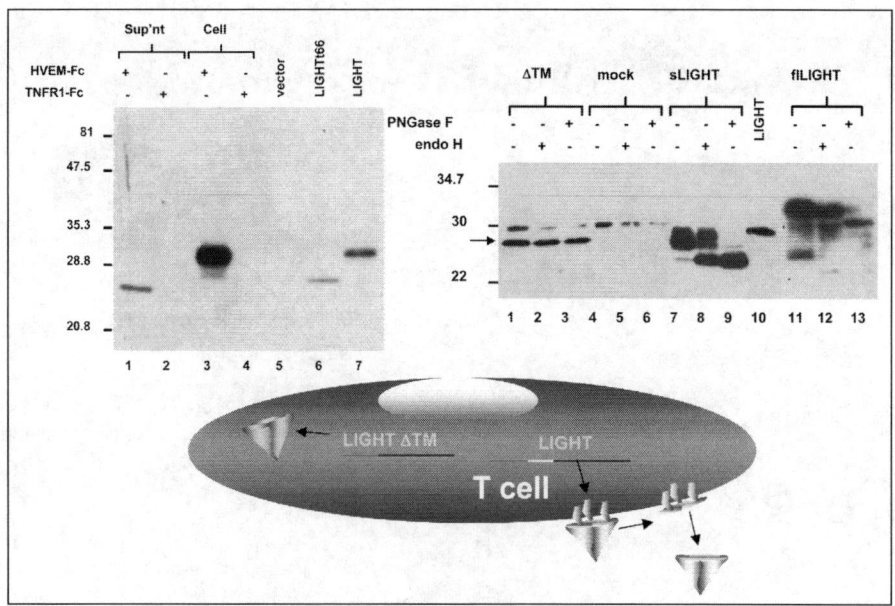

Figure 4. Processing pathway and isoforms of LIGHT Left panel, 293T-Cells were transiently transfected with plasmids encoding either membrane LIGHT or empty pCDNA3.1(+). HVEM-Fc was used to precipitate LIGHT from the tissue culture supernatant (lane 1) or cell lysate (lane 3) of full length LIGHT transfected 293T-Cells. The precipitates were resolved by SDS-PAGE and Western blot analysis using a rat anti-LIGHT polyclonal serum as a probe. TNFR1-Fc was used to control for nonspecific binding to membrane LIGHT (lane 2) or supernatants (lane 4). An equivalent amount (5x10⁴ cell equivalents) from each transfected cell lysate was loaded in lanes 5 and 7. Purified recombinant soluble LIGHTt66 (10 ng)(lane 6) used as a molecular mass marker. Right panel, LIGHTΔTM is not glycosylated. Immunoprecipitates from the NP40 cell lysates of 293T-Cells transfected with soluble LIGHTΔTM (lanes 1-3), pCDNA3.1(+) alone (lane 4-6), LIGHTt66 (lanes 7-9) or full length LIGHT (lanes 11-13) encoding plasmids are shown. Detergent lysates were precleared with an isotype control and then immunoprecipitated with mouse anti-human LIGHT antibody and protein G. The immunoprecipitates were digested with either endoglycosidase H (lanes 2, 5, 8,12), PNGaseF (lanes 3, 6, 9,13) or left untreated (lanes 1,4, 7,11); purified soluble LIGHT (lane 10). The cartoon depicts the alternate spliced forms of LIGHT and LIGHT shedding from the membrane. Reproduced with permission from: Granger SW, Butrovich KD, Houshmand P et al. J Immunol. 2001;167:5122-5128.

have an extracellular domain comprised of four CRD. LIGHT is also bound by a soluble decoy receptor (DcR3) providing a posttranslational control mechanism to turn off signaling[12](DcR3) also binds TL1A and FasL reemphasizing the common functional links of these ligands. LIGHT can also be proteolytically cleaved (shed) into a soluble form that retains receptor-binding activity. Interestingly, an alternate transcript of LIGHT encodes a deletion of the transmembrane region, which is directed into the cytosol in a nonglycosylated form of unknown function (Fig. 4).

The LIGHT-HVEM-BTLA Switch

A new paradigm emerged with the discovery that HVEM is an activating signal for an inhibitory coreceptor known as B and T-lymphocyte attenuator (BTLA)[13](Fig. 5). BTLA has an intermediate type Ig fold[14] making it structurally diverse from other cosignaling molecules such as CD28, CTLA4, ICOS, or PD1[15,16] and providing the basis for specific interaction with HVEM. The cytoplasmic domain of BTLA contains an inhibitory tyrosine-based motif (ITIM) that counteracts

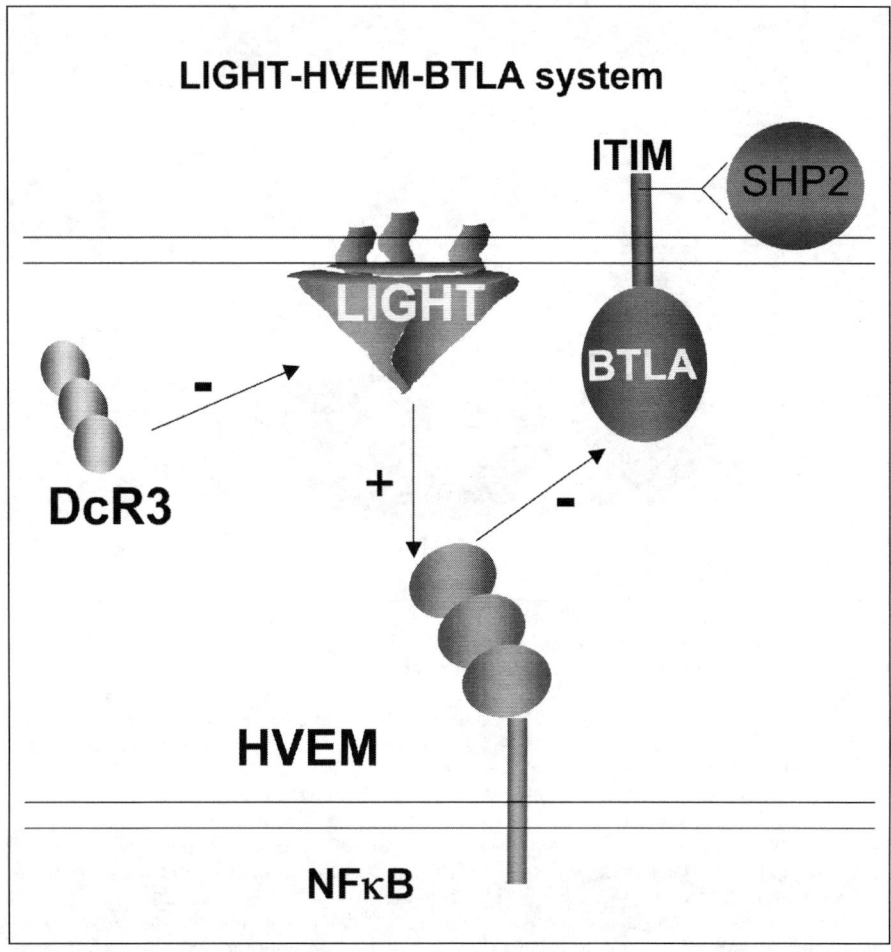

Figure 5. The LIGHT-HVEM-BTLA system. The arrows indicate the ligand-receptor binding interactions. LIGHT-HVEM activates NFκB as part of its positive signaling activity, where as HVEM activates BTLA to recruit tyrosine phosphatase SHP2, which attenuates signaling in T- and B-cells. Decoy receptor-3 binds LIGHT and can inhibit signaling.

kinases via recruitment of tyrosine phosphatases (SHP-1 and SHP-2) attenuating proliferation signals in antigen activated lymphocytes.[17-19] BTLA engages the N-terminal, first CRD of HVEM in the same topographical site occupied by Herpes Simplex virus glycoprotein D.[14,20] In contrast, LIGHT occupies a topographically distinct site in CRD2 and 3 on the opposite face of HVEM from where BTLA binds. Thus, HVEM can mediate both positive and negative signaling though different mechanisms. BTLA has a strong inhibitory effect on T- and B- cells, which is thought to function as a control for tolerance to self tissues and homeostasis.

LIGHT-Mechanism of Action

LIGHT is a key factor in the HVEM-BTLA switch between positive and inhibitory signaling.[20-22] Studies indicate that LIGHT in its membrane-anchored position disrupts the binding interaction between HVEM and BTLA.[20] This feature provides LIGHT with three functional attributes: (1) activation of LTβR, (2) activation of HVEM and (3) disruption of the HVEM-BTLA

Table 1. LIGHT in experimental pathogenesis models

Model	Result	References
Transgenic LIGHT		
LIGHT Tg in T-Cells	Acute onset, autoimmune like disease. Inflamed intestines, reproductive organs, skin and liver; abnormal lymphoid tissues	48,49
LIGHT-Tg T-Cell transfer	Atherosclerosis	46
LIGHT-Tg T-Cell transfer	Inflammatory bowel disease	50
LIGHT tumor transgene	LIGHT induced tumor rejection by CD8 T-Cells	51
Decoy Receptor		
MHC II disparte GVHD	HVEM-Fc or LTβR-Fc decreased inflammation	52,53
EAE experimental autoimmune encephalitis	LTβR-Fc suppressed paralysis	54
Cuperizone-induced demyelination	LTβR-Fc decreased demyelination and enhanced remyelination	55
CIA collagen-induced arthritis	LTβR-Fc suppressed	56
LIGHT-/- mice		
Cardiac allograft rejection	Rejection was minimized	57
Graft vs host disease	Reduced inflammation	58
Superantigen	CD8 T-Cell proliferation defect	25
Mitogen induced hepatitis	increased survival and decreased hepatic inflammation mediated by CD4 T or NK cells	30

complex, all of which act to promote immune and inflammatory processes.[20] Thus, targeting LIGHT may block signaling via its two receptors, HVEM and LTβR and leave intact the inhibitory HVEM-BTLA pathway. Interestingly, supportive evidence for this mechanism is found in a viral pathogen. A BTLA binding protein encoded by human cytomegalovirus (UL144 orf) competes with HVEM for binding BTLA and effectively inhibits human T-Cell proliferation.[20]

Expression patterns of the ligand and receptor determine the physiological cellular response. LIGHT is expressed transiently in activated T- and B-cells, but constitutively in lymphoid tissue resident dendritic cells. HVEM is expressed on T- and B-lymphocytes and other hematopoietic cells and on mucosal epithelium, whereas LTβR is broadly distributed on stroma and parenchyma cells of most organs, dendritic cells and tissue macrophages, but is conspicuously absent on T and B-lymphocytes. BTLA is also broadly expressed in all hematopoietic cells. This complex expression pattern suggests that intercellular interactions between multiple cell types will be involved in determining whether the response is ultimately stimulatory and/or inhibitory.

As a cosignaling system, LIGHT expression on antigen presenting dendritic cells is thought to engage HVEM on the surface of naïve T-Cells, enhancing proliferation and differentiation into effector cells following antigen recognition. Both HVEM and BTLA are constitutively expressed on naïve DC, B and T-Cells, thus the action of HVEM-BTLA pathway may keep naïve cells in a resting state by controlling the extent of kinase activity emanating spontaneously from antigen receptor complex on T- and B-cells. As part of the cosignaling process, the LTβR controls the proliferation of dendritic cells within lymphoid organs after binding LTαβ or LIGHT expressed on activated cells.[23] Thus, blockade of LTαβ or LIGHT may decrease the numbers of DC involved in activating T-Cells, thus dampening inflammation.

Immunobiology of LIGHT

In vivo analyses of transgenic, knockout and pharmacological models in mice indicate that LIGHT and LTαβ play a crucial role in immune regulation and targeting these molecules may impact disease processes (Table 1). An inflammatory role for LIGHT has emerged from studies of transgenic mice with constitutive LIGHT expression in the T-Cell lineage. T-Cells that express human or mouse LIGHT displayed a profound multi-organ inflammatory phenotype. LIGHT is normally transiently expressed and highly regulated at multiple steps during transcriptional and posttranslational (shedding and DcR3) stages of its expression. Although enforced expression might not replicate the physiological action of LIGHT, the model clearly demonstrates the potential of LIGHT as a potent inducer of tissue damaging inflammation. The proinflammatory action of LIGHT to induce an immune response is further underscored by the rejection of tumors engineered to express LIGHT. Additionally, some of the phenotypes within these LIGHT transgenic mice may mimic the action normally provided by LTαβ-LTβR system, or the nonphysiological disruption of inhibitory signals mediated by the HVEM-BTLA pathway needed to maintain immune homeostasis.

The use of purified receptor-Fc fusion proteins (LTβR-Fc or HVEM-Fc) as decoys to pharmacologically block the interactions of LIGHT or LTαβ with cellular receptors has provided complementary results to the genetic models (Table 1). Delineating the role of LIGHT by pharmacologic methods alone is complicated by the multiple ligand specificities of these decoy receptors.

Alternately, mice deficient in *LIGHT* provide a genetic model for understanding more directly the physiological role of this cytokine.[24-26] LIGHT deficient mice are developmentally normal, with wild type lymphoid subsets and tissues, unlike animals deficient in components of the LTαβ-LTβR pathway or the offspring of pregnant mice treated in utero with LTβR-Fc, which lack most of their secondary lymphoid tissues (intestinal Peyer's patches and lymph nodes).[27] Although both LTαβ and LIGHT can signal via the LTβR, the difference in phenotype is due in part to preferential expression of LTαβ during embryogenesis by lymphoid tissue inducer cells.[28] Deficiency in LIGHT enhanced cardiac allograft survival and decreased tissue damage in graft vs host disease, both CD8 T-Cell effector models (Table 1). CD4 T-Cells may also use LIGHT as a mediator of inflammation. LTβR-Fc blocked intestinal inflammation in the CD4 T-Cell transfer model[29] and in a hepatitis model mediated by CD4 T and NK cells, LIGHT-/- mice had significantly increased survival and decreased hepatic inflammation.[30]

Evolutionary pressures have guided multiple viral families (pox, herpes, adeno) to target the immediate TNF family as part of the pathogen's strategy to modulate host defenses.[31] For instance, poxviruses utilize soluble TNF receptors as virulence factors in controlling host defenses,[32] providing a prototype of TNFR2-Fc (etanercept). Two distinct human herpesviruses, Herpes Simplex and Cytomegalovirus, target the LIGHT-HVEM-BTLA switch, which strengthens the notion that this pathway is an important control point for regulating immunity.[20,33] Thus, viruses provide additional hints at potential pathways for controlling unwanted immune responses. Interestingly, LIGHT is dispensable for host defense to some viral pathogens indicating that genetic inactivation of LIGHT was not overwhelmingly immunosuppressive.[34,35]

Clinical Indications for LIGHT

The concept that LIGHT provides a critical proinflammatory signal during cellular immune responses is reinforced by the studies of patients with inflammatory bowel disease (IBD).[36,37] Cell surface LIGHT is expressed on human mucosal T-Cells and NK cells and a subpopulation of gut-homing CD4+ T-Cells in the periphery, but not by naïve T-Cells in blood. Quantitative analysis of LIGHT mRNA in a cohort of inflammatory bowel disease patients indicated elevated expression in biopsies from small bowel and from inflamed sites, implicating LIGHT as a mediator of mucosal inflammation. In addition, CD2-mediated stimulation induced LIGHT expression on intestinal CD4+ T-Cells, but not on peripheral blood T-Cells, suggesting a gut-specific, Ag-independent mechanism can regulate LIGHT expression. A susceptibility locus for IBD (*IBD6*) is found on

Chr19p13,[38-40] although this region is gene dense, the status of *LIGHT* as disease candidate is significant and is consistent with observations in experimental animal models.

LIGHT has been implicated as a key mediator in atherosclerosis and rheumatoid arthritis. In atherosclerosis, oxidized HDL induced LIGHT in vitro and LIGHT expression was detected in atherosclerotic plaques with elevated serum levels in patients with angina.[41] In a mouse model of allograft arterial disease (class II mismatch), blockade of the LIGHT pathway with HVEM-Fc attenuated luminal occlusion, decreased intragraft cytokine expression and reduced smooth muscle cell proliferation.[42] In a potentially related observation, an allelic variant of LTα (252 A—>G) is linked to dislipidemia[43] and risk for myocardial infarction[44] although the latter observation was not replicated in all populations.[45] The shared binding of LIGHT and LTα to HVEM provides a potential mechanistic link, however LTα is a low affinity ligand for HVEM[10] (high affinity for TNFR1 and TNFR2) and LTα is also part of the LTαβ-LTβR signaling pathway. Recent studies in mice support a role for LIGHT and LTαβ in regulating lipid metabolism during inflammation.[46] Moreover, LTβR-Fc reduced the dyslipidemia in mice deficient in low-density lipoprotein receptor, which lack the ability to control lipid levels in the blood, an important risk factor for coronary heart disease. Additionally, LIGHT is expressed in inflamed joints and patients with rheumatoid arthritis accumulated elevated serum levels, consistent with a role of LIGHT in bone resorption.[47]

Together, the genetic evidence, animal models, pathogen targeting and expression patterns in human disease provides evidence that therapy directed at antagonizing LIGHT or LTαβ may be effective in inflammation driven mucosal and arterial diseases and similar autoimmune disorders. Early clinical trials of LTβR-Fc in rheumatoid arthritis revealed promising results at low doses, reinforcing the idea that LIGHT and LTαβ may play a role in joint disease.

Directed Therapeutics

The discovery of the LIGHT-HVEM-BTLA switch provides three novel targets for modulating immunity that may be useful in treatment of autoimmune diseases, cancer and infections. The extracellular position of the ligands and receptors in the TNF family provides a direct route to biologic-based therapeutics. Antibodies or decoy receptors antagonize the ligand-receptor interaction, thus interfering in cellular communication. However, antibodies may have secondary effects, such as activating effector systems like complement and cellular cytotoxicity, which may eliminate disease causing cells that express LIGHT or LTαβ on their surface. By contrast, antibody based agonists to individual receptors may be useful in activating specific receptors, in contrast to polygamous ligands, thus selectively enhancing cellular responses required to help resolve persistent infections or eliminate tumors. Blockade of LIGHT and LTαβ may be useful in limiting inflammation in autoimmune diseases. Agonists directed at BTLA may be useful in preventing activation of initial immune responses for instance in allograft rejection or graft vs host disease. By contrast, agonists directed at LTβR or HVEM may be useful in promoting immune responses against tumors and pathogens causing persistent infections.

Historically, no single criterion stood out as a predictor of the relevant clinical indication to apply TNF modulators. Presently, integration of the all available data including experimental animal models and human studies coupled with a mechanistic understanding is required to identify the relevant clinical situation to apply a given inhibitor.

Acknowledgements

The author thanks the assistance of April Kinkade, Mick Croft and Steve Granger for helpful comments. This work was supported in part by grants from the National Institutes of Health (R37AI33068, AI067890 and AI048073).

References

1. Locksley RM, Killeen N, Lenardo MJ. The TNF and TNF receptor superfamilies: Integrating mammalian biology. Cell 2001; 104:487-501.
2. Feldmann M, Brennan FM, Paleolog E et al. Anti-TNFalpha therapy of rheumatoid arthritis: what can we learn about chronic disease? Novartis Found Symp 2004; 256:53-69; discussion 69-73, 106-111, 266-109.

3. Granger SW, Ware CF. Commentary: Turning on LIGHT. J Clinical Investigation 2001; 108:1741-1742.
4. Watts TH. TNF/TNFR family members in costimulation of T-Cell responses. Annu Rev Immunol 2005; 23:23-68.
5. So T, Lee SW, Croft M. Tumor necrosis factor/tumor necrosis factor receptor family members that positively regulate immunity. Int J Hematol 2006; 83(1):1-11.
6. Ware CF. NETWORK COMMUNICATIONS: Lymphotoxins, LIGHT and TNF. Annu Rev Immunol 2005; 23:787-819.
7. Chaplin D, Fu YX. Cytokine regulation of secondary lymphoid organ development. Curr Opin Immunol 1998; 10:289-297.
8. Gommerman JL, Browning JL. Lymphotoxin/light, lymphoid microenvironments and autoimmune disease. Nat Rev Immunol 2003; 3(8):642-655.
9. Drayton DL, Liao S, Mounzer RH, Ruddle NH. Lymphoid organ development: from ontogeny to neogenesis. Nat Immunol 2006; 7(4):344-353.
10. Mauri DN, Ebner R, Montgomery RI et al. LIGHT, a new member of the TNF superfamily and lymphotoxin a are ligands for herpesvirus entry mediator. Immunity 1998; 8:21-30.
11. Rooney IA, Butrovich KD, Glass AA et al. The lymphotoxin-beta receptor is necessary and sufficient for LIGHT-mediated apoptosis of tumor cells. J Biol Chem 2000; 275:14307-14315.
12. Yu KY, Kwon B, Ni J et al. A newly identified member of tumor necrosis factor receptor superfamily (TR6) suppresses LIGHT-mediated apoptosis. J Biol Chem 1999; 274(20):13733-13736.
13. Sedy JR, Gavrieli M, Potter KG et al. B and T-lymphocyte attenuator regulates T-Cell activation through interaction with herpesvirus entry mediator. Nat Immunol 2005; 6(1):90-98.
14. Compaan DM, Gonzalez LC, Tom et al. Attenuating lymphocyte activity: the crystal structure of the BTLA-HVEM complex. J Biol Chem 2005; 280(47):39553-39561.
15. Garapati VP, Lefranc MP. IMGT Colliers de Perles and IgSF domain standardization for T-Cell costimulatory activatory (CD28, ICOS) and inhibitory (CTLA4, PDCD1 and BTLA) receptors. Dev Comp Immunol 2007.
16. Keir ME, Sharpe AH. The B7/CD28 costimulatory family in autoimmunity. Immunol Rev 2005; 204:128-143.
17. Riley JL, June CH. The CD28 family: a T-cell rheostat for therapeutic control of T-cell activation. Blood 2005; 105(1):13-21.
18. Chemnitz JM, Lanfranco AR, Braunstein I et al. B and T-lymphocyte attenuator-mediated signal transduction provides a potent inhibitory signal to primary human CD4 T-Cells that can be initiated by multiple phosphotyrosine motifs. J Immunol 2006; 176(11):6603-6614.
19. Wu TH, Zhen Y, Zeng C et al. B and T-lymphocyte attenuator interacts with CD3zeta and inhibits tyrosine phosphorylation of TCRzeta complex during T-cell activation. Immunol Cell Biol 2007.
20. Cheung TC, Humphreys IR, Potter KG et al. Evolutionarily divergent herpesviruses modulate T-Cell activation by targeting the herpesvirus entry mediator cosignaling pathway. Proc Natl Acad Sci USA 2005; 102(37):13218-13223.
21. Croft M. The evolving crosstalk between co-stimulatory and co-inhibitory receptors: HVEM-BTLA. Trends Immunol 2005; 26(6):292-294.
22. Watts TH, Gommerman JL. The LIGHT and DARC sides of herpesvirus entry mediator. Proc Natl Acad Sci USA 2005; 102(38):13365-13366.
23. Kabashima K, Banks TA, Ansel KM et al. Intrinsic lymphotoxin-beta receptor requirement for homeostasis of lymphoid tissue dendritic cells. Immunity 2005; 22(4):439-450.
24. Scheu S, Alferink J, Potzel T et al. Targeted Disruption of LIGHT Causes Defects in Costimulatory T-Cell activation and reveals cooperation with lymphotoxin beta in mesenteric lymph node genesis. J Exp Med 2002; 195:1613-1624.
25. Tamada K, Ni J, Zhu G et al. Cutting Edge: Selective Impairment of CD8(+) T-Cell Function in Mice Lacking the TNF Superfamily Member LIGHT. J Immunol 2002; 168(10):4832-4835.
26. Liu J, Schmidt CS, Zhao F et al. LIGHT-deficiency impairs CD8+ T-Cell expansion, but not effector function. Int Immunol 2003; 15(7):861-870.
27. Rennert P, Browning JL, Hochman PS. Normal development of lymphnodes is disrupted by soluble LT beta receptor-Ig fusion protein Europe Cytokine Network 1996; 7.
28. Nishikawa S, Honda K, Vieira P. Organogenesis of peripheral lymphoid organs. Immunol Rev 2003; 195:72-80.
29. Mackay F, Browning JL, Lawton P et al. Both the lymphotoxin and tumor necrosis factor pathways are involved in experimental murine models of colitis. Gastroenterology 1998; 115(6):1464-1475.
30. Anand S, Wang P, Yoshimura K et al. Essential role of TNF family molecule LIGHT as a cytokine in the pathogenesis of hepatitis. J Clin Invest 2006; 116(4):1045-1051.

31. Rahman MM, McFadden G. Modulation of tumor necrosis factor by microbial pathogens. PLoS Pathog 2006; 2(2):e4.
32. Smith CA, Davis T, Anderson D et al. A receptor for tumor necrosis factor defines an unusual family of cellular and viral proteins Science 1990; 248:1019-1024.
33. Kinkade A, Ware CF. The DARC conspiracy—virus invasion tactics. Trends Immunol 2006; 27(8):362-367.
34. Sedgmen BJ, Dawicki W, Gommerman JL et al. LIGHT is dispensable for CD4+ and CD8+ T-Cell and antibody responses to influenza A virus in mice. Int Immunol 2006; 18(5):797-806.
35. Banks TA, Rickert S, Benedict CA et al. A-lymphotoxin-IFN-beta axis essential for lymphocyte survival revealed during cytomegalovirus infection. J Immunol 2005; 174(11):7217-7225.
36. Cohavy O, Zhou J, Granger SW et al. LIGHT expression by mucosal T-Cells may regulate IFN-gamma expression in the intestine. J Immunol 2004; 173(1):251-258.
37. Cohavy O, Zhou J, Ware CF et al. LIGHT is constitutively expressed on T and NK cells in the human gut and can be induced by CD2-Mediated signaling. J Immunol 2005; 174(2):646-653.
38. Rioux JD, Silverberg MS, Daly MJ et al. Genomewide search in Canadian families with inflammatory bowel disease reveals two novel susceptibility loci. Am J Hum Genet 2000; 66:1863-1870.
39. Low JH, Williams FA, Yang X et al. Inflammatory bowel disease is linked to 19p13 and associated with ICAM-1. Inflamm Bowel Dis 2004; 10(3):173-181.
40. Tello-Ruiz MK, Curley C, DelMonte T et al. Haplotype-based association analysis of 56 functional candidate genes in the IBD6 locus on chromosome 19. Eur J Hum Genet 2006; 14(6):780-790.
41. Scholz H, Sandberg W, Damas JK et al. Enhanced plasma levels of LIGHT in unstable angina: possible pathogenic role in foam cell formation and thrombosis. Circulation 2005; 112(14):2121-2129.
42. Kosuge H, Suzuki JI, Kakuta T et al. Attenuation of graft arterial disease by manipulation of the LIGHT Pathway. Arterioscler Thromb Vasc Biol 2004.
43. Padovani JC, Pazin-Filho A, Simoes MV. Gene polymorphisms in the TNF locus and the risk of myocardial infarction. Thromb Res 2000; 100(4):263-269.
44. Tanaka T, Ozaki K. Inflammation as a risk factor for myocardial infarction. J Hum Genet 2006; 51(7):595-604.
45. Clarke R, Xu P, Bennett D et al. Lymphotoxin-alpha gene and risk of myocardial infarction in 6,928 cases and 2,712 controls in the ISIS case-control study. PLoS Genet 2006; 2(7):e107.
46. Lo JC, Wang Y, Tumanov AV et al. Lymphotoxin beta receptor-dependent control of lipid homeostasis. Science 2007; 316(5822):285-288.
47. Edwards JR, Sun SG, Locklin R et al. LIGHT (TNFSF14), a novel mediator of bone resorption, is elevated in rheumatoid arthritis. Arthritis Rheum 2006; 54(5):1451-1462.
48. Shaikh R, Santee S, Granger SW et al. Constitutive expression of LIGHT on T-Cells leads to lymphocyte activation, inflammation and tissue destruction. J Immunol 2001; 167:6330-6337.
49. Wang J, Lo JC, Foster A et al. The regulation of T-Cell homeostasis and autoimmunity by T-Cell derived LIGHT. J Clin Invest 2001; 108:1771-1780.
50. Wang J, Anders RA, Wang Y et al. The critical role of LIGHT in promoting intestinal inflammation and Crohn's disease. J Immunol 2005; 174(12):8173-8182.
51. Fan Z, Yu P, Wang Y et al. NK-cell activation by LIGHT triggers tumor-specific CD8+ T-cell immunity to reject established tumors. Blood 2006; 107(4):1342-1351.
52. Brown GR, Lee EL, El-Hayek J et al. IL-12-independent LIGHT signaling enhances MHC class II disparate CD4+ T-Cell alloproliferation, IFN-gamma responses and intestinal graft-versus-host disease. J Immunol 2005; 174(8):4688-4695.
53. Wu Q, Fu YX, Sontheimer RD. Blockade of lymphotoxin signaling inhibits the clinical expression of murine graft-versus-host skin disease. J Immunol 2004; 172(3):1630-1636.
54. Gommerman JL, Giza K, Perper S et al. A role for surface lymphotoxin in experimental autoimmune encephalomyelitis independent of LIGHT. J Clin Invest 2003; 112(5):755-767.
55. Plant SR, Iocca HA, Wang Y et al. Lymphotoxin beta receptor (Lt betaR): dual roles in demyelination and remyelination and successful therapeutic intervention using Lt betaR-Ig protein. J Neurosci 2007; 27(28):7429-7437.
56. Fava RA, Notidis E, Hunt J et al. A role for the lymphotoxin/LIGHT axis in the pathogenesis of murine collagen-induced arthritis. J Immunol 2003; 171(1):115-126.
57. Ye Q, Fraser CC, Gao W et al. Modulation of LIGHT-HVEM costimulation prolongs cardiac allograft survival. J Exp Med 2002; 195(6):795-800.
58. Xu Y, Flies AS, Flies DB et al. Selective targeting of the LIGHT-HVEM costimulatory system for the treatment of graft-versus-host disease. Blood 2007; 109(9):4097-4104.

CHAPTER 11

GITR:
A Modulator of Immune Response and Inflammation

Giuseppe Nocentini and Carlo Riccardi*

Abstract

Glucocorticoid-Induced TNFR-Related (GITR) protein belongs to Tumor Necrosis Factor Receptor Superfamily (TNFRSF) and stimulates both the acquired and innate immunity. It is expressed in several cells and tissues, including T and Natural Killer (NK) cells and is activated by its ligand, GITRL, mainly expressed on Antigen Presenting Cells (APCs) and endothelial cells. GITR/GITRL system participates in the development of autoimmune/inflammatory responses and graft vs. host disease and potentiates response to infection and tumors. These effects are due to several concurrent mechanisms including: co-activation of effector T-cells, inhibition of regulatory T (Treg) cells, NK-cell co-activation, activation of macrophages, modulation of DC function and regulation of the extravasation process. In this chapter we describe: 1) the main structural features of GITR and GITRL, 2) the transduction pathways activated by GITR triggering, 3) the effects derived from GITR/GITRL system interaction, considering the interplay between the different cells of the immune system. Moreover, the potential use of GITR/GITRL modulators in disease treatment is discussed.

Introduction

The immune system is the main player in protection against pathogens and against transformed cells. Thus, immunodepression is an important cause of infection (peculiar of chronic infections) and probably plays a role in the development of tumors. On the other hand, exaggerated immune responses are responsible for autoimmune diseases, lesions deriving from chronic inflammation (e.g., fibrosis) or even death (e.g., shock). Modulation of the immune system response is useful in the treatment and/or prevention of several pathological conditions, including persistent infections, chronic inflammation, graft vs. host disease, transplant rejection and tumors. However, current treatments are not completely satisfactory and new therapeutic approaches should be developed to reach cure for disease.

The immune response derives from a complex interplay between the cells of innate immunity including monocytes/macrophages, neutrophils (PMNs), natural killer (NK) cells and dendritic cells (DCs), the vascular system actively participating in recruitment of inflammatory cells and the cells of acquired immunity including T- and B-lymphocytes. T-cell response is due to activation of effector T-cells (CD4[+] and CD8[+]) following triggering by an antigen, associated to antigen presenting cells (APCs) and costimulatory signals (e.g., through activation of CD28 receptor) that allows an efficient and potent activation. The expansion of activated effector T-cells is controlled by some specialized subsets of T-lymphocytes with suppressor activity. The naturally occurring thymus-derived regulatory T-cells (Treg cells, CD4[+]CD25[+]) are the most studied cells[1] but other

*Corresponding Author: Carlo Riccardi—Dipartimento di Medicina Clinica e Sperimentale, Sezione di Farmacologia, Università di Perugia, Via del Giochetto, 06100 Perugia. Email: riccardi@unipg.it

Therapeutic Targets of the TNF Superfamily, edited by Iqbal S. Grewal.

suppressor cells such as CD8+CD25+, CD8+CD28- or CD4-CD8-CD3+ T-cells, have been shown to play an important role.[2] A sophisticated interplay among effector T-cells, suppressor T-cells and APCs (either immmunogenic and/or tolerogenic) determines the final outcome of the immune response.

Proteins belonging to the tumor necrosis factor receptor superfamily (TNFRSF), characterized by the presence of cysteine pseudo-repeats in the extracellular region, are deeply involved in the activation, differentiation and survival of cells of the immune system.[3] Their ligands, belonging to the tumor necrosis factor superfamily (TNFSF), are type II transmembrane proteins that are not only able to specifically stimulate the respective receptors but can also signal inside the cells where they are expressed. This chapter describes the role of Glucocorticoid-Induced TNFR-Related (GITR) protein, in the development of acquired and innate response. Recent data, outlining a potential role of GITR in the homeostasis of other systems, will be briefly considered.

GITR: Structure, Transduction Pathway and Tissue Distribution

GITR Gene and GITR Splicing Variants

GITR is a type I transmembrane glycoprotein, cloned in 1997[4] and selectively activated by its ligand (GITRL).[5-11] GITR gene comprises 5 exons, the first 3 encoding the extracellular domain; exon 4 encoding a small part of the extracellular domain, the transmembrane domain and part of the cytoplasmic domain and exon 5 encoding the cytoplasmic domain.[12] Both murine and human GITR genes originate alternatively spliced products.[13] Among them, soluble spliced products of the GITR gene: mGITRD, mGITRD2 and hGITR variant 2.[13] These soluble proteins may function as a decoy receptor, inhibiting GITR-GITRL interaction, and if they are expressed at high levels in physiological or pathological conditions, it becomes difficult to predict the in vivo effect of administering anti-GITR Abs and other GITR or GITRL soluble proteins.

The extracellular domain of GITR is formed by 3 cysteine-rich domains (CRDs) that appear to be noncanonical. However, the first CRD of GITR is incomplete and badly conserved among mammalian species, suggesting it may have a low functional meaning (Krautz et al submitted). The cytoplasmic domain of GITR shows good homology with the cytoplasmic domains of OX40, 4-1BB and CD27 (similarity between 45 and 50%).[12] The homologies span the complete cytoplasmic domain but are centered in 2 segments called domain 1 and 2.[12] Domain 1 (R-[KR] -x(0,2)-[KHR]-x(0,2)-[PY]) is next to transmembrane region. Domain 2 (S-[CF]-x(0,2)-P-x(0,1)- [QE]-E-E-x(2,7)-[ED]) is close to the –COOH terminus of the proteins and we have proposed to call it "life domain" opposite to the "death domain" present in other TNFRSF members whose triggering activates apoptosis.[4,12] In conclusion, the good homology in the cytoplasmic domain between GITR, CD27, OX40 and 4-1BB and a quite good homology with CD40,[14] together with some functional similarity, led us to define a new subfamily inside TNFRSF.[4,12]

GITR Transduction Pathways

There is clear evidence that, following activation, GITR binds and activates several TNF Receptor Associated Factors (TRAFs)[6,7,15] and that the domain responsible for TRAF binding is the PEEE motif, present in the domain 2. GITR triggering activates Nuclear Factor κB (NF-κB), but the correlation among NF-κB activation (through both canonical and noncanonical pathways), TRAFs and GITR is still under investigation (Krautz et al submitted). In particular, some studies have described TRAF2-induced NF-κB activation following GITR activation, while another study described TRAF2-induced NF-κB inactivation.[6,16]

GITR has no death domain in its structure. However, it can induce apoptosis by binding a protein, that has a death domain homology region in its central region, called Siva.[14,17] Siva modulates Bcl-2 family members and caspase activation.[18] In vitro binding studies and sequence alignment support the conclusion that P-[IE]-[QE]-E (inside domain 2) is the main binding motif for Siva.[14] This domain is also capable of TRAF2 binding. Thus, it is possible that, depending on the functional status of the cell, GITR triggering may lead to different effects. Indeed, a Casein

Kinase II phosphorilation (CKII) site is present in GITR and we have evidence that phosphorilation modulates TRAF2 and Siva binding in an opposite way (Nocentini et al unpublished).

In vitro data suggest that GITR also binds the protein arginine N-methyltransferase (PRMT1) in analogy with BTG2,[19] a cytoplasmic protein with antiproliferative activity showing homology with GITR (Krautz et al submitted). PRMT1, the enzyme that catalyses most of the type-I methylation reactions, is involved in protein trafficking, signal transduction and transcriptional regulation[20] and is able to activate NF-κB.[21] The functional meaning of the GITR/PRMT1 interaction is at present unknown.

GITR Tissue distribution

GITR mRNA is mainly expressed in naïve and activated T- and NK-cells, where it is upregulated for several days following cell activation (Table 1). On the contrary, immature thymic CD4$^+$CD8$^+$ cells do not express mGITR.[27]

CD4$^+$CD25$^+$ Treg cells and other regulatory cells such as CD4$^+$CD25$^-$, CD8$^+$CD25$^+$ and CD8$^+$CD28$^-$ express GITR at high levels (Table 1). This observation has suggested that GITR is a marker of suppressor cells. However, activated effector T-cells express similar high levels of GITR.

GITR is also expressed in hematological cells, other than T- or NK-cells, including mast cells, PMNs, B-cells, macrophages and other APCs (Table 1). Moreover, GITR expression has also been detected on osteoclast precursor cells, keratinocytes and retinal pigment epithelial cells (RPE)(Table 1).[36,38,39]

Table 1. GITR expression in mouse and human cells

Cell Type	Level of GITR Expression	Ref.
Naïve CD4$^+$CD25$^-$ T-cells (effector function)	Intermediate	11, 22-26
Naïve CD8$^+$ T-cells (effector function)	Intermediate/low	11, 24, 25, 27
T-cells with suppressor function, including Treg cells	High	11, 22-24, 26, 28-30
Natural killer (NK) cells	Intermediate	31
B-cells	Low	27
Monocytes/macrophages	Low	27, 32-34
Plasmacytoid dendritic cells (DCs)	No expression	32
Mature DCs	No expression	32
Mast cells	Intermediate	35
Polymorphonucleated leukocytes (PMNs)	Intermediate	32, 34
Eosinophils	Intermediate/low	32
Basophils	Intermediate/low	32
Activated T-cells with effector function	High/very high	22-24, 26
Activated T-cells with suppressor function	Very high	22-24, 26, 27, 29
Activated NK-cells	High	31
Activated B-cells	Intermediate/low	27
Activated monocytes/macrophages	Intermediate/low	27, 33, 34
Activated plasmacytoid DCs	Intermediate	32
Activated DCs	Intermediate	32
Activated mast cells	Intermediate	35
Activated PMNs	High	34
Endothelial cells (ECs)	No expression	33
Activated ECs	Intermediate/low	33
Keratinocytes	Intermediate	36
Osteoclasts	Low	37

Table 2. GITRL expression in mouse and human cells

Cell Type	Level of GITRL Expression	Ref.
Dendritic cells (DCs)	Medium/low	6, 8-10, 32, 42
Activated plasmacytoid DCs (2-48 h)	Very high	32
Monocytes/macrophages	Medium/low	6, 8-10, 32, 42
Activated monocytes/macrophages (2-48 h)	High	43, 44
B-cells	Medium/low	6, 8-10, 32, 42
Naïve T-cells	No expression/low	9, 32, 45
Activated T-cells (3-24 h)	Medium/low	25, 32
Glucocorticoid treated T-cells (3 h)	Medium/low	Krautz et al submitted
Eosinophils	Low	32
Basophils	Low	32
Endothelial cells (ECs)	High	7, 46
IFN-activated ECs	Very high	46

GITRL: Tissue Distribution and Function

GITRL is a recently cloned type II glycoprotein, belonging to the TNF superfamily (TNFSF).[6-11] This protein is formed by an N-terminal cytoplasmic domain, a transmembrane domain and a –COOH terminal extracellular domain.[8] The cytoplasmic domain of GITRL shows a high homology with OX40L[40] and, despite its shortness (21 amino acidic residues), may activate an intracellular signal following GITR/GITRL binding.[38,41] This possibility is further suggested by the high similarity among GITRL cytoplasmic domains of mammals, showing the conserved motif E-x-M-P-L-x(2)-S-x(2)-Q-x-A-x-R-x(2)-K-x-W-L.

GITRL is expressed in professional and nonprofessional APCs, including unstimulated myeloid DC subsets, plasmacytoid DC precursors (pDC), B-cells and monocytes (Table 2).[6,8-10,32,42] High levels of GITRL expression have been detected in endothelial cells (ECs) and in particular in microvascular-derived ECs.[46] Other cells, reported in Table 2, express GITRL at lower levels,[32] but it must still be ascertained if the low mRNA level observed determines sufficient protein expression to have a functional meaning.

In response to pro-inflammatory stimuli, GITRL is rapidly upregulated in APCs and ECs and declines in 1-2 days to the initial or even lower levels (Table 2). However, not all pro-inflammatory stimuli promote GITRL upregulation. For example, in ECs, GITRL is upregulated by IFNα and IFNβ and not by proinflammatory cytokines and LPS.[46] In addition, GITRL is upregulated in T-cells after activation[25] or glucocorticoid treatment (Krautz et al submitted).

GITR/GITRL System Modulates T-Lymphocyte Activation

GITR modulates effector T-cell activation. In fact, several studies using mice in which GITR expression was deleted (GITR-/-) or mice treated with agonist anti-GITR antibody, demonstrate that GITR participates in the activation of the immune response. As detailed in Table 3, physiological or pharmacological GITR triggering exacerbates autoimmune diseases, graft vs. host reaction and potentiates anti-tumor and antiviral responses. Moreover, inhibiting GITR triggering by using GITR-Fc fusion protein (the extracellular domain of GITR fused with Fc fragment) ameliorates autoimmune and inflammatory diseases (Table 4).

How GITR triggering modulates activation of effector T-cells is reported in the paragraphs below and summarized in Figure 1. This aspect has recently been summarized in some review papers.[45,65,66]

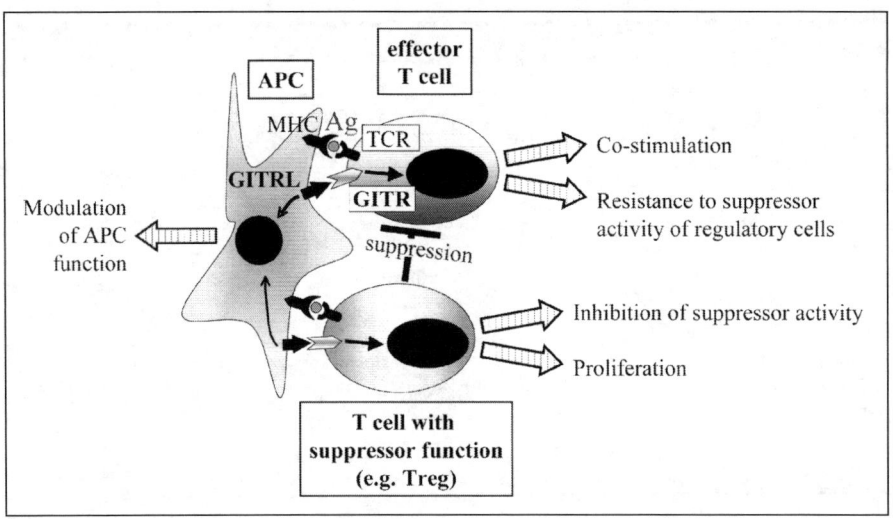

Figure 1. Effects of GITR/GITRL system activation in the modulation of responder T-cell activation. During antigen (Ag) presentation GITR is triggered in responder and regulatory T-cells (e.g., Treg). Triggering of GITRL modulates APC (e.g., dendritic cell) function.

Co-Activating Function on Effector T-Lymphocytes

GITR is a co-activating molecule. In fact, GITR costimulation increases activation and proliferation of TCR-triggered CD4$^+$ and CD8$^+$ T-cells.[9,11,15,24,25] This effect is evident when GITR is triggered by agonist anti-GITR Abs, soluble GITRL or GITRL-transfected cells.[9,11,23-25] It is also evident when T-cells from wild type and GITR$^{-/-}$ mice are compared. Among several activation-related effects, anti-GITR and anti-CD3 Ab cotreatment caused higher IL-2 and IFNγ production and induced higher expression of T-cell activation markers, compared to treatment with anti-CD3 Ab alone.[11]

The costimulatory power of GITR seems to be lower than that of CD28 but qualitatively different.[11,24,27,67] In fact, studies on total lymph node cell populations of GITR$^{-/-}$ and CD28$^{-/-}$ mice demonstrated that in the presence of weak CD3 triggering (soluble anti-CD3 in the absence of feeder) and IL-2, the lack of CD28 impaired only in part T-cell activation, while the lack of GITR completely abolished T-cell activation.[25] Moreover, studying the effect of RPE cells on T-cell proliferation, it was demonstrated that GITR triggering abrogated RPE-mediated immunosuppression, while a weaker effect was seen with CD28 triggering,[67] confirming the different effects of CD28 and GITR.

Some studies suggest a specific role for GITR in CD4$^+$ and CD8$^+$ cells in relation to CD28. During the activation process of CD4$^+$CD25$^-$ cells, GITR upregulation is mainly dependent on CD28 stimulation, as demonstrated by an increased expression of GITR after CD28 triggering and a substantial inhibition of GITR upregulation when physiological CD28 engagement was inhibited by anti-CD80/86 Abs.[25,68] Thus, in CD4$^+$ cells, GITR should be regarded as one of the pathways activated by CD28 triggering. In CD8$^+$ T-cells, the relation GITR/CD28 is somewhat different. In fact, our unpublished studies indicate that in the absence of GITR, CD8$^+$ cells cannot be stimulated by CD28 when suboptimal doses of anti-CD3 Ab are used while in the absence of CD28, GITR can normally exert its co-activating functions (Fig. 2)(Ronchetti et al manuscript in preparation). Thus, in CD8$^+$ cells, GITR seems to be a molecule necessary for CD28 costimulatory activity. These findings may explain why GITR activation potentiates more the response of CD8$^+$ cells than that of CD4$^+$ effector cells in some in vivo studies.[51,53]

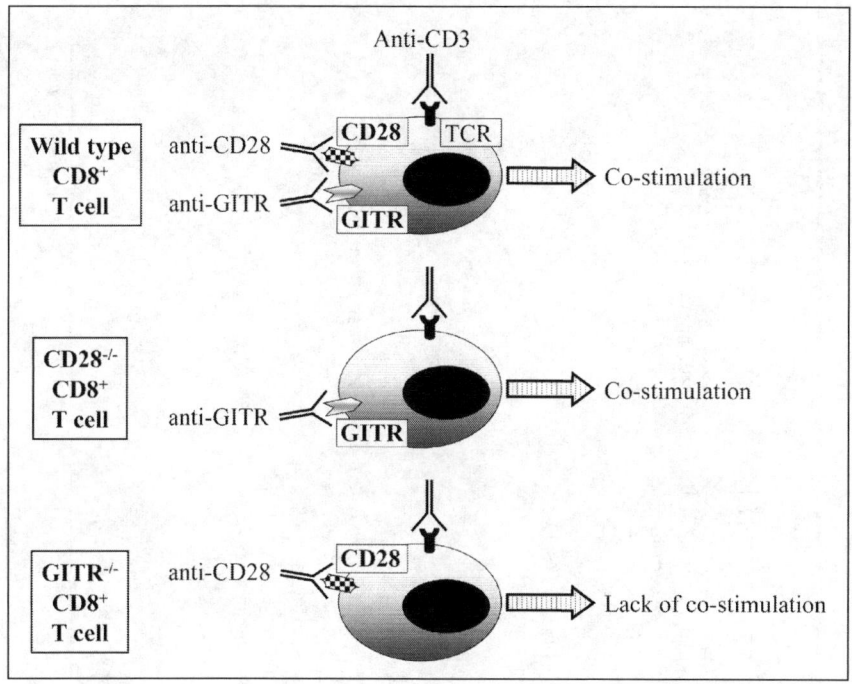

Figure 2. GITR triggering is necessary for costimulation of CD8⁺ responder T-cells, while CD28 triggering is dispensable, as demonstrated in GITR⁻/⁻ mice (unpublished data).

Modulation of the Interplay Regulatory/Effector T-Cells

GITR triggering enhances T-cell activation also through mechanisms different from co-stimulation of effector T-cells. One of these mechanisms is inhibition of regulatory T-cell activity (including Treg cells). In fact, two studies, aimed at evaluating the possible effect of agonist Abs directed towards several TNFRSF members, demonstrated that anti-GITR Ab was the only one capable of reverting the suppressor effect of Treg cells.[22,27] Other studies have demonstrated the same effect when GITR triggering was exerted by GITRL expressed on APCs.[8,9,11,69] GITR triggering is also effective in abolishing the activity of other suppressor cells such as RPE cells,[67] or CD4⁺CD25⁻ T-cells present in aged mice[70] and in old human donors.[71] The most obvious mechanism explaining the lower suppressor activity of Treg cells is that GITR engagement in Treg cells inhibits their activity.[65] However, it is also possible that GITR triggering in effector T-cells makes them more resistant to Treg cell suppression.[45] Our current opinion is that both mechanisms are effective. In fact, two studies suggest that in effector T-cells GITR triggering activates a pathway (still undisclosed) distinct from that activated by CD28, specifically antagonizing the immuno-suppression.[25,67] Others studies demonstrate that GITR triggering activates a signaling pathway in Treg cells, as directly demonstrated by modulation of granzyme B in GITR-cotriggered Treg cells[72] or by in vitro and in vivo experiments, demonstrating that triggering of GITR expressed in Treg cells is responsible for the increased activation of effector T-cells.[11,27,47,73]

After GITR triggering, the inhibition of Treg cell suppressor activity (and of other T subsets with suppressor activity) is transient. Moreover, GITR-cotriggered Treg cells lose their anergic state and proliferate.[11,24,69] The physiological role of GITR for Treg cell expansion is also suggested by a decreased amount of Treg cells in GITR⁻/⁻ mice.[11,25] Thus, the transient inhibition of suppressor activity could be countered by an increased Treg cell proliferation and could explain why in vivo

Table 3. Effect of GITR activation in mouse disease models

Disease Model	GITR Stimulation*	Effect	Ref.
Normal mouse	Anti-GITR mAb	Pharmacological GITR stimulation promotes development of autoimmune gastritis	27
Experimental Autoimmune Encephalomyelitis (EAE)	Anti-GITR mAb	Pharmacological GITR stimulation exacerbates EAE clinical disease progression as suggested by: • decreased survival • heavier disease	23
Collagen-Induced Arthritis (CIA), GITR^{-/-} mice	Physiologic GITR activation	Lack of GITR reduced CIA severity as suggested by: • reduced erythema and edema • reduced bone erosion	47
CIA and OVA-induced allergic airway inflammation	Anti-GITR mAb	Pharmacological GITR stimulation exacerbated CIA severity as suggested by: • increase of articular index disease • increased of affected paws • earlier onset of arthritis Pharmacological GITR stimulation exacerbated murine allergic airway inflammation	48
Carrageenan-induced lung inflammation (pleurisy), GITR^{-/-} mice	Physiologic GITR activation	Lack of GITR reduced pleurisy severity as suggested by: • decreased production of turbid exudate containing a lower number of leukocytes • reduction of inflammatory markers.	33
Bleomycin-induced chronic lung injury, GITR^{-/-} mice	Physiologic GITR activation	Lack of GITR reduced chronic lung injury severity as suggested by: • increased survival • body weight gain • reduction of edema formation • reduction of lung injury • reduction of PMN infiltration	49

continued on next page

Table 3. *Continued*

Disease Model	GITR Stimulation*	Effect	Ref.
TNBS-induced inflammatory bowel diseases (IBD), GITR-/- mice	Physiologic GITR activation	Lack of GITR reduced TNBS-induced colitis severity by reducing innate immune responses and effector T-cell activition as suggested by: • increased survival • body weight gain • amelioration of clinical and histological score • reduction of PMN infiltration • lower level of cytokines • amelioration of clinical score • lower level of inflammatory cytokines	34
TNBS-induced IBD	Anti-GITR mAb	Pharmacological GITR stimulation exacerbated the TNBS-induced colitis severity as suggested by: • decreased survival • increased histological injury	50
Acute Graft Vs Host Disease (GVHD)	Anti-GITR mAb	Pharmacological GITR stimulation • exacerbated GVHD induced by: CD8+CD25- T-cells • decreased GVHD induced by: CD4+CD25- T-cells	51
Chronic GVHD	Anti-GITR mAb	Pharmacological GITR stimulation • increased survival • blocked the progression of cGVHD • inhibited glomerulonephritis • decreased levels of IgG1 anti-DNA autoantibody	52

continued on next page

Table 3. *Continued*

Disease Model	GITR Stimulation*	Effect	Ref.
GVHD	Anti-GITR mAb	Pharmacological GITR stimulation converted chronic GVHD in acute GVHD as suggested by: • body weight loss • increased intestinal damage • lymphopenia	53
Autoimmune diabetes in SCID recipients	Anti-GITR mAb	Pharmacological GITR stimulation promoted development of autoimmune diabetes in SCID recipients mice when transferred with diabetogenic BDC2.5 CD4$^+$ T and protected by OVA-specific DO11.10 CD4$^+$ T-cells following stimulation with soluble OVA	54
Experimental autoimmune thyroiditis (EAT)	Anti-GITR mAb	Pharmacological GITR stimulation interfered with EAT tolerance by: enabling thyroiditogenic T-cells as suggested by: • increased cell infiltration • increased histological injury	55
Acute Friend virus infection	Anti-GITR mAb	Pharmacological GITR stimulation increased immune response as suggested by: • reductions in both acute virus loads and CD4$^+$ T-cell-related pathology • long-term improvement of CD8$^+$ T-cell-mediated antitumor responses (tumor size)	56
Chronic Friend virus infection	Anti-GITR mAb	Pharmacological GITR stimulation increased immune response as suggested by: • improved IFNγ production • reduction of viral loads	57
Herpes simplex virus (HSV) infection	Anti-GITR mAb	Pharmacological GITR stimulation increased immune response • enhanced HSV-specific CD4$^+$ T-cell immunity • diminished T-cell mediated ocular lesions	44
Human immunodeficiency virus (HIV) DNA vaccines	GITRL 4-trimer	Multimeric soluble GITRL enhanced immune response to DNA vaccination as suggested by: • increased CD8$^+$ T-cell • increased CD4$^+$ T-cell • increased antibody responses	58

continued on next page

Table 3. *Continued*

Disease Model	GITR Stimulation*	Effect	Ref.
α-galagtosylceramide treatment, hypersensitivity pneumonitis	Anti-GITR mAb	Pharmacological GITR stimulation induced NKT-cell activation in α-galagtosylceramide-treated mice as suggested by: • increased cytokine production The adoptive transfer of GITR pretriggered NKT-cells into CD1d$^{-/-}$ mice attenuated hypersensitivity pneumonitis	31
Filariasis	Anti-GITR mAb	Pharmacological GITR stimulation increased immune response as suggested by: • increased parasite killing	59
Candida albicans infection, GITR$^{-/-}$ mice	Physiologic GITR activation	Lack of GITR decreased *C. albicans* induced disease as suggested by: • increased survival • decreased yeast load in kidneys and brain	40
B16 melanoma	Anti-GITR mAb	Pharmacological GITR stimulation increased immune response as suggested by • tumor diameter reduction	60
B16 melanoma	GITRL over expression	Increased GITR stimulation inhibited tumor growth as suggested by: • increased survival • reduction of tumor volume	61
MethA-induced fibrosarcoma	Anti-GITR mAb	Pharmacological GITR stimulation increased immune response as suggested by: • eradication of established tumors (90%) without eliciting overt autoimmune disease • potent tumor-specific immunity promoting 100% rejection of reinoculated tumors	62

continued on next page

Table 3. *Continued*

Disease Model	GITR Stimulation*	Effect	Ref.
Antitumor vaccine with differentiation antigens	Anti-GITR mAb	Pharmacological GITR stimulation enhanced immune response to vaccination with tumor differentiation antigens as suggested by: • increased tumor-free survival • enhanced primary CD8+ T-cell responses against tumors • prolonged persistence of the antigen-specific CD8+ T-cells It was associated with a modest increase of focal autoimmunity	63
Splanchnic artery occlusion (SAO) shock, GITR−/− mice	Physiologic GITR activation	Lack of GITR partially protected from SAO as suggested by: • increased survival • significant decrease of marker of histological injury	64
UV light-induced inflammation	Physiologic GITR activation	Lack of GITR increase UVB light-induced apoptosis in keratinocytes	36

*The effects of GITR stimulation were studied by comparing GITR−/− with GITR+/+ mice (physiologic GITR activation), by using an antiGITR mAb (DTA1) or by GITRL (soluble or overexpressed in cells).

Table 4. Effect of GITR inhibition and/or GITRL activation in mouse disease models

Disease Model	Inhibition of GITR Stimulation or GITRL Triggering*	Effect	Ref.
Carrageenan-induced lung inflammation (pleurisy)	GITR-Fc	Cotreatment with carrageenan and GITR-Fc fusion protein decreased pleurisy severity as suggested by: • decreased number of inflammatory cells in pleural space • decreased PMN lung infiltration	33
Bleomycin-induced chronic lung injury	GITR-Fc	Continuous infusion of GITR-Fc fusion protein in bleomycin-treated mice decreased chronic lung injury severity as suggested by: • increased survival • body weight gain • reduction of edema formation • reduction of lung injury • reduction of PMN infiltration • reduction of cytokine production	49
TNBS-induced inflammatory bowel diseases (IBD)	GITR-Fc	Repeated treatment with GITR-Fc fusion protein in TNBS-treated mice weakened IBD in normal mice and in lymphocyte-deficient SCID mice as suggested by: • body weight gain • amelioration of clinical and histological score • reduction of PMN infiltration • lower level of IFNγ	34
Normal mouse	Soluble GITR	Pharmacological treatment caused: • enlarged spleen • increased percentage of PMNs and monocytes in peripheral blood	42

*By using the extracellular domain of GITR (in dimeric form, GITR-Fc; as a monomer, soluble GITR) two effects can be obtained: (1) inhibition of physiologic GITR stimulation by endogenous ligand, (2) GITRL triggering. Data do not clarify which is the prominent effect.

GITR stimulation does not cause overt autoimmunity,[62,74] suggesting that it may have a physiological role in the control of inflammation.

In conclusion, GITR triggering has 3 effects on Treg/effector cell interplay: (1) transient inhibition of Treg cell suppressor activity, (2) decreased sensitivity of effector T-cells to Treg suppression, (3) promotion of proliferation and expansion of the Treg cell compartment.

Modulation of the Interplay DCs/Regulatory/Effector T-Cells

Evidence for modulation of DC function by the GITR/GITRL system was first obtained studying *C. albicans* infection in GITR[-/-] mice.[40] In particular, a higher level of IL-12 in DCs of GITR[-/-] mice due to the lack of GITR and the consequent activation of GITRL has been detected. Thus, GITRL can modulate the immune response not only by triggering GITR expressed by effector and Treg cells, but also by modulating DC activity through reverse signaling.

GITR/GITRL System Modulates Innate Immune Response

Physiological or pharmacological GITR triggering exacerbates acute and chronic inflammatory response and shock in mouse models (Table 3). Moreover, inhibiting GITR triggering by using GITR-Fc fusion protein ameliorates inflammation (Table 4). These effects are due not only to modulation of T-cell activation but also to modulation of extravasation and innate immunity, as summarized in Table 5.

GITR-GITRL System in Leukocyte Extravasation and Edema

In GITR[-/-] mice, the extravasation process following pro-inflammatory stimuli is hampered and the presence of pro-inflammatory cells, including macrophages and PMNs, is decreased compared to wild type mice.[33,64] Moreover, in wild type mice, the co-administration of GITR-Fc which blocks GITR triggering by GITRL, decreases the extravasation process following pro-inflammatory treatments.[33,49] Adhesion molecules ICAM-1, P-selectin and E-selectin are upregulated in ECs following inflammation, but in GITR[-/-] mice their upregulation is almost completely abolished.[33,64] Since during the inflammatory response both GITR and GITRL are expressed in ECs, the mechanisms potentially responsible for the results observed are more than one, including GITR and/or GITRL signaling. Since a recent study demonstrated that GITR-activated signals are able to modulate expression of P-selectin and E-selectin in T-cells,[67] the more likely mechanism is that GITR

Table 5. Effect of GITR/GITRL activation on cells of innate immunity and endothelial cells

Cell Type	Mechanism Underlined	Effect	Ref.
Macrophages	GITRL activation	Increased expression of COX-2 and increased production of PGE$_2$	37,75
	GITR (and/or GITRL) activation*	Increased expression of COX-2 and increased production of PGE$_2$	33,47
	GITRL activation	Increased expression of iNOS and increased production of NO	75,76
	GITR (and/or GITRL) activation*	Increased expression of iNOS and increased production of NO	33,47
	GITRL activation	Increased production of MMP-2, -9, -13	44,77,78
	GITR activation	Decreased production of MMP-9	44
	GITR activation	Increased production of MMP-9	79
	GITR (and/or GITRL) activation*	Increased production of TNFα, IFNγ, IL-1β, IL-6, IL-12, MIP-1, MIP-2	33,47,49,64
	GITR activation	Increased production of TNFα, IL-8, MCP-1	79
NK-cells	GITR activation	Increased production of IFNγ	32
NKT-cells	GITR activation	Increased production of IL-4, IL-10, IL-13, IFNγ	31
Endothelial cells	GITR (and/or GITRL) activation*	Increased expression of adhesion molecules (ICAM-1, P-selectin, E-selectin)	33,64

*These studies were performed using GITR[-/-] mice. Therefore, both GITR and GITRL triggering lack. However, results obtained treating GITR[+/+] mice with GITR-Fc suggest that GITR more than GITRL triggering is involved.

(expressed on ECs), triggered by GITRL (expressed on PMNs and monocytes), participates in the upregulation of adhesion molecules.

Another feature regulated by ECs is edema, an event due to several mechanisms, including tight junction changes. In some inflammatory models, there were less edema and exudate formation in GITR[-/-] mice than in GITR[+/+] mice.[33,47,49] Staining of ZO-1, a marker of tight junction integrity, showed much higher degree of immunostaining disruption in lungs of carrageenan-treated GITR[+/+] mice compared to carrageenan-treated GITR[-/-] mice, suggesting a role of GITR/GITRL system in tight junction integrity.[33]

GITR-GITRL System and Activation of Innate Immunity

GITR triggering plays a role in NK and NKT-cell activation. Mouse NKT-cells are costimulated by GITR at a level comparable to that obtained with CD28 cotriggering, both in vitro and in vivo, as assessed by cytokine production.[31] GITR triggering in NK-cells promotes NK-cell cytotoxicity and IFNγ production.[32] Moreover, NK lytic activity induced by activated DCs is decreased by neutralizing anti-GITRL Abs suggesting that GITRL expressed in DCs has a physiologic role in activating NK-cells.

The activation level of macrophages is higher in wild type mice than in GITR[-/-] mice.[33,47] This phenomenon could be due to several mechanisms including higher density of inflammatory cells and higher concentration of pro-inflammatory cytokines in the inflammatory site of wild type mice due to a more efficient extravasation process. However, it is possible that GITR/GITRL system participates in macrophage activation. For example, it favors production of the inducible isoform of cyclo-oxigenase (COX-2) as suggested by lower COX-2 levels in the joints of GITR[-/-] mice following collagen-induced arthritis[47] or in the lungs following carrageenan-induced pleurisy.[33] This effect may be due to GITRL triggering as suggested by in vitro studies, where GITRL was stimulated by sGITR (the extracellular domain of GITR produced in *E. coli* as a monomer) or GITR-Fc (produced in eukaryotic cells as a dimer) and induced COX-2 and PGE_2 production in bone-marrow stromal cells, peritoneal macrophages and RAW 264,7 cell line.[37,75] Similar in vitro and in vivo results were obtained with the pro-inflammatory molecule NO produced by the inducible isoform nitric oxide synthase (iNOS).[33,47,76,80]

Matrix metalloproteinases (MMPs) are synthesized in response to diverse stimuli including cytokines, growth factors, hormones and oxidative stress and are involved in the development of several diseases, including inflammatory and vascular diseases. GITR/GITRL interaction causes modulation of some MMPs but contrasting data have been published so that it is not clear if either an increase or decrease of MMPs is induced. In fact, Kim et al showed that GITR stimulation by anti-GITR Ab induces MMP-9 in mouse and human macrophages from different tissues and monocyte/macrophage cell lines[79] while other studies have demonstrated that GITRL triggering by sGITR upregulates MMP-9 and MMP-2 in murine peritoneal macrophages[78] and anti-GITRL Ab upregulates MMP-9 secretion in CD11b[+] cells isolated from virus-infected corneas.[44] It has been suggested that this could be due to the block of GITR/GITRL interaction instead of GITRL triggering. In fact, anti-GITR treatment negatively modulated MMP-9 expression both in vitro (CD11[+] cells) and in vivo (corneal extract of mice with herpes simplex virus infection). Finally, human GITRL triggering (shGITR) induces MMP-13 secretion in fibroblast-like synovial cells and may promote tissue destruction in rheumatoid arthritis.[77]

Cytokine production is also modulated by GITR/GITRL system. For example, in GITR[-/-] mice, the partial resistance to CIA, is accompanied by less IFNγ, IL-6, TNFα, macrophage inflammatory protein-1 (MIP-1) and MIP-2 secretion[47] and the partial resistance to TNBS-induced colitis is correlated with less IL-12, TNF-α and IL-6 produced by lamina propria mononuclear cells. Moreover, CD4[+] lamina propria lymphocytes released less IL-2 and more IL-10 and TGF-β than GITR[+/+] controls. SAO shock is less aggressive and carrageenan- and bleomycin-induced lung injury are less damaging in GITR[-/-] mice and this correlates with lower TNFα and IL-1β production as compared to GITR[+/+] controls.[33,49,64]

Concluding Remarks

Presented data clearly indicate that autoimmune/inflammatory diseases and reaction towards antigens are modulated through GITR/GITRL system interfering with acquired immunity (including effector T-lymphocytes, Treg cells and APCs), innate immunity (including NK-cells and macrophages) and ECs. The relevance of GITR- and GITRL-mediated signals in different cells of the immune system determines the final outcome of response and varies depending on the experimental model analyzed. However, the implementation of biological tools able to modulate the GITR/GITRL system deserves effort and appears to be potentially useful.

In this context, the relevance of GITRL requires further investigations. In fact, GITRL can function as a stimulus for GITR and can also signal in the cells. This potential double role is a confusing factor because several cells, including macrophages, PMNs, DCs and activated T-cells express both GITR and GITRL and every time an antibody or a fusion protein, specific for GITR or GITRL, is used it can elicit opposite effects on GITR and GITRL. For example, when an agonistic GITR-Fc is used, 2 effects are possible: (1) inhibition of GITR activation by endogenous GITRL, (2) activation of GITRL. In GITR$^{-/-}$ mice, cells lack both GITR and GITRL signaling, since GITRL, present in GITR$^{-/-}$ mice, is not activated by GITR. Therefore, in order to approach modulation of GITR and GITRL in clinical settings it is of utmost interest to understand the specific role of GITR and its ligand in disease models. A better characterization of the agonistic and antagonistic properties of antibodies and fusion proteins is required. Moreover, preparation and study of GITRL$^{-/-}$ mice would be of help.

Apart from their role in immunity, recent data suggest that GITR and GITRL play a role in other systems. For example, they participate in protection of the skin from the pro-apoptotic effects of UVB light and in osteoclast differentiation.[36,38] The expression of GITR in other tissues, such as lung, kidney and brain, suggest that GITR may play further undisclosed roles. These findings, while open a way to new therapeutic approaches, also raise the possibility that in vivo modulation of GITR-GITRL system could lack sufficient specificity and favor adverse events. Therefore, modulators of GITR-GITRL system have to be tested also from this point of view, before planning their use in humans for the treatment of inflammatory/autoimmune diseases, transplant rejection, persistent infection and tumors.

Acknowledgements

This work was supported by Associazione Italiana per la Ricerca sul Cancro (AIRC), Milan and MURST, Rome, Italy.

References

1. Sakaguchi S, Sakaguchi N, Asano M et al. Immunologic self-tolerance maintained by activated T-cells expressing IL-2 receptor alpha-chains (CD25). Breakdown of a single mechanism of self-tolerance causes various autoimmune diseases. J Immunol 1995; 155(3):1151-1164.
2. Beissert S, Schwarz A, Schwarz T. Regulatory T-cells. J Invest Dermatol 2006; 126(1):15-24.
3. Watts TH. TNF/TNFR family members in costimulation of T-cell responses. Annu Rev Immunol 2005; 23:23-68.
4. Nocentini G, Giunchi L, Ronchetti S et al. A new member of the tumor necrosis factor/nerve growth factor receptor family inhibits T-cell receptor-induced apoptosis. Proc Natl Acad Sci USA 1997; 94(12):6216-6221.
5. Bossen C, Ingold K, Tardivel A et al. Interactions of Tumor Necrosis Factor (TNF) and TNF Receptor Family Members in the Mouse and Human. J Biol Chem 2006; 281(20):13964-13971.
6. Kwon B, Yu KY, Ni J et al. Identification of a novel activation-inducible protein of the tumor necrosis factor receptor superfamily and its ligand. J Biol Chem 1999; 274(10):6056-6061.
7. Gurney AL, Marsters SA, Huang RM et al. Identification of a new member of the tumor necrosis factor family and its receptor, a human ortholog of mouse GITR. Curr Biol 1999; 9(4):215-218.
8. Kim JD, Choi BK, Bae JS et al. Cloning and characterization of GITR ligand. Genes Immun 2003; 4(8):564-569.
9. Tone M, Tone Y, Adams E et al. Mouse glucocorticoid-induced tumor necrosis factor receptor ligand is costimulatory for T-cells. Proc Natl Acad Sci USA 2003; 100(25):15059-15064.

10. Yu KY, Kim HS, Song SY. USA. Identification of a ligand for glucocorticoid-induced tumor necrosis factor receptor constitutively expressed in dendritic cells. Biochem Biophys Res Commun 2003; 310(2):433-438.

11. Ronchetti S, Zollo O, Bruscoli S et al. GITR, a member of the TNF receptor superfamily, is costimulatory to mouse T-lymphocyte subpopulations. Eur J Immunol 2004; 34(3):613-622.

12. Nocentini G, Bartoli A, Ronchetti S et al. Gene structure and chromosomal assignment of mouse GITR, a member of the tumor necrosis factor/nerve growth factor receptor family. DNA Cell Biol 2000; 19(4):205-217.

13. Nocentini G, Ronchetti S, Bartoli A et al. Identification of three novel mRNA splice variants of GITR. Cell Death Differ 2000; 7(4):408-410.

14. Spinicelli S, Nocentini G, Ronchetti S et al. GITR interacts with the pro-apoptotic protein Siva and induces apoptosis. Cell Death Differ 2002; 9(12):1382-1384.

15. Esparza EM, Arch RH. Glucocorticoid-induced TNF receptor functions as a costimulatory receptor that promotes survival in early phases of T-cell activation. J Immunol 2005; 174(12):7869-7874.

16. Esparza EM, Arch RH. Glucocorticoid-induced TNF receptor, a costimulatory receptor on naive and activated T-cells, uses TNF receptor-associated factor 2 in a novel fashion as an inhibitor of NF-kappa B activation. J Immunol 2005; 174(12):7875-7882.

17. Prasad KV, Ao Z, Yoon Y et al. CD27, a member of the tumor necrosis factor receptor family, induces apoptosis and binds to Siva, a proapoptotic protein. Proc Natl Acad Sci USA 1997; 94(12):6346-6351.

18. Py B, Slomianny C, Auberger P et al. Siva-1 and an alternative splice form lacking the death domain, Siva-2, similarly induce apoptosis in T-lymphocytes via a caspase-dependent mitochondrial pathway. J Immunol 2004; 172(7):4008-4017.

19. Lin WJ, Gary JD, Yang MC et al. The mammalian immediate-early TIS21 protein and the leukemia-associated BTG1 protein interact with a protein-arginine N-methyltransferase. J Biol Chem 1996; 271(25):15034-15044.

20. An W, Kim J, Roeder RG. Ordered cooperative functions of PRMT1, p.300 and CARM1 in transcriptional activation by p.53 Cell 2004; 117(6):735-748.

21. Ganesh L, Yoshimoto T, Moorthy NC et al. Protein methyltransferase 2 inhibits NF-kappaB function and promotes apoptosis. Mol Cell Biol 2006; 26(10):3864-3874.

22. McHugh RS, Whitters MJ, Piccirillo CA et al. CD4(+)CD25(+) immunoregulatory T-cells: gene expression analysis reveals a functional role for the glucocorticoid-induced TNF receptor. Immunity 2002; 16(2):311-323.

23. Kohm AP, Williams JS, Miller SD. Cutting edge: ligation of the glucocorticoid-induced TNF receptor enhances autoreactive CD4+ T-cell activation and experimental autoimmune encephalomyelitis. J Immunol 2004; 172(8):4686-4690.

24. Kanamaru F, Youngnak P, Hashiguchi M et al. Costimulation via glucocorticoid-induced TNF receptor in both conventional and CD25+ regulatory CD4+ T-cells. J Immunol 2004; 172(12):7306-7314.

25. Stephens GL, McHugh RS, Whitters MJ et al. Engagement of glucocorticoid-induced TNFR family-related receptor on effector T-cells by its ligand mediates resistance to suppression by CD4+CD25+ T-cells. J Immunol 2004; 173(8):5008-5020.

26. Zelenika D, Adams E, Humm S et al. Regulatory T-cells overexpress a subset of Th2 gene transcripts. J Immunol 2002; 168(3):1069-1079.

27. Shimizu J, Yamazaki S, Takahashi T et al. Stimulation of CD25(+)CD4(+) regulatory T-cells through GITR breaks immunological self-tolerance. Nat Immunol 2002; 3(2):135-142.

28. Uraushihara K, Kanai T, Ko K et al. Regulation of murine inflammatory bowel disease by CD25+ and CD25-CD4+ glucocorticoid-induced TNF receptor family-related gene+regulatory T-cells. J Immunol 2003; 171(2):708-716.

29. Scotto L, Naiyer AJ, Galluzzo S et al. Overlap between molecular markers expressed by naturally occurring CD4+CD25+ regulatory T-cells and antigen specific CD4+CD25+ and CD8+CD28-T suppressor cells. Hum Immunol 2004; 65(11):1297-1306.

30. Cosmi L, Liotta F, Lazzeri E et al. Human CD8+CD25+ thymocytes share phenotypic and functional features with CD4+CD25+ regulatory thymocytes. Blood 2003; 102(12):4107-4114.

31. Kim HJ, Kim HY, Kim BK et al. Engagement of glucocorticoid-induced TNF receptor costimulates NKT-cell activation in vitro and in vivo. J Immunol 2006; 176(6):3507-3515.

32. Hanabuchi S, Watanabe N, Wang YH et al. Human plasmacytoid predendritic cells activate NK-cells through glucocorticoid-induced tumor necrosis factor receptor-ligand (GITRL). Blood 2006; 107(9):3617-3623.

33. Cuzzocrea S, Nocentini G, Di Paola R et al. Proinflammatory role of glucocorticoid-induced TNF receptor-related gene in acute lung inflammation. J Immunol 2006; 177(1):631-641.

34. Santucci L, Agostini M, Bruscoli S et al. GITR modulates innate and adaptive mucosal immunity during the development of experimental colitis in mice. Gut 2006.

35. Nakae S, Suto H, Iikura M et al. Mast cells enhance T-cell activation: importance of mast cell costimulatory molecules and secreted TNF. J Immunol 2006; 176(4):2238-2248.

36. Wang J, Devgan V, Corrado M et al. Glucocorticoid-induced tumor necrosis factor receptor is a p21Cip1/WAF1 transcriptional target conferring resistance of keratinocytes to UV light-induced apoptosis. J Biol Chem 2005; 280(45):37725-37731.

37. Shin HH, Kim SJ, Kang SY et al. Soluble glucocorticoid-induced tumor necrosis factor receptor stimulates osteoclastogenesis by down-regulation of osteoprotegerin in bone marrow stromal cells. Bone 2006.

38. Shin HH, Kim SJ, Lee DS et al. Soluble glucocorticoid-induced tumor necrosis factor receptor (sGITR) stimulates osteoclast differentiation in response to receptor activator of NF-kappaB ligand (RANKL) in osteoclast cells. Bone 2005; 36(5):832-839.

39. Kim BJ, Li Z, Fariss RN et al. Constitutive and cytokine-induced GITR ligand expression on human retinal pigment epithelium and photoreceptors. Invest Ophthalmol Vis Sci 2004; 45(9):3170-3176.

40. Agostini M, Cenci E, Pericolini E et al. The glucocorticoid-induced tumor necrosis factor receptor-related gene modulates the response to Candida albicans infection. Infect Immun 2005; 73(11):7502-7508.

41. Shin HH, Kim SJ, Lee HS et al. The soluble glucocorticoid-induced tumor necrosis factor receptor causes cell cycle arrest and apoptosis in murine macrophages. Biochem Biophys Res Commun 2004; 316(1):24-32.

42. Shin HH, Kim SG, Lee MH et al. Soluble glucocorticoid-induced TNF receptor (sGITR) induces inflammation in mice. Exp Mol Med 2003; 35(5):358-364.

43. Cardona ID, Goleva E, Ou LS et al. Staphylococcal enterotoxin B inhibits regulatory T-cells by inducing glucocorticoid-induced TNF receptor-related protein ligand on monocytes. J Allergy Clin Immunol 2006; 117(3):688-695.

44. Suvas S, Kim B, Sarangi PP et al. In vivo kinetics of GITR and GITR ligand expression and their functional significance in regulating viral immunopathology. J Virol 2005; 79(18):11935-11942.

45. Shevach EM, Stephens GL. The GITR-GITRL interaction: costimulation or contrasuppression of regulatory activity? Nat Rev Immunol 2006; 6(8):613-618.

46. Nardelli B, Zaritskaya L, McAuliffe W et al. Osteostat/tumor necrosis factor superfamily 18 inhibits osteoclastogenesis and is selectively expressed by vascular endothelial cells. Endocrinology 2006; 147(1):70-78.

47. Cuzzocrea S, Ayroldi E, Di Paola R et al. Role of glucocorticoid-induced TNF receptor family gene (GITR) in collagen-induced arthritis. FASEB J 2005; 19(10):1253-1265.

48. Patel M, Xu D, Kewin P et al. Glucocorticoid-induced TNFR family-related protein (GITR) activation exacerbates murine asthma and collagen-induced arthritis. Eur J Immunol 2005; 35(12):3581-3590.

49. Cuzzocrea S, Ronchetti S, Genovese T et al. Genetic and pharmacological inhibition of GITR-GITRL interaction reduces chronic lung injury induced by bleomycin instillation. FASEB J 2007; 21(1):117-129.

50. Lee SK, Choi BK, Kim YH et al. Glucocorticoid-induced tumour necrosis factor receptor family-related receptor signalling exacerbates hapten-induced colitis by CD4+ T-cells. Immunology 2006; 119(4):479-487.

51. Muriglan SJ, Ramirez-Montagut T, Alpdogan O et al. GITR activation induces an opposite effect on alloreactive CD4(+) and CD8(+) T-cells in graft-versus-host disease. J Exp Med 2004; 200(2):149-157.

52. Kim J, Choi WS, Kim HJ et al. Prevention of chronic graft-versus-host disease by stimulation with glucocorticoid-induced TNF receptor. Exp Mol Med 2006; 38(1):94-99.

53. Kim J, Choi WS, Kang H et al. Conversion of alloantigen-specific CD8+ T-cell anergy to CD8+ T-cell priming through in vivo ligation of glucocorticoid-induced TNF receptor. J Immunol 2006; 176(9):5223-5231.

54. Suri A, Shimizu J, Katz JD et al. Regulation of autoimmune diabetes by non-islet-specific T-cells—a role for the glucocorticoid-induced TNF receptor. Eur J Immunol 2004; 34(2):447-454.

55. Morris GP, Kong YC. Interference with CD4+CD25+ T-cell-mediated tolerance to experimental autoimmune thyroiditis by glucocorticoid-induced tumor necrosis factor receptor monoclonal antibody. J Autoimmun 2006; 26(1):24-31.

56. He H, Messer RJ, Sakaguchi S et al. Reduction of retrovirus-induced immunosuppression by in vivo modulation of T-cells during acute infection. J Virol 2004; 78(21):11641-11647.

57. Dittmer U, He H, Messer RJ et al. Functional impairment of CD8(+) T-cells by regulatory T-cells during persistent retroviral infection. Immunity 2004; 20(3):293-303.

58. Stone GW, Barzee S, Snarsky V et al. Multimeric soluble CD40 ligand and GITR ligand as adjuvants for human immunodeficiency virus DNA vaccines. J Virol 2006; 80(4):1762-1772.

59. Taylor MD, LeGoff L, Harris A et al. Removal of regulatory T-cell activity reverses hyporesponsiveness and leads to filarial parasite clearance in vivo. J Immunol 2005; 174(8):4924-4933.

60. Turk MJ, Guevara-Patino JA, Rizzuto GA et al. Concomitant tumor immunity to a poorly immunogenic melanoma is prevented by regulatory T-cells. J Exp Med 2004; 200(6):771-782.

61. Calmels B, Paul S, Futin N et al. Bypassing tumor-associated immune suppression with recombinant adenovirus constructs expressing membrane bound or secreted GITR-L. Cancer Gene Ther 2005; 12(2):198-205.

62. Ko K, Yamazaki S, Nakamura K et al. Treatment of advanced tumors with agonistic anti-GITR mAb and its effects on tumor-infiltrating Foxp3+CD25+CD4+ regulatory T-cells. J Exp Med 2005; 202(7):885-891.

63. Cohen AD, Diab A, Perales MA et al. Agonist anti-GITR antibody enhances vaccine-induced CD8(+) T-cell responses and tumor immunity. Cancer Res 2006; 66(9):4904-4912.

64. Cuzzocrea S, Nocentini G, Di Paola R et al. Glucocorticoid-induced TNF receptor family gene (GITR) knockout mice exhibit a resistance to splanchnic artery occlusion (SAO) shock. J Leukoc Biol 2004; 76(5):933-940.

65. Nocentini G, Riccardi C. GITR: a multifaceted regulator of immunity belonging to the tumor necrosis factor receptor superfamily. Eur J Immunol 2005; 35(4):1016-1022.

66. Esparza EM, Arch RH. Signaling triggered by glucocorticoid-induced tumor necrosis factor receptor family-related gene: regulation at the interface between regulatory T-cells and immune effector cells. Front Biosci 2006; 11:1448-1465.

67. Mahesh SP, Li Z, Liu B et al. Expression of GITR ligand abrogates immunosuppressive function of ocular tissue and differentially modulates inflammatory cytokines and chemokines. Eur J Immunol 2006; 36(8):2128-2138.

68. Kohm AP, Podojil JR, Williams JS et al. CD28 regulates glucocorticoid-induced TNF receptor family-related gene expression on CD4+ T-cells via IL-2-dependent mechanisms. Cell Immunol 2005; 235(1):56-64.

69. Ji HB, Liao G, Faubion WA et al. Cutting edge: the natural ligand for glucocorticoid-induced TNF receptor-related protein abrogates regulatory T-cell suppression. J Immunol 2004; 172(10):5823-5827.

70. Shimizu J, Moriizumi E. CD4+CD25−T-cells in aged mice are hyporesponsive and exhibit suppressive activity. J Immunol 2003; 170(4):1675-1682.

71. Tsaknaridis L, Spencer L, Culbertson N et al. Functional assay for human CD4+CD25+ Treg cells reveals an age-dependent loss of suppressive activity. J Neurosci Res 2003; 74(2):296-308.

72. Gondek DC, Lu LF, Quezada SA et al. Cutting edge: contact-mediated suppression by CD4+CD25+ regulatory cells involves a granzyme B-dependent, perforin-independent mechanism. J Immunol 2005; 174(4):1783-1786.

73. Valzasina B, Guiducci C, Dislich H et al. Triggering of OX40 (CD134) on CD4(+)CD25+ T-cells blocks their inhibitory activity: a novel regulatory role for OX40 and its comparison with GITR. Blood 2005; 105(7):2845-2851.

74. Ramirez-Montagut T, Chow A, Hirschhorn-Cymerman D et al. Glucocorticoid-Induced TNF Receptor Family Related Gene Activation Overcomes Tolerance/Ignorance to Melanoma Differentiation Antigens and Enhances Antitumor Immunity. J Immunol 2006; 176(11):6434-6442.

75. Shin HH, Kwon BS, Choi HS. Recombinant glucocorticoid induced tumour necrosis factor receptor (rGITR) induced COX-2 activity in murine macrophage Raw 264.7 cells. Cytokine 2002; 19(4):187-192.

76. Shin HH, Lee HW, Choi HS. Induction of nitric oxide synthase (NOS) by soluble glucocorticoid induced tumor necrosis factor receptor (sGITR) is modulated by IFN-gamma in murine macrophage. Exp Mol Med 2003; 35(3):175-180.

77. Kim SJ, Shin HH, Park SY et al. Induction of MMP-13 expression by soluble human glucocorticoid-induced tumor necrosis factor receptor in fibroblast-like synovial cells. Osteoarthritis Cartilage 2006; 14(2):146-153.

78. Lee HS, Shin HH, Kwon BS et al. Soluble glucocorticoid-induced tumor necrosis factor receptor (sGITR) increased MMP-9 activity in murine macrophage. J Cell Biochem 2003; 88(5):1048-1056.

79. Kim WJ, Bae EM, Kang YJ et al. Glucocorticoid-induced tumour necrosis factor receptor family related protein (GITR) mediates inflammatory activation of macrophages that can destabilize atherosclerotic plaques. Immunology 2006; 119(3):421-429.

80. Shin HH, Lee MH, Kim SG et al. Recombinant glucocorticoid induced tumor necrosis factor receptor (rGITR) induces NOS in murine macrophage. FEBS Lett 2002; 514(2-3):275-280.

CHAPTER 12

Targeting CD30/CD30L in Oncology and Autoimmune and Inflammatory Diseases

Ezogelin Oflazoglu, Iqbal S. Grewal and Hanspeter Gerber*

Abstract

The transmembrane receptor CD30 (TNFRSF8) and its ligand CD30L (CD153, TNFSF8) are members of the tumor necrosis factor (TNF) superfamily and display restricted expression in subpopulations of activated T-and B-cells in nonpathologic conditions. CD30 expression is upregulated in various hematological malignancies, including Reed-Sternberg cells in Hodgkin's disease (HD), anaplastic large cell lymphoma (ALCL) and subsets of Non-Hodgkin's lymphomas (NHLs). Increased CD30L expression was found on mast cells within HD tumors and preclinical and clinical studies with compounds targeting the CD30/CD30L system in HD and ALCL demonstrated therapeutic benefit. Upregulation of CD30 and CD30L is also linked to leukocytes in patients with chronic inflammatory diseases, including lupus erythematosus, asthma, rheumatoid arthritis and atopic dermatitis (AD). Preclinical studies conducted with transgenic mice or biologic compounds suggested important regulatory functions of the CD30-CD30L system in various aspects of the immune system. Such key regulatory roles and their low expression in normal conditions combined with increased expression in malignant tissues provided a strong rationale to investigate CD30 and CD30L as therapeutic targets in hematologic malignancies, autoimmune and inflammatory diseases. In this report, we review the pharmacodynamic effects of specific therapeutic compounds targeting the CD30/CD30L system in preclinical- and clinical studies.

Gene Structure and Expression of CD30

CD30 is a member of the tumor necrosis factor receptor (TNFR) superfamily that includes TNFR, CD40, Fas (CD95) and OX-40 (CD134), among others (reviewed in).[1] Human CD30 is a type 1 glycoprotein, containing both N- and O-linked sugars, with a molecular weight ranging from 105-120 kDa.[2] The intracellular portion of the protein contains several serine/threonine phosphorylation sites, which regulate cell signaling following receptor ligation. Mature human CD30 is comprised of 577 amino acids, including a 365 amino acid residue extracellular region, a 24 amino acid transmembrane segment and a 188 amino acid cytoplasmic domain.[2] The preprocessed form of the transmembrane protein includes an additional 18 amino acid signal sequence. Structurally, human CD30 is composed of six cysteine-rich repeats in the extracellular domain, characteristic of this family, interposed with a 60 amino acid partial repeat.[3] An 85 kDa form of CD30, a product of proteolytic cleavage (sCD30) can be found in the blood of patients with CD30

*Corresponding Author: Hanspeter Gerber—Seattle Genetics, Inc, 21823 30th Drive, Southeast, Bothell, Washington 9802, USA. Email: hgerber@seagen.com

Therapeutic Targets of the TNF Superfamily, edited by Iqbal S. Grewal.
©2009 Landes Bioscience and Springer Science+Business Media.

positive lymphomas or autoimmune diseases.[4] An alternatively spliced transcript (isoform 2) was described, encoding a 132 amino acid N-terminal fragment located in the cytoplasm. Between species, the CD30 coding regions are relatively well conserved, with 64%, 58% and 97% sequence identity between human and mouse, rat and chimpanzee, respectively.

In nonpathological conditions, CD30 expression is generally limited to activated B and T-lymphocytes and NK cells and generally lower levels of expression were reported for activated monocytes and eosinophils.[5] In addition, CD30 is found on a small percentage of CD8 positive T-cells and negligible expression on naïve or resting lymphocytes was described (Table 1).[6] CD30 expression is induced on T-cells following mitogen activation, antigen receptor cross-linking or as a result of viral infection.[7] Histological examination of CD30 expression in normal tissues

Table 1. Cells expressing CD30 and/or CD30L

CD30 Expressing Cells	CD30L Expressing Cells
Activated T-cells	T-cells
Activated B-cells	B-cells
NK-cells	Mast cells
Activated monocytes	Neutrophils
Macrophages	
Eosinophils	

Table 2. Tumor cells expressing CD30 and/or CD30L

CD30 Expressing Cells	CD30L Expressing Cells
R-S cells in HD	B-cell lymphoma
ALCL	
Subset of NHL	
Embryonal carcinoma	
Seminoma	

Table 3. Reported CD30 expression in immunologic diseases

Disease	sCD30	CD30+ Cells in Blood	CD30+ Cells in Tissues
Atopic dermatitis	+	+	+
Atopic asthma	+	+	+
Allergic rhinitis	+	mRNA	+
Scleroderma	+	-	+
SLE	+	-	+
Sjogren's syndrome	+	-	+
Rheumatoid arthritis	+	-	+
Hashimoto thyroiditis	+	-	-
Wegener's granulomatosis	+	-	-
Primary biliary cirrhosis	+	-	+

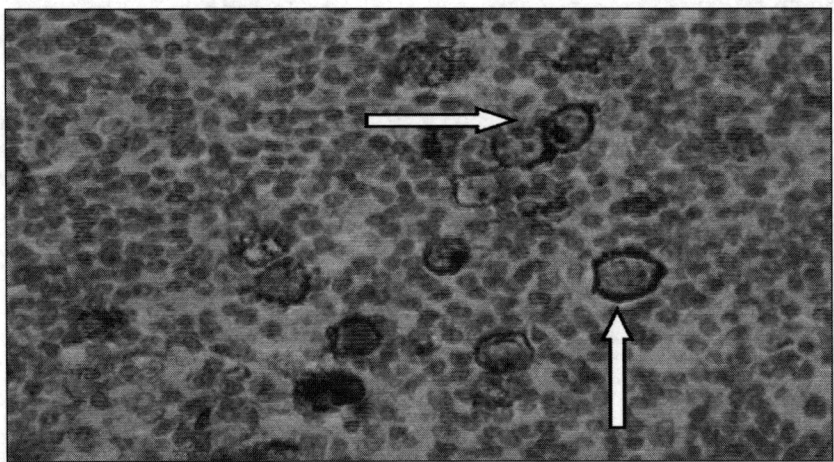

Figure 1. Immunohistochemical analysis of tumor sections from HD patient for CD30 expression. Tumor sample derived from the lymph node of a patient with HD were stained with an anti-hCD30 antibody (Clone HRS4). CD30 staining is restricted to Reed Sternberg cells and is not present on tumor stroma as indicated by arrows.

identified a rare population of large lymphoid cells in sections of lymph node, tonsil, thymus and endometrial cells with decidual changes.[8] Importantly, CD30 expression is absent on most cells outside the immune system (Table 1).

CD30 was originally identified based on its strong cell surface expression on Reed-Sternberg (R-S) cells (Fig. 1), the malignant cell-type in HD and CD30 is now used as a diagnostic marker for this disease.[9] CD30 is also expressed on ALCL tumor cells, on subsets of Non-Hodgkins Lymphomas (NHL) and on some rare solid tumors, including embryonal carcinomas and seminomas[10] (reviewed in Table 2).[11-13] A correlation between the elevated levels of sCD30 in the sera of patients with ALCL[14] or HD[9,15] and poor disease prognosis was also reported.

In autoimmune diseases, CD30 is expressed at high levels on activated lymphocytes in multiple sclerosis and systemic sclerosis patients. Similar to the findings in hematologic malignancies, elevated levels of the soluble form (sCD30) were detectable in their sera and the levels frequently correlated with disease severity (Table 3).[16,17] Increased serum levels of sCD30 were also found in individuals infected with one of several different viruses, including hepatitis B and C, human immunodeficiency virus (HIV) and Epstein-Barr virus (EBV). Finally, increased levels of sCD30 were detectable in sera of individuals with chronic inflammatory diseases such as systemic lupus erythematosis or rheumatoid arthritis,[18-24] atopic dermatitis (AD),[25-28] asthma,[29,30] allergic rhinitis[31] and scleroderma.[16] In conclusion, high serum levels of sCD30 represent an independent predictor of disease progression and poor prognosis for patients with CD30-positive lymphomas, autoimmune diseases or viral infections.

Gene Structure and Expression of CD30L

CD30L is a 234-amino-acid type II, single pass transmembrane protein with a calculated molecular weight of 26 kDa. CD30L belongs to the TNF family[2] and is the only known ligand for CD30. The human CD30L gene has been mapped to chromosome 9q33.[32] CD30L has significant structural similarities to TNF-α, TNF-β, CD40 ligand (CD40L) and Fas ligand (FasL).[1] RNA transcripts encoding CD30L are detected in B-cells, activated T-cells, macrophages, granulocytes, eosinophils and some HTLV-1-positive T-cell lines.[33-40] At the protein level, CD30L is expressed on activated peripheral blood T-cells, B-cells, neutrophils, mast cells, monocytes and macrophages (Table 1).[41] Interspecies sequence comparison of CD30L genes revealed a high level of sequence identity of, with 86, 99.5 and 78% identity between human and dog, chimpanzee and mouse orthologs, respectively. Only one isoform has been described for CD30L and this sequence lacks the consensus proteolytic cleavage motif found in many TNF family members.

Signaling and Biological Functions of the CD30/CD30L System

Activation of the CD30 receptor in response to ligand stimulation or cross-linking by immobilized antibodies induces trimerization and recruitment of signaling proteins. Due to the lack of an intrinsic enzymatic domain within the cytoplasmic tail of CD30, signal transduction is exclusively mediated by members of the TNFR-associated factor (TRAF) family and various TRAF-binding proteins. The intracellular levels and sub-cellular localization of TRAF2 is altered upon binding of CD30 to its ligand.[42,43] CD30-mediated signaling engages multiple pathways, including MAP kinases and NF-κB.[44,45] Depending on the cell types and costimulatory signals involved, CD30 mediated signal transduction events are capable of promoting cell proliferation, cell survival or anti-proliferative effects and cell death. For example, induction of CD30 signaling in ALCL cells by an anti-CD30 antibody leads to apoptotic cell death with selective reduction of TRAF2 and an impaired ability to activate NF-κB.[46] In contrast, the same anti-CD30 antibody induced proliferation of HD and other tumor cell lines.[34] The molecular mechanism underlying such differential responses of different tumor cell types to anti-CD30 antibodies is not completely understood. However, constitutive activation of the NF-κB signaling pathway present in some tumor cell lines was suggested to dictate the outcome of the response.[46] In support of this model, stimulation of CD30 on HD target cells and concomitant inhibition of NF-κB by bortezomib resulted in enhanced therapeutic effects in both, in vitro and in vivo systems.[47]

In the immune system, ligation of CD30 by CD30L has been associated with 4 basic biological functions: a) CD30 can act as a costimulatory molecule in synergism with the CD3/TCR complex;[48,49] b) CD30 is involved in the regulation of immune cell memory functions as demonstrated by experiments conducted with CD30-deficient mice. CD30 deficiency was associated with impaired capacity to sustain follicular germinal center responses and substantially reduced recall memory antibody responses in mice;[50,51] c) down-regulation of the cellular immune response on activated T- and B-cells and activation-induced cell death of thymocytes in the negative selection process of autoreactive T-cells;[10,48,49] and d) although reverse signaling via TNF family ligands is not well established, a few examples in the literature provided evidence to suggest the possibility for reverse signaling via CD30L. For example, cross-linking of CD30L on neutrophils resulted in an oxidative burst and the production of the pro-inflammatory chemokine IL-8 by these cells. Similarly, peripheral T-cells activated to express CD30L responded to cross-linking by ligand with increased proliferation and secretion of IL-6.[39] In another report, triggering of CD30L on mast cells via CD30 was shown to result in degranulation-independent secretion of chemokines, including IL-8, macrophage inflammatory protein-1alpha (MIP-1alpha) and MIP-1beta.[52]

Combined, these findings suggest that CD30 signaling induces pleiotropic responses, which in addition to the cell type, are dependent on the activation- and/or transformation status. Furthermore, CD30 signaling is context dependent and can be affected by extracellular factors such as extracellular matrix composition at the sites where CD30 and/or CD30L positive cells are interacting (reviewed in 53). Finally, the signaling mechanisms described above were found to be associated with paracrine, juxtacrine and autocrine regulatory loops[54] between cells expressing the respective ligand/receptors (Table 1).

Development of Therapeutic Compounds Targeting CD30/CD30L

Antibodies targeting TNF family members can exert antagonist or agonistic signaling effects, depending on their ability to induced receptor/ligand oligomerization and/or blocking of ligand-receptor interactions. In addition to such direct effects on cell signaling, therapeutic antibodies can induce cell death of target antigen expressing cells by engaging effector cells via antigen dependent cellular cytotoxicity (ADCC), complement dependent cytotoxicity (CDC) or antigen dependent cellular phagocytosis (ADCP). Based on the differing abilities of antibodies to interfere with cell signaling and to engage effector cell functions, it is likely that different therapeutic compounds will induce unique sets of pharmacodynamic responses, which may additionally be influenced by intrinsic characteristics of the experimental models employed. These circumstances may help to better understand some of the controversial findings regarding the therapeutic effects of antibodies acting on the CD30/CD30L pathway in oncology,[54] as reviewed below. Some of the variability in the pharmacodynamic properties of compounds may be additionally explained by differences in their epitope recognition and binding affinities.

Preclinical Development of Therapeutic Antibodies Targeting CD30 or CD30L in Hematological Malignancies

In 1994, Gruss et al generated a monoclonal anti-CD30 antibody (M67) that inhibited growth of ALCL tumor cells. However, this antibody stimulated the growth of HD cell lines in vitro and had no effects on the growth of human HD cell lines implanted in mice.[34,35] While most of the therapeutic compounds targeting CD30 were active in models of ALCL, some of them failed to induce cell death when tested on human HD tumor cell lines.[34] A correlation between the antitumor effects of the M67 antibody and the differences in the constitutive NF-κB signaling in ALCL and HD cell lines was proposed as the basis of the difference in the outcome.[46] Data from in vitro studies suggested that ALCL cells undergo apoptosis following exposure to immobilized M67, a finding that was attributed to the inability of these cells to activate the transcription factor NF-κB. In contrast, HD cell lines (L428, KM-H2, L591), which constitutively expressed NF-κB, were not sensitive to M67 treatment.

A chimeric anti-CD30 antibody cAC10 (also called SGN-30), a derivative of the mouse mono-clonal antibody AC10, was tested for its ability to target CD30 positive tumor cells. The SGN-30 prolonged survival of mice bearing chemotherapy resistant human CD30 positive ALCL tumor cells.[55,56] Furthermore, the pharmacological effects of SGN-30 were evaluated in disseminated and subcutaneous models of HD disease. Treatment with SGN-30 resulted in significantly improved survival rates of mice or in the inhibition of tumor growth in these models.[57] In addition, synergis-tic antitumor activities were achieved when SGN-30 was combined with conventional cytotoxic drugs such as bleomycin. In vitro, doxorubicin, vinblastin, etoposide, cisplatin, cytarabine and chlorambucil increased antitumor activity when combined with SGN-30.[58]

In addition to SGN-30, an antibody drug conjugate consisting of monomethyl auristatin E (MMAE) conjugated to the anti-CD30 monoclonal antibody cAC10 (SGN-35), was tested in preclinical models of HD and ALCL in SCID mice and showed promising initial results.[59-61] The mechanism of action employed by naked antibodies is different from antibody drug conjugates which can destroy tumor cells by delivering a toxic compound into the cells via target mediated cellular internalization. Improved efficacy of SGN-35 relative to the unconjugated antibody (cAC10/SGN-30) was demonstrated and complete tumor regressions were obtained at doses as low as 1 mg/kg.[62,63]

Clinical Studies Conducted with Compounds Targeting CD30 in Hematological Malignancies

In 1992, Falini et al tested the murine anti-CD30 mAb Ber-H2 clinically in HD patients.[64] Despite the successful in vivo targeting of malignant tumor cells as assessed by immunohistological analysis of tumor biopsies and immunoscintigraphy, there was no evidence of tumor regression. To enhance the efficacy in HD and ALCL, modified murine anti-CD30 mAbs were developed with improved potency to kill tumor cells. These approaches included the covalent conjugation of saporin (SO6), a type-1 ribosome-inactivating protein, to Ber-H2,[61] Ki-4.dgA,[65] or bispecific constructs HRS-3/A9[66,67] and H22xKi-4.[68] Alternatively, murine MAbs were conjugated with radionucleotides to generate radioimmunoconjugates such as[131]I-Ki-4 and tested clinically in HD patients.[69] The pharmacological effects of these compounds were only transient (≤2 months) and no objective responses were reported. These early trials were conducted using murine antibodies and high levels of human anti-mouse antibodies (HAMA) were identified in the sera of most patients.

Bi-specific antibodies targeting two cell surface antigens (anti-CD16 / anti-CD30) were also tested clinically in early stage trials involving 15 patients with HD. Four out of nine patients displayed a clinical response, among them, one complete response, one partial response and two patients with stable disease were reported. However 9 out of 15 patient sera were positive for HAMA.[67,70] Overall, these early attempts to target CD30 positive hematologic-malignancies in clinical trials failed, possibly due to the induction of neutralizing HAMA antibodies.

Safety and tolerability of this chimeric anti-CD30 antibody of SGN-30 was assessed in phase I and phase I/II dose escalation studies in patients with refractory or relapsed CD30+ hematologic malignancies, including HD and NHL.[71,72] SGN-30 was tested at doses of up to 15 mg/kg (single dose) and up to 12 mg/kg (multiple dose) and both regiments were well tolerated in most patients and a maximum tolerated dose was not reached.[73] SGN-30 was also tested in a single agent phase II study in patients with HD[74] and ALCL.[75] Encouraging response rates were achieved in patients with CD30 positive ALCL, particularly in patients with cutaneous ALCL. Four of five patients with cutaneous ALCL responded to therapy with SGN-30 and four out of 20 systemic ALCL patients achieved tumor remissions.[76] Phase II studies combining SGN-30 with chemotherapy have been initiated in HD and systemic ALCL. The National Cancer Institute (NCI) is currently sponsoring a phase II trial of SGN-30 in combination with GVD chemotherapy (gemcitabine, vinorelbine and doxil) in relapsed/refractory HD patients. The NCI is also sponsoring a phase II trial of SGN-30 plus CHOP (cyclophosphamide, doxorubicin, vincristine and prednisone) in newly diagnosed patients with systemic ALCL.[76]

A phase I dose-escalation trial of SGN-35 for relapsed or refractory Hodgkin's disease and other CD30-positive hematologic malignancies is currently ongoing. The study is designed to evaluate the safety, pharmacokinetic profile and antitumor activity of SGN-35.

Therapeutic Effects of Targeting CD30/CD30L in Preclinical Models of Autoimmune and Inflammatory Diseases

The pharmacodynamic effects of a rat anti-mouse CD30L mAb (clone RM153;[77] were evaluated in models of diabetes,[78] skin allograft rejection,[79] infectious disease setting[80] and graft versus host disease (GVHD).[81] RM153 was shown to not only block CD30/CD30L interaction but also to induce ablation of CD30L positive cells in mice.[79] In NOD mice, prevention or delayed onset of diabetes was observed following RM153 treatment, which was explained by the failure of NOD splenocytes to transfer diabetes into NOD-SCID mice. Positive therapeutic effects were also reported when RM153 was tested in a model of graft versus host disease (GVHD), where prolonged survival of allografted mice was observed.[81] In this model, RM153 treatment blocked the ability of antigen-induced, adoptively transferred T-regulatory cells (Tregs) to delay skin allograft rejection. When tested in an infectious disease model, RM153 treatment increased bacterial burden in rodents,[80] suggesting anti-inflammatory activities. Interestingly, experiments conducted with mice lacking CD30 (CD30[(-/-)] mice) revealed impaired thymic negative selection and augmented T-cell autoreactivity. However, these effects were shown to be strain specific. Tregs derived from CD30[(-/-)] knock-out mice were significantly less effective in preventing lethality in an experimental model of graft versus host disease (GVHD). In the same model, blockade of the CD30/CD30L pathway with the neutralizing anti-CD30L mAb RM153 induced a reduction of Treg mediated protection from pro-inflammatory cytokine accumulation and donor-type T-cell apoptosis. Combined, these data demonstrate that early CD30 signaling is critical for Treg mediated GVHD protection after major-MHC mismatch bone marrow transplantation.[82]

The role of CD30 in a murine asthma model was investigated by using CD30-deficient mice, which were immunized with ovalbumin (OVA) to induce an asthma-like phenotype. The results from the genetic experiments were similar to the pharmacological effects observed when testing mAbs blocking either CD30 receptor or its ligand, CD30L/CD153. All three approaches resulted in significantly reduced airway inflammation, serum IgE levels and Th2 cytokine levels, demonstrating that CD30/CD30L interactions play important roles in the induction of Th2 cell-mediated allergic asthma.[83] For autoimmune indications, it is worth noting that the key findings regarding the biological role of the CD30/CD30L system, as determined by pharmacological intervention studies with monoclonal antibodies, are supported by recent findings from gene ablation experiments involving CD30- knock-out mice[51,84] or from CD30-transgenic mice (reviewed in ref. 85). In conclusion, targeting the CD30/CD30L system in experimental models of autoimmune diseases induced positive therapeutic effects. However, at this time, it remains unclear whether this activity can be attributed to interference with ligand-receptor interaction, depletion of CD30L positive cells or a combination of both.

Additional evidence in support of a potential role of the CD30/CD30L system in inflammatory diseases is provided by studies conducted with atopic dermatitis (AD) patients. AD is a chronic relapsing skin disease most commonly found in young children with a lifetime prevalence of 10-20% in developed countries but is also affecting 1-3% of adults.[86] AD is a complex disorder and in the most common "extrinsic" form, it is associated with increased IgE levels which have specificity for common environmental allergens (reviewed by ref. 87).

In a study investigating the expression of CD30 by infiltrating T-cells in lesional skin of patients with active, acute AD, a significant proportion of T-cells was identified to strongly expressed CD30. In contrast, CD30 was undetectable in patients with acute contact dermatitis.[27] The predominance of CD30+ lymphocytes in the skin of patients with AD and their ability to produce cytokines such as IL-3, IL-4 and IL-5 suggested that these cell may play a role in the pathogenesis of this disease.[95] Interestingly, sCD30 is released into the blood after chronic lymphocyte activation and elevated levels of sCD30 have been reported in patients with AD,[25] but not in healthy controls or in patients with acute contact dermatitis or respiratory atopic disorders.[25,95] Soluble CD30 plasma concentrations have been shown to correlate with disease severity of AD patients. In support of potential utility of sCD30 to monitor AD disease progression, sCD30 plasma levels were diminished following topical steroid treatment to reduce disease activity scores.[88,95] In this study with patients suffering from severe refractory AD and treated with cyclosporine, all patients displayed elevated sCD30 at baseline which became significantly reduced after 6 weeks of treatment and a correlation with diminished disease activity was noted.[89] Similar results were obtained in a study wherein severe AD patients were treated with cyclosporine for 12 weeks and the improvements in clinical symptoms correlated with reduction of serum IL-4 and sCD30 levels.[90]

The presence of activated CD30+ lymphocytes in the skin and elevated serum levels of sCD30 in the serum of patients with AD indirectly suggested potential regulatory functions of CD30 positive cells in disease pathogenesis and potential utility of compounds interfering with CD30 functions. The presence of high levels of sCD30 in patients with active disease renders further support for an important role of CD30 as an activation marker, useful for evaluation of a T-cell driven immune responses. However, despite encouraging evidence for therapeutic benefit in preclinical studies and correlative expression studies with patient samples, clinical trials with compounds targeting CD30/CD30L in inflammatory disease indication have not been reported.

Diagnostic Utility of sCD30 Level in Serum of Patients with Inflammatory Diseases

Several studies identified positive correlations between CD30 expression in tissue samples and/or serum levels of soluble CD30 and the severity of allergic diseases. In patients with systemic lupus erythematosus (SLE), the serum levels of sCD30 were compared with the classic parameters used to determine SLE activity. In patients with active disease, the serum levels of sCD30 were increased approximately 2 fold when compared to healthy controls and significant correlations between the levels of sCD30 and the SLE disease activity index, the C4 component of the complement system and anti-C1q antibodies, were identified. These findings suggested potential utility for sCD30 levels to determine and monitor SLE disease activity during treatment.

Soluble CD30 levels were also assessed in patients with localized scleroderma and a significant increase was identified when compared to healthy controls. The sCD30 serum concentrations correlated with the number of sclerotic lesions, the number of involved areas, levels of anti-histone antibody IgM and levels of interleukin 6. These results indicated that serum sCD30 levels may be helpful to assess disease stage of scleroderma and the response to treatment.[16] Additional studies looking at sCD30 serum levels were conducted with children suffering from atopic dermatitis (AD) or bronchial asthma and their relation to disease severity was investigated. In these patients, serum sCD30 levels correlated with the severity of AD and bronchial asthma, suggesting potential utility for sCD30 as an objective biomarker for the management of this autoimmune disease.[29]

In RA patients, high levels of sCD30 were found in peripheral blood and synovial fluids. In addition, CD30/CD3 double positive cells were present at significantly increased levels in synovial fluids, but not in peripheral blood of these patients. Serum values of sCD30 were higher in active than inactive RA patients and directly correlated with rheumatoid factor serum titers. Combined, these data strongly support an involvement of CD30+ T-cells in the immune processes of rheumatoid synovitis.[23] A counter regulatory role for CD30 on CD4+ T-cells has been suggested at sites of inflammation in Th1-mediated conditions, such as rheumatoid arthritis.[91,92] The correlation between disease severity and CD30/30L expression levels provided indirect evidence for potential therapeutic benefit when using compounds interfering with the CD30/CD30L system in several autoimmune diseases. However, a more comprehensive validation of the diagnostic value of sCD30 levels in patients with autoimmune disease, including direct comparison with standard diagnostic methods, is required.[29,93]

Future Directions

Analysis of human tissues or blood samples revealed a correlation between CD30 or sCD30 expression levels and disease progression in patients with rheumatoid arthritis,[94] multiple sclerosis, systemic sclerosis,[16,17] systemic lupus erythematosis and in CD30 positive, lymphoproliferative diseases such as HD and ALCL.[9] The correlations between disease stages and sCD30 levels suggested utility of CD30 as diagnostic tool and provided correlative evidence for a potential causative role for CD30 in disease progression.

While CD30 and CD30L represent only two components out of the many factors known to contribute to disease pathology of hematological and autoimmune disorders, preclinical and clinical data suggest that therapeutic intervention strategies targeting this pathway can achieve significant improvements. Preclinical experiments testing therapeutic compounds targeting the CD30/CD30L signaling pathway demonstrated beneficial therapeutic effects when tested in models of hematopoietic malignancies, autoimmune and inflammatory diseases. Data from early clinical trials demonstrated therapeutic benefit when targeting CD30 in sALCL and HD with therapeutic antibodies in single agent settings. Dose escalation studies in humans showed anti-CD30 mAbs to be safe and well tolerated, as dose limiting toxicities have not been reported. Dose escalation studies of the anti-CD30 ADC SGN-35 is currently ongoing and holds great promise for the improvement of therapeutic options in single agent settings or in combination with standard of care chemotherapy. Future development of anti-CD30 compounds in oncology indications will likely include combination of targeted therapeutic compounds with standard of care or combinations with other experimental anti-cancer compounds. Better understanding of the biological functions of the CD30/30L pathway and the mechanism of action by which these therapeutic compounds induce antitumor activity may help to identify the most effective combination treatments or to identify the patients that benefit most.

The preclinical data generated using anti-CD30 antibodies demonstrated therapeutic benefit in autoimmune indications. The immune-suppressive effects observed when targeting the CD30/CD30L system with therapeutic antibodies were supported by more recent experiments conducted in knock-out or transgenic mice, respectively. However, despite the strong preclinical data demonstrating therapeutic benefit, clinical trials in autoimmune indications have yet to be initiated to validate these preclinical observations in human diseases.

The search for predictive markers for response to treatment to anti-CD30 or CD30L compounds may help to accelerate their clinical development in oncology and autoimmune indications. Analysis of patient samples identified several correlations between disease severity and serum sCD30 levels in oncology and autoimmune diseases. Further validation of sCD30 levels as prognostic marker for disease severity in humans and their utility as potential surrogate markers for response to treatment in clinical trials is of highest value. Better understanding of the mechanism of action of therapeutic compounds targeting CD30 will be helpful in the rational design of future therapeutics and in the selection of combination treatments with the goal to improve efficacy and therapeutic benefit. From preclinical experiments, a role for NF-κB signaling in hematologic malignancies was suggested. Therefore, combination studies of anti-CD30 compounds with agents affecting NF-κB signaling in HD represent a promising combination treatment strategy. In this respect, CD30-CD30L is likely to remain the focus of intense preclinical and clinical investigation over the next several years.

Acknowledgements

We would like to thank Che-Leung Law, Mark Sandbaken and Nathan Ihle for critical reading of the manuscript.

References

1. Smith CA et al. CD30 antigen, a marker for Hodgkin's lymphoma, is a receptor whose ligand defines an emerging family of cytokines with homology to TNF. Cell 1993; 73(7):1349-60.
2. Gruss H J, Duyster J, Herrmann. Structural and biological features of the TNF receptor and TNF ligand superfamilies: interactive signals in the pathobiology of Hodgkin's disease. Ann Oncol 1996; 7 Suppl 4:19-26.
3. Durkop H et al. Molecular cloning and expression of a new member of the nerve growth factor receptor family that is characteristic for Hodgkin's disease. Cell 1992; 68(3):421-7.
4. Cabanillas F et al. Lymphomatoid papulosis: a T-cell dyscrasia with a propensity to transform into malignant lymphoma. Ann Intern Med 1995; 122(3):210-7.
5. Berro AI, Perry GA, Agrawal DK. Increased expression and activation of CD30 induce apoptosis in human blood eosinophils. J Immunol 2004; 173(3):2174-83.
6. Agrawal B, Reddish M, Longenecker BM. CD30 expression on human CD8+ T-cells isolated from peripheral blood lymphocytes of normal donors. J Immunol 1996; 157(8):3229-34.
7. Romagnani S et al. Role for CD30 in HIV expression. Immunol Lett 1996; 51(1-2):83-8.
8. Durkop H et al. Expression of the CD30 antigen in nonlymphoid tissues and cells. J Pathol 2000; 190(5):613-8.
9. Kaudewitz P et al. Atypical cells in lymphomatoid papulosis express the Hodgkin cell-associated antigen Ki-1. J Invest Dermatol 1986; 86(4):350-4.
10. Chiarle R et al. CD30 in normal and neoplastic cells. Clin Immunol 1999; 90(2):157-64.
11. Granados S, Hwang ST. Roles for CD30 in the biology and treatment of CD30 lymphoproliferative diseases. J Invest Dermatol 2004; 122(6):345-7.
12. Stein H et al. CD30(+) anaplastic large cell lymphoma: a review of its histopathologic, genetic and clinical features. Blood 2000; 96(12):3681-95.
13. Younes A, ME Kadin. Emerging applications of the tumor necrosis factor family of ligands and receptors in cancer therapy. J Clin Oncol 2003; 21(18):3526-34.
14. Zinzani PL et al. Anaplastic large-cell lymphoma: clinical and prognostic evaluation of 90 adult patients. J Clin Oncol 1996; 14(3):955-62.
15. Pizzolo G, Romagnani S. CD30 molecule (Ki-1 Ag): more than just a marker of CD30+ lymphoma. Haematologica 1995; 80(4):357-66.
16. Ihn H et al. Circulating levels of soluble CD30 are increased in patients with localized scleroderma and correlated with serological and clinical features of the disease. J Rheumatol 2000; 27(3):698-702.
17. McMillan SA et al. Evaluation of the clinical utility of cerebrospinal fluid (CSF) indices of inflammatory markers in multiple sclerosis. Acta Neurol Scand 2000; 101(4):239-43.
18. Horn-Lohrens O et al. Shedding of the soluble form of CD30 from the Hodgkin-analogous cell line L540 is strongly inhibited by a new CD30-specific antibody (Ki-4). Int J Cancer 1995; 60(4):539-44.
19. Nadali G et al. Serum level of the soluble form of the CD30 molecule identifies patients with Hodgkin's disease at high risk of unfavorable outcome. Blood 1998; 91(8):3011-6.
20. Pizzolo G et al. Serum levels of soluble CD30 molecule (Ki-1 antigen) in Hodgkin's disease: relationship with disease activity and clinical stage. Br J Haematol 1990; 75(2):282-4.
21. Pizzolo G et al. High serum level of soluble CD30 in acute primary HIV-1 infection. Clin Exp Immunol 1997; 108(2):251-3.
22. Caligaris-Cappio F et al. Circulating levels of soluble CD30, a marker of cells producing Th2-type cytokines, are increased in patients with systemic lupus erythematosus and correlate with disease activity. Clin Exp Rheumatol 1995; 13(3):339-43.

23. Gerli R et al. High levels of the soluble form of CD30 molecule in rheumatoid arthritis (RA) are expression of CD30+ T-cell involvement in the inflamed joints. Clin Exp Immunol 1995; 102(3):547-50.

24. Okumura M et al. Increased serum concentration of soluble CD30 in patients with Graves' disease and Hashimoto's thyroiditis. J Clin Endocrinol Metab 1997; 82(6):1757-60.

25. Bengtsson A et al. Elevated serum levels of soluble CD30 in patients with atopic dermatitis (AD). Clin Exp Immunol 1997; 109(3):533-7.

26. Dummer W, Brocker EB, Bastian BC. Elevated serum levels of soluble CD30 are associated with atopic dermatitis, but not with respiratory atopic disorders and allergic contact dermatitis. Br J Dermatol 1997; 137(2):185-7.

27. Caproni M et al. In vivo relevance of CD30 in atopic dermatitis. Allergy 1997; 52(11):1063-70.

28. Frezzolini A et al. Soluble CD30 in pediatric patients with atopic dermatitis. Allergy 1997; 52(1):106-9.

29. Heshmat NM, El-Hadidi ES. Soluble CD30 serum levels in atopic dermatitis and bronchial asthma and its relationship with disease severity in pediatric age. Pediatr Allergy Immunol 2006; 17(4):297-303.

30. Leonard C et al. Allergen-induced CD30 expression on T-cells of atopic asthmatics. Clin Exp Allergy 1997; 27(7):780-6.

31. Nogueira JM et al. Soluble CD30, dehydroepiandrosterone sulfate and dehydroepiandrosterone in atopic and non-atopic children. Allerg Immunol (Paris) 1998; 30(1):3-8.

32. Croager EJ, Abraham LJ. Characterisation of the human CD30 ligand gene structure. Biochim Biophys Acta 1997; 1353(3):231-5.

33. Gattei V et al. CD30 ligand is frequently expressed in human hematopoietic malignancies of myeloid and lymphoid origin. Blood 1997; 89(6):2048-59.

34. Gruss HJ et al. Pleiotropic effects of the CD30 ligand on CD30-expressing cells and lymphoma cell lines. Blood 1994; 83(8):2045-56.

35. Gruss HJ et al. Expression and regulation of CD30 ligand and CD30 in human leukemia-lymphoma cell lines. Leukemia 1994; 8(12):2083-94.

36. Nicod LP, Isler P. Alveolar macrophages in sarcoidosis coexpress high levels of CD86 (B7.2), CD40 and CD30L. Am J Respir Cell Mol Biol 1997; 17(1):91-6.

37. Pinto A et al. Human eosinophils express functional CD30 ligand and stimulate proliferation of a Hodgkin's disease cell line. Blood 1996; 88(9):3299-305.

38. Shanebeck KD et al. Regulation of murine B-cell growth and differentiation by CD30 ligand. Eur J Immunol 1995; 25(8):2147-53.

39. Wiley SR, Goodwin RG, Smith CA. Reverse signaling via CD30 ligand. J Immunol 1996; 157(8):3635-9.

40. Younes A et al. CD30 ligand is expressed on resting normal and malignant human B-lymphocytes. Br J Haematol 1996; 93(3):569-71.

41. Molin D et al. Mast cells express functional CD30 ligand and are the predominant CD30L-positive cells in Hodgkin's disease. Br J Haematol 2001; 114(3):616-23.

42. Duckett CS, Thompson CB. CD30-dependent degradation of TRAF2: implications for negative regulation of TRAF signaling and the control of cell survival. Genes Dev 1997; 11(21):2810-21.

43. Aizawa S et al. Tumor necrosis factor receptor-associated factor (TRAF) 5 and TRAF2 are involved in CD30-mediated NFkappaB activation. J Biol Chem 1997; 272(4):2042-5.

44. Duckett CS et al. Induction of nuclear factor kappaB by the CD30 receptor is mediated by TRAF1 and TRAF2. Mol Cell Biol 1997; 17(3):1535-42.

45. Horie R et al. A novel domain in the CD30 cytoplasmic tail mediates NFkappaB activation. Int Immunol 1998; 10(2):203-10.

46. Mir SS, Richter BW, Duckett CS. Differential effects of CD30 activation in anaplastic large cell lymphoma and Hodgkin disease cells. Blood 2000; 96(13):4307-12.

47. Boll B et al. The fully human anti-CD30 antibody 5F11 activates NF-{kappa}B and sensitizes lymphoma cells to bortezomib-induced apoptosis. Blood 2005; 106(5):1839-42.

48. Chiarle R et al. CD30 overexpression enhances negative selection in the thymus and mediates programmed cell death via a Bcl-2-sensitive pathway. J Immunol 1999; 163(1):194-205.

49. Gilfillan MC et al. Expression of the costimulatory receptor CD30 is regulated by both CD28 and cytokines. J Immunol 1998; 160(5):2180-7.

50. Podack ER et al. CD30-governor of memory T-cells? Ann N Y Acad Sci 2002; 975:101-13.

51. Gaspal FM et al. Mice deficient in OX40 and CD30 signals lack memory antibody responses because of deficient CD4 T-cell memory. J Immunol 2005; 174(7):3891-6.

52. Fischer M et al. Mast cell CD30 ligand is upregulated in cutaneous inflammation and mediates degranulation-independent chemokine secretion. J Clin Invest 2006; 116(10):2748-56.

53. Schneider C, Hubinger G. Pleiotropic signal transduction mediated by human CD30: a member of the tumor necrosis factor receptor (TNFR) family. Leuk Lymphoma 2002; 43(7):1355-66.

54. Hsu PL, Hsu SM. Autocrine growth regulation of CD30 ligand in CD30-expressing Reed-Sternberg cells: distinction between Hodgkin's disease and anaplastic large cell lymphoma. Lab Invest 2000; 80(7):1111-9.
55. Tian ZG et al. In vivo antitumor effects of unconjugated CD30 monoclonal antibodies on human anaplastic large-cell lymphoma xenografts. Cancer Res 1995; 55(22):5335-41.
56. Pfeifer W et al. A murine xenograft model for human CD30+ anaplastic large cell lymphoma. Successful growth inhibition with an anti-CD30 antibody (HeFi-1). Am J Pathol 1999; 155(4):1353-9.
57. Wahl AF et al. The anti-CD30 monoclonal antibody SGN-30 promotes growth arrest and DNA fragmentation in vitro and affects antitumor activity in models of Hodgkin's disease. Cancer Res 2002; 62(13):3736-42.
58. Cerveny, CG et al. Signaling via the anti-CD30 mAb SGN-30 sensitizes Hodgkin's disease cells to conventional chemotherapeutics. Leukemia 2005; 19(9):1648-55.
59. Klimka A et al. An anti-CD30 single-chain Fv selected by phage display and fused to Pseudomonas exotoxin A (Ki-4(scFv)-ETA') is a potent immunotoxin against a Hodgkin-derived cell line. Br J Cancer 1999; 80(8):1214-22.
60. Pasqualucci L et al. Antitumor activity of anti-CD30 immunotoxin (Ber-H2/saporin) in vitro and in severe combined immunodeficiency disease mice xenografted with human CD30+ anaplastic large-cell lymphoma. Blood 1995; 85(8):2139-46.
61. Falini B et al. Response of refractory Hodgkin's disease to monoclonal anti-CD30 immunotoxin. Lancet 1992; 339(8803):1195-6.
62. Hamblett KJ et al. Effects of drug loading on the antitumor activity of a monoclonal antibody drug conjugate. Clin Cancer Res 2004; 10(20):7063-70.
63. Francisco JA et al. cAC10-vcMMAE, an anti-CD30-monomethyl auristatin E conjugate with potent and selective antitumor activity. Blood 2003; 102(4):1458-65.
64. Falini B et al. In vivo targeting of Hodgkin and Reed-Sternberg cells of Hodgkin's disease with monoclonal antibody Ber-H2 (CD30): immunohistological evidence. Br J Haematol 1992; 82(1):38-45.
65. Schnell R et al. Clinical evaluation of ricin A-chain immunotoxins in patients with Hodgkin's lymphoma. Ann Oncol 2003; 14(5):729-36.
66. Hartmann F et al. Anti-CD16/CD30 bispecific antibody treatment for Hodgkin's disease: role of infusion schedule and costimulation with cytokines. Clin Cancer Res 2001; 7(7):1873-81.
67. Hartmann F et al. Treatment of refractory Hodgkin's disease with an anti-CD16/CD30 bispecific antibody. Blood 1997; 89(6):2042-7.
68. Borchmann P et al. Phase 1 trial of the novel bispecific molecule H22xKi-4 in patients with refractory Hodgkin lymphoma. Blood 2002; 100(9):3101-7.
69. Schnell R et al. Treatment of refractory Hodgkin's lymphoma patients with an iodine-131-labeled murine anti-CD30 monoclonal antibody. J Clin Oncol 2005; 23(21):4669-78.
70. Hartmann F et al. Treatment of Hodgkin's disease with bispecific antibodies. Ann Oncol 1996; 7 Suppl 4:143-6.
71. Bartlett NL et al. Phase I study of SGN-30, a chimeric monoclonal antibody (mAB) in patients with refractory or recurrent CD30+ hematologic malignancies. Blood 2002; 100(11):Abs 1403.
72. Carabasi M et al. Pharmacokinetics, safety and tolerability of SGN-30, a chimeric monoclonal antibody (mAb), administered as a single dose to patients with CD30+ hematologic malignancies. Proc Am Soc Clin Oncol 2003; 22:Abs 722.
73. Bartlett NL et al. Safety, antitumor activity and pharmacokinetics of six weekly doses of SGN-30 (anti-CD30 monoclonal antibody) in patients with refractory or recurrent CD30+ hematologic malignancies. Blood 2003; 102(11):Abs 2390.
74. Leonard J et al. Phase II study to SGN-30 (Anti-CD30 monoclonal antibody) in patients with refractory or recurrent Hodgkin's disease. Blood 2004; 104(11):Abs 2635.
75. Forero A et al. Initial phase II results of SGN-30 (anti-CD30 monoclonal antibody) in patients with refractory or recurrent systemic anaplastic large cell lymphoma (ALCL). J Proc Am Soc Clin Oncol 2005; 24: Abs 6601.
76. Schnell R, Borchmann P. SGN-30 (Seattle genetics). Curr Opin Mol Ther 2006; 8(2):164-72.
77. Shimozato O et al. Expression of CD30 ligand (CD153) on murine activated T-cells. Biochem Biophys Res Commun 1999; 256(3):519-26.
78. Chakrabarty S et al. Critical roles of CD30/CD30L interactions in murine autoimmune diabetes. Clin Exp Immunol 2003; 133(3):318-25.
79. Beckmann J et al. The role of CD30 in skin and heart allograft rejection in the mouse. Transplant Proc 2001; 33(1-2):140-1.
80. Florido M et al. Contribution of CD30/CD153 but not of CD27/CD70, CD134/OX40L, or CD137/4-1BBL to the optimal induction of protective immunity to Mycobacterium avium. J Leukoc Biol 2004; 76(5):1039-46.

81. Blazar BR et al. CD30/CD30 ligand (CD153) interaction regulates CD4+ T-cell-mediated graft-versus-host disease. J Immunol 2004; 173(5):2933-41.

82. Zeiser R et al. Early CD30 signaling is critical for adoptively transferred CD4+CD25+ regulatory T-cells in prevention of acute graft versus host disease. Blood 2006.

83. Polte T, Behrendt AK, Hansen G. Direct evidence for a critical role of CD30 in the development of allergic asthma. J Allergy Clin Immunol 2006; 118(4):942-8.

84. Lane PJ et al. CD4+CD3– cells regulate the organization of lymphoid tissue and T-cell memory for antibody responses. Int J Hematol 2006; 83(1):12-6.

85. Kennedy MK, Willis CR, Armitage RJ. Deciphering CD30 ligand biology and its role in humoral immunity. Immunology 2006; 118(2):143-52.

86. Leung DY, Bieber T. Atopic dermatitis. Lancet 2003; 361(9352):151-60.

87. Simpson EL, Hanifin JM. Atopic dermatitis. Med Clin North Am 2006; 90(1):149-67, ix.

88. Folster-Holst R et al. Soluble CD30 plasma concentrations correlate with disease activity in patients with atopic dermatitis. Acta Derm Venereol 2002; 82(4):245-8.

89. Caproni M et al. Soluble CD30 and cyclosporine in severe atopic dermatitis. Int Arch Allergy Immunol 2000; 121(4):324-8.

90. Bottari V et al. Cyclosporin A (CyA) reduces sCD30 serum levels in atopic dermatitis: a possible new immune intervention. Allergy 1999; 54(5):507-10.

91. Gerli R et al. Role of CD30+ T-cells in rheumatoid arthritis: a counter-regulatory paradigm for Th1-driven diseases. Trends Immunol 2001; 22(2):72-7.

92. Okamoto A et al. Pathophysiological functions of CD30+ CD4+ T-cells in rheumatoid arthritis. Acta Med Okayama 2003; 57(6):267-77.

93. Ciferska H et al. The levels of sCD30 and of sCD40L in a group of patients with systemic lupus erythematodes and their diagnostic value. Clin Rheumatol 2006.

94. Gerli R et al. CD30+ T-cells in rheumatoid synovitis: mechanisms of recruitment and functional role. J Immunol 2000; 164(8):4399-407.

95. Oflazoglu E et al. CD30 expression on CD10a+ and CD8+ cells in atopic dermatitis and correlation with disease severity. Eur J Dermatol. 2008; 18:41-49.

CHAPTER 13

Tumor Necrosis Factor Receptor Superfamily Member 21:
TNFR-Related Death Receptor-6, DR6

Robert Benschop, Tao Wei and Songqing Na*

Abstract

TNFRSF21 (death receptor-6, DR6) is an orphan TNF receptor superfamily member and belongs to a subgroup of receptors called death receptors. DR6 is expressed ubiquitously with high expression in lymphoid organs, heart, brain and pancreas. Ectopic expression of DR6 in some cell lines leads to apoptosis and activation of the JNK and NF-κB pathways. Some tumor cells overexpress DR6, typically in conjunction with elevated anti-apoptosis molecules. DR6 deficient mice (DR6$^{-/-}$) show normal development with no gross pathology in any major organs. In the absence of DR6, ligation of the TCR results in enhanced T-cell proliferation, activation and skewed Th2 cytokine production. Similarly, B-cells lacking DR6 show increased proliferation, cell division and cell survival upon mitogenic stimulation (anti-CD40 and LPS) or BCR ligation. As a result, DR6$^{-/-}$ mice show increased Th2 immune responses to both T-dependent and -independent antigens. All those data indicate that DR6 plays an important regulatory role for the generation of adaptive immunity. More importantly, DR6$^{-/-}$ mice are resistant to EAE and allergic airway hypersensitivity, possibly as a result of a deficiency in the migration of antigen specific T-cells. Therefore, DR6 is a potential therapeutic target for treating inflammatory and autoimmune disease by means of biological intervention. In addition, DR6 is highly expressed in many tumor cell lines and tumor samples. Interestingly, both of its transcriptional and cell surface expression are regulated by the NF-κB pathway and metalloproteinase in some tumor cell lines, respectively. The role of DR6 as an apoptosis-inducing receptor is less clear and perhaps cell type dependent. Therefore, in addition to its roles in regulating immune responses, DR6 may also be involved in tumor cell survival and immune evasion, which is subject to future investigations.

Introduction

Tumor necrosis factor (TNF) family members and their receptors have been recognized as the key players in normal cellular functions in mediating the growth, differentiation, apoptosis and survival in both immune and non-immune cell types. The abnormal expression, activation or functional changes of many of the family members has led to diseases such as rheumatoid arthritis,[1] inflammatory bowel disease,[2] osteoporosis[3] and cancer.[4,5] Understanding the interaction between ligand and receptor and the signal transduction pathway is the key to reveal their physiological functions and provide for potential therapeutic applications.

The TNF receptor family members are characterized by several extracellular, cysteine-rich motifs which contains the ligand-binding domain.[6] Compared with their extracellular domains,

---

*Corresponding Author: Songqing Na—Lilly Research Laboratories, Eli Lilly and Co, Indianapolis, IN 46285 USA. Email: na_songqing@lilly.com

Therapeutic Targets of the TNF Superfamily, edited by Iqbal S. Grewal.
©2009 Landes Bioscience and Springer Science+Business Media.

the intracellular domains of the receptors show more diversity. Among them, there is a subgroup which has a cytoplasmic death domain and activation of those receptors by their ligand leads to receptor-mediated Caspase activation and cellular apoptosis. In 1998, Pan et al[7] identified a new family member that they named death receptor-6 (DR6) by searching the EST database using the protein sequence of the extracellular, cysteine-rich ligand binding domain of TNFR2. During the same period time, we used a similar approach by taking the extracellular cysteine-rich domain of osteoprotegerin (OPG) and identified the same molecule. In the recent nomenclature, DR6 has been designated as tumor necrosis factor receptor superfamily member 21 (TNFRSF21) and is just one of the few orphan receptors in the family. Extensive efforts to identify the ligand for DR6 have been without success. As a result, our ability to study the physiological function of DR6 has been limited. Using the genetic approach by deleting the DR6 gene in the mouse genome has proved fruitful and revealed several functions for DR6 in cancer and especially in immune regulation. In this chapter, we will discuss the DR6 sequence and structure, expression, signaling pathway and regulatory roles in immune modulation and its possible role in cancer.

DR6: Sequence, Structure and Expression

Human DR6 is a type I transmembrane protein and has a total of 655 amino acids and similar to other TNFR family members has a common structural framework defined by the presence of cysteine residues in highly conserved locations within the extracellular cysteine-rich domains. DR6 has a putative signal sequence at its N-terminus (amino acids 1-41). Unlike DR4 and DR5, DR6 has four extracellular cysteine-rich domains that are most related to those of osteoprote-gerin (OPG) and TNFR2 with 36% and 42% amino acid identities, respectively. Within its cytoplasmic domain, DR6 contains a death domain which is related to those of all known death domain-containing TNFR family members. Based on its amino sequence, the death domain of DR6 is most related to that of TNFR1 (27.2% identity) and least to that of DR5 (19.7% identity). Interestingly, the position of the DR6 death domain differs from the other family members and is directly adjacent to the transmembrane domain followed by a 150 amino acid tail. In addition, following the death domain is a putative leucine zipper sequence overlapping with a proline-rich domain.[7] We searched several major genome databases and identified DR6 genes from 17 differ-ent species including fish, chicken, rodent to monkey and human (Table 1). Based on sequence similarity (Fig. 1) and phylogenetic analysis, the known DR6 genes appear to be divided into two main clusters: mammals and fishes (Fig. 2). Within each cluster, the DR6 sequences share 73-99% and 51-68% identity, respectively; DR6 of human, monkey and mouse are highly homologous and share 89-99% sequence identity. The DR6 sequence of Chicken and frog is closer to the mammals than to the fishers, but the paucity of data regarding DR6 sequence in additional avians and amphibians/reptiles prevents assignment of these sequences to either of the well represented clusters or the identification of a different cluster. The DR6 sequences between the mammal and fish clusters exhibit only 44-54% sequence identity.

Based on mRNA expression, DR6 has been found in most tissues and the transcript is es-pecially abundant in heart, brain, placenta, pancreas and immune lymphoid organs including spleen, thymus, lymph nodes and bone marrow. The expression of DR6 in mouse shows a similar pattern to that in human tissues except that DR6 expression in kidney is higher in mouse than in human.[9] Interestingly, DR6 transcripts are also found at high levels in some cancer cell lines including colorectal adenocarcinoma (SW480, HA1233, HT-29), nonsmall lung carcinoma (A549, HA188), melanoma (G361), breast cancer (MDA-MB-231) and prostate tumor cell lines includ-ing DU145 and PC3.[8] Furthermore, these authors found that the expression of DR6 is increased in cancerous tissue biopsies from patients with late stage prostate or breast cancer compared with levels in normal tissue. Expression is particularly high in prostate tumors with Gleason score of 9 to 10 compared with prostate tumor score obtained from early stage disease.

There is some evidence suggesting that expression of DR6 is regulated in activation and differentiation processes. We showed that the activation of mature B lymphocytes by BCR or anti-CD40 Ab or LPS leads to a profound downregulation of cell surface DR6 expression.[10] In

Table 1. DR6 family proteins from different species used for phylogenetic tree (Fig. 1) and multiple sequence alignment (Fig. 2)

Species Name	Common Name	Ensembl ID	Refseq ID
Bos taurus	cow	ENSBTAP00000026719	
Homo sapiens	human	ENSP00000296861	NP_055267
Canis familiaris	dog	ENSCAFP00000003059	
Mus musculus	house mouse	ENSMUSP00000024708	NP_848704
Rattus norvegicus	Norway rat	ENSRNOP00000015918	XP_236992
Echinops telfairi	small Madagascar hedgehog	ENSETEP00000006116	
Gasterosteus aculeatus	three spined stickleback	ENSGACP00000005616	
Danio rerio	zebrafish	ENSDARP00000036002	
Macaca mulatta	rhesus monkey	ENSMMUP00000015624	
Monodelphis domestica	gray short-tailed opossum	ENSMODP00000030255	
Oryctolagus cuniculus	rabbit	ENSOCUP00000014212	
Oryzias latipes	Japanese medaka	ENSORLP00000019568	
Pan troglodytes	chimpanzee	ENSPTRP00000031175	XP_001145645
Takifugu rubripes	torafugu	NEWSINFRUP00000153994	
Xenopus tropicalis	western clawed frog	ENSXETP00000024705	
Tetraodon nigroviridis	bony fishes 2	GSTENP00035511001	
Gallus gallus	chicken	ENSGALP00000026931	

T lymphocytes, the differentiation of T-cells also affects DR6 expression: naïve Th0 T-cells have higher levels of DR6 transcript which is decreased after T-cells are committed to either Th1 or Th2 differentiation.[11] In tumor cells, the expression of DR6 seems to be regulated by TNF-α induced NF-κB activation pathway. Upon treatment with TNF-α, DR6 expression is increased in a time dependent fashion in LnCAP cells. TNF-α also moderately increases DR6 expression in endothelial cells. The increased DR6 expression induced by TNF-α stimulation is dependent on NF-κB activation, since both the NF-κB nuclear translocation inhibitory peptide and nonsteroidal anti-inflammatory drugs (NSAIDs) inhibited the effect of TNF-α on the induction of DR6 expression.[8] Interestingly, high DR6 expression in tumor cells also correlates with constitutive high basal level of NF-κB activation,[8] suggesting that the expression of DR6 is dependent on the NF-κB pathway activation mediated by either external stimuli such as extrinsic TNF-α stimulation or intrinsic constitutive activation in those cancer cells.

Signaling of DR6

Ectopic overexpression of TNFR members can mimic ligand activation and triggers ligand-independent receptor activation and downstream signaling events. Using this system, Pan et al demonstrated that overexpression of DR6 in Hela cells induces apoptosis, although the apoptosis induced by DR6 is about 50% less effective than other death receptors such as DR4.[7] In a coexpression system it was found that DR6 does not form protein-protein complexes with the adaptor molecule FADD.[7] However, DR6 expression together with another adaptor protein, TRADD, does lead to the formation of DR6-TRADD complexes. The interaction between DR6 and TRADD seems to be specific, since other adaptor molecules such as RAIDD and RIP, which are involved in binding to other TNFR family members, do not interact with DR6 in this cell assay system.[7] Not surprisingly, overexpression of DR6 in HEK293 cells also induces NF-κB activation, which requires the cytoplasmic domain of DR6 and presumably adaptor proteins such as TRADD, since deletion of the cytoplasmic domain of DR6 completely abolishes NF-κB activation and apoptosis. Interestingly, high basal level of NF-κB activation in tumor cells leads

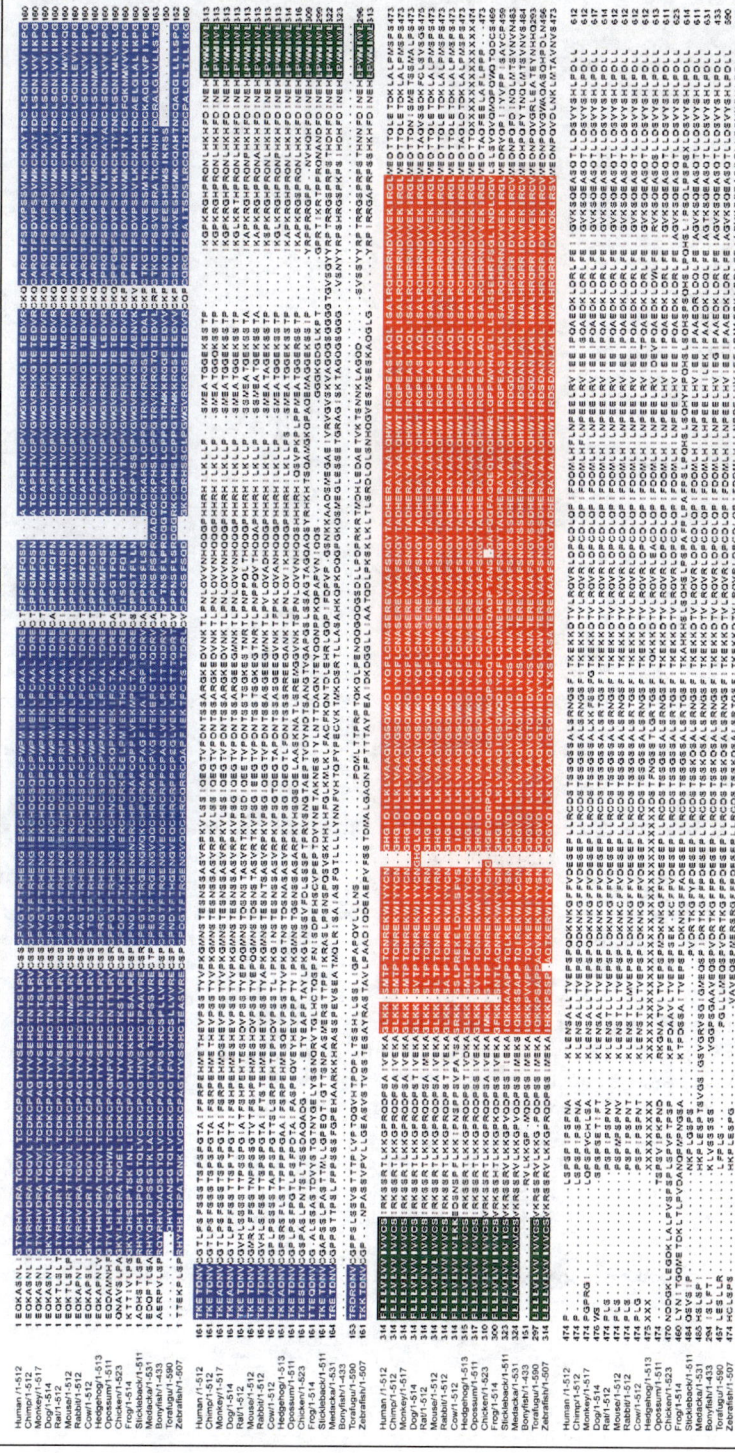

Figure 1. Alignment of DR6 protein family sequences. The alignment was generated by Clustalx with Blosum matrix and default gap penalties and rendered using Jalview. DR6 protein family was computed by Markov Clustering method[22] and annotated in Ensembl database (http://www.ensembl. org). Sequence ID of each species is shown in Table 1. Four consecutive cysteine-rich domains (CRDs), transmembrane helix and death domain are colored in blue, green and red respectively. Signal peptides were removed from the figure.

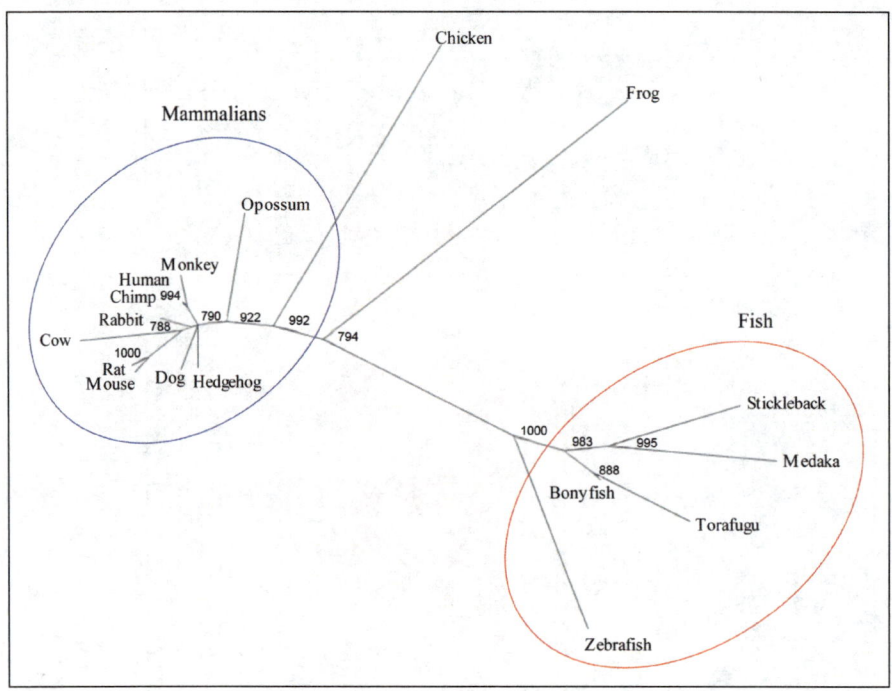

Figure 2. An unrooted distance tree of DR6 family proteins, displaying the number of replications in 1000 bootstrappings. Phylogenetic analysis based on the multiple sequence alignment in Figure 1 was carried out in PHYLIP package. Sequence ID of each species are listed in Table 1.

to the increased DR6 expression,[8] suggesting that DR6 is a potential target gene regulated by NF-κB. Whether the regulation of DR6 expression is controlled by an autocrine mechanism is subject to further investigation. In addition, overexpression of DR6 also leads to JNK activation as evidenced in vitro by cytoplasmic JNK kinase-mediated c-Jun phosphorylation. Clearly, the definitive signaling components from DR6 to either NF-κB or JNK are still missing and need to be further explored.

Another approach to explore the signaling pathway of DR6 in the absence of a known DR6 ligand comes from studying cell signaling from DR6[-/-] mice. In the absence of DR6, activation of CD4[+] T-cells by TCR ligation leads to rapidly increased nuclear accumulation of the transcriptional factor, NF-ATc.[9] As a result, the nuclear NF-ATc from DR6 deficient T-cells demonstrates higher specific DNA binding activity. Interestingly, another family member, NF-ATp, is not affected by the lack of DR6 in T-cells. Furthermore, in contrast to NF-ATc activation and NF-κB activation in HEK293 cells shown previously by Pan et al,[7] NF-κB activation upon TCR ligation is identical in CD4[+] T-cells from both WT and DR6[-/-] mice as evidenced by similar nuclear translocation of NF-κB p50.[12] Together, these data suggest that DR6 specifically modulates NF-ATc transcription activity. Consistent with the activation of the JNK pathway by DR6 overexpression in HEK293 cells, JNK activation is decreased in CD4[+] T-cells of DR6[-/-] mice upon TCR ligation.[11] Both the increased NF-ATc nuclear translocation and decreased JNK activation in DR6 deficient CD4[+] T-cells are consistent with the fact that the phosphorylation of NF-ATc regulates its nuclear translocation and JNK has been demonstrated to inhibit targeting of the protein phosphatase calcineurin to NF-ATc.[12] Therefore, the absence of DR6 may, to some extent, reverse the inhibitory effect of JNK on calcineurin to NF-ATc and promote its nuclear translocation.

In contrast to T-cells, DR6 is involved in regulating the NF-κB signaling pathway in mouse B-cells.[10] In the absence of DR6, stimulation of B-cells with anti-CD40 Ab or IgM leads to the rapid and marked increase of the nuclear accumulation of NF-κB transcription factor, c-Rel. Consistent with those observations, the increased nuclear translocation of c-Rel also correlates with increased c-Rel DNA binding capacity as evidenced by gel mobility shift assays. Furthermore, the increased c-Rel transcriptional activity in the absence of DR6 leads to the increased expression of its target gene, Bcl-X$_L$ and reduces cell apoptosis upon treatment with anti-CD40 and IgM in B-cells,[10] suggesting that DR6 is involved in activating the NF-κB pathway. Together, the current evidence suggests that the modulation of NF-κB activation by DR6 is cell type- and stimulus-dependent, which could be explained by the differential expression of cofactors involved in DR6 signaling in different lymphocytes.

Biological Functions of DR6

Most of our knowledge around the functions of DR6 is derived from studying the effects of DR6 gene ablation in mice. Both V. Dixit, et al and our group independently generated DR6-deficient (DR6$^{-/-}$) mice with largely similar initial findings.[9-11] DR6$^{-/-}$ mice are viable, fertile and no gross pathology is observed in any of the major organs. Also no differences are observed in immunoglobulin levels, numbers of neutrophils, monocytes/macrophages, NK cells, or B-cells in the major lymphoid organs. A slight elevation is observed in the number of T-cells in the thymus and peripheral blood of DR6$^{-/-}$ mice, but T-cell numbers in the spleen and lymph nodes are comparable between WT and KO mice. Therefore, DR6 does not seem to be required for embryonic or immune lineage development.

DR6 Regulates CD4$^+$ T-Cell Proliferation and Th Cell Differentiation

Although DR6 does not appear to affect development, DR6 exhibits multiple levels of immune modulatory effects as demonstrated in DR6$^{-/-}$ mice. These differences between DR6$^{-/-}$ and WT littermates become apparent only upon stimulation of the immune system. In the absence of DR6, T-cell proliferation in vitro is greatly enhanced in response to mitogenic stimulation including TCR and costimulatory factors. Furthermore, the cytokine secretion profile is skewed, favoring production of Th2-type cytokines (IL-4, IL-5, IL-10, IL-13). Interestingly, there is no distinction of CD4$^+$ T-cells in their ability to produce the Th1 cytokine, IFN-γ, between WT and DR6$^{-/-}$ mice. Subsequent experiments inducing Th differentiation in vitro clearly demonstrated enhanced Th2 differentiation in T-cells lacking DR6. It should be noted that Th1 differentiation was equally successful in CD4$^+$ T-cells of WT and DR6$^{-/-}$ mice. In addition, the enhanced T-cell proliferation and Th2 cytokine production in T-cells of DR6$^{-/-}$ mice are recapitulated ex vivo using T-cells from mice immunized with the T-cell dependent antigen, keyhole limpet hemocyanin (KLH). Production of Th1 cytokines (IL-2 and IFN-γ) is also slightly higher compared to WT mice, but this difference was not nearly as pronounced as observed for the Th2 cytokines.[9,11] Taken together, these studies demonstrate that DR6 plays important roles in regulating T-cell activation responses as well as Th cell differentiation.

DR6 Regulates B-Cell Expansion, Survival and Humoral Response

In addition to its function in T-cell proliferation and differentiation, DR6 also affects B-cellular functions including cell expansion and humoral responses.[10-11] Upon BCR and B-cell mitogenic (LPS, anti-CD40) stimulations in vitro, B-cells from DR6$^{-/-}$ mice exhibit dramatically increased proliferation primarily due to a combination of increased cell division and reduced apoptosis. In addition, the B7 family costimulatory molecules, CD80 and CD86, are also significantly upregulated in B-cells from DR6$^{-/-}$ after stimulation compared to DR6 WT cells. This might have important consequences for the efficacy with which T- and B-cells interact. Indeed, germinal center formation is greatly enhanced in DR6$^{-/-}$ mice upon immunization. As a result, T-cell-dependent antigen-specific immunoglobulin titers in vivo are significantly elevated in DR6$^{-/-}$ mice after immunization. In addition, the immunoglobulin production in response to T-independent antigens was also enhanced in DR6$^{-/-}$ mice, demonstrating that the lack of DR6 affects intrinsic B-cell responses.[10]

Role for DR6 in Inflammatory and Autoimmune Diseases

The in vitro studies of both T- and B-cells using DR6$^{-/-}$ mice clearly demonstrate that DR6 is a critical regulator for adaptive immunity. To further test this, a number of pathologically relevant disease models have been tested using DR6$^{-/-}$ mice. Transferring T-cells from DR6$^{-/-}$ mice in a model for acute graft-versus-host disease (GVHD) results in a more rapid onset and severe pathology than when WT T-cells are transferred. Mice receiving T-cells from DR6$^{-/-}$ mice exhibit a more rapid weight loss and earlier organ damage in the thymus, spleen and intestines. Subsequently, this accelerated course of GVHD leads to the earlier mortality.[13] The severe GVHD symptoms following transfer of T-cells from DR6$^{-/-}$ mice is primarily due to the enhanced activation and expansion of CD4^{+} and CD8^{+} T-cells from DR6$^{-/-}$ mice in vivo.[13] This result is in line with the hyper-proliferation of T-cells from DR6$^{-/-}$ mice to stimuli observed in vitro and further support the idea of DR6 as a negative regulator of immune activation.

Multiple sclerosis is an autoimmune demyelinating disease characterized by inappropriate host immune response to self central nervous system (CNS) antigens. Although no true preclinical model of MS exists, experimental autoimmune encephalomyelitis (EAE) is a widely used animal model of antigen-driven T-cell autoimmunity that is targeted at CNS. Upon immunization with myelin oligodendrocyte glycoprotein (MOG) peptide, the mouse myelin-specific T-cells infiltrate into the CNS and the resulting damage causes paralysis. After immunization with MOG peptide, WT mice exhibit a high grade of paralysis as expected in this model. In contrast, DR6$^{-/-}$ mice are highly resistant to both onset and progression of disease.[14] Interestingly, antigen recall responses show increased proliferation of splenic CD4^{+} T-cells from DR6$^{-/-}$ mice ex vivo. Also in line with the previous studies, Th2 cytokine responses are elevated in CD4^{+} T-cells of DR6$^{-/-}$ mice without any difference in their ability to produce Th1 cytokines. In contrast, mononuclear cell (including CD4^{+} T-cells) infiltration in the CNS is markedly reduced in DR6$^{-/-}$ mice immunized with MOG. Transfer of myelin-specific T-cells from DR6$^{-/-}$ mice into WT does not result in disease, but DR6$^{-/-}$ mice receiving myelin-specific WT T-cells do develop EAE symptoms.[14] This demonstrates that despite immune recognition of the antigen, there is an intrinsic inability of DR6$^{-/-}$ T-cells to induce disease. Recent studies have revealed that an IL-23 –induced subset of CD4 T-cells, Th17 cells, are critical pathogenic cells in inducing EAE (see reviews in refs. 15-17). Therefore, it would be interesting to study whether DR6 plays a role in Th17 cell differentiation and IL-17 production in CD4^{+} T helper cells. In additional studies, we found a reduced induction of the key integrin VLA-4 upon activation of T-cells from DR6$^{-/-}$ mice. It is known that VLA-4 is critical for T-cell infiltration into the CNS and this suggests a mechanism for the apparent resistance of DR6$^{-/-}$ mice to EAE induction. Therefore, blocking DR6 can be a potential strategy for modulating the migration of pathogenic T-cells in patients with multiple sclerosis.

In the allergic airway hypersensitivity model for asthma, mice are immunized first and then challenged in the lungs with antigen (typically ovalbumin).[18] Hallmarks of the disease are broncho-constriction and hyper eosinophilia with Th2 cytokine production. Surprisingly, airway lung inflammation was attenuated in DR6$^{-/-}$ mice, as evidenced by reduced numbers of eosinophils and lower IL-5 and IL-13 in the broncho-alveolar lavage fluids.[19] Histological examination demonstrates a reduction in the number of inflammatory cells in the lung of DR6$^{-/-}$ mice compared to WT mice. These results are somewhat unexpected since the previous studies demonstrated a hyper-activation profile and Th2 skewing following stimulation in DR6$^{-/-}$ mice.[9-11] Differences in the immunization protocol and method of challenge might account for this. Alternatively, cells lacking DR6 could have a relative defect in their ability to travel to the site of antigen (i.e., the lung). This hypothesis is supported by the observations in the EAE model where T-cell activation takes place in DR6$^{-/-}$ mice, but cells do not infiltrate into the area where the antigen is expressed (i.e., the CNS). Therefore, additional research seems warranted to investigate the effects of DR6 on expression of adhesion molecules and chemokine receptors on T-cells.

Is DR6 a Death Receptor?

DR6 belongs to a subgroup of TNFR called death receptors due to the presence of a death domain within its cytoplasmic portion. Since the ligand for DR6 is unknown, experimental confirmation of a direct role for DR6 in the induction of apoptosis is difficult. Nevertheless, mimicking ligand-induced receptor activation by overexpressing DR6 in certain cells such as Hela cells provided evidence that DR6 can induce apoptosis, albeit with relative impotency.[7] This depends on the full intracellular domain (including the death domain)[7] and can be inhibited by the caspase inhibitor Z-VAD and intracellular expression of anti-apoptotic genes such as Bcl-X_L and survivin.[8] Interestingly, the DR6-induced apoptosis also seems to be cell type dependent. For example, expression of DR6 in LnCAP induces significant apoptosis, but expression of DR6 does not induce apoptosis in PC3 and DU145. This differential apoptosis-inducing ability of DR6 appears to be related to the cellular expression level of anti-apoptotic genes.[8] However, gene ablation of DR6 did not result in pathology or tissue abnormality in vivo, suggesting a minor role for DR6 in apoptosis at best in vitro. Furthermore, no evidence for altered apoptosis has been found in $CD4^+$ T-cells of DR6$^{-/-}$ mice, which could be due to the redundancy by other death receptors.[9-11] On the other hand, B-cells from DR6$^{-/-}$ mice have a significantly lower percentage of apoptotic cells following stimulation,[10] suggesting that at least in B-cells DR6 may enhance the apoptosis process. Taken together, with the possible exception of B-cells, there does not appear to be a major role for DR6 in regulation of apoptotic processes in normal cells. Cancer cells in which DR6 is upregulated can escape apoptosis by increasing expression of anti-apoptotic proteins.

Alternative Function of DR6

A number of tumor cell lines are found to express DR6 on their cell surface.[8] If overexpression of DR6 on tumor cells can potentially induce apoptosis, then why do some tumor cells overexpress DR6 on their cell surface? Recently, it has been shown that DR6 is a substrate of the membrane associated matrix metalloproteinase 14 (MMP-14).[20] In fact, MMP-14 mediated cleavage leads to the release of the full extracellular domain of DR6 in the supernatant (Benschop et al, unpublished observations). The extracellular domain of DR6 inhibits cytokine-driven monocyte differentiation into dendritic cells in vitro. Furthermore, the extracellular domain of DR6 can lead to cell death in differentiating monocytes (Benschop et al, unpublished observations). We hypothesize that this is one of the tumor evasion mechanisms by which emerging tumors inhibit the development of local immunity. This data also implies that monocytes express a potential counterpart for DR6, by which the soluble extracellular portion of DR6 binds and triggers signaling events that lead to the increased cell death and impaired dendritic cell differentiation.

Conclusion

Upon ligand binding and activation, the TNF receptor superfamily members trigger cell signaling and mediate cell proliferation, survival, apoptosis and differentiation. DR6 (TNFRSF21) belongs to a subgroup of this family called death receptors, based on a cytoplasmic death domain sequence. Despite extensive efforts to identify the ligand for DR6, DR6 still remains as an orphan TNF receptor superfamily member. The lack of a known ligand for DR6 has hampered the ability to fully understand the functions and the mechanism of action of DR6. The limited numbers of studies, but notably those using DR6$^{-/-}$ mice, have revealed potentially significant regulatory roles for DR6 in adaptive immunity and provided impetus for a continued search for its ligand and additional physiological functions of DR6 in the future. Understanding the effects of modulating DR6 expression and function could provide a potential new pathway for therapeutic applications for treating inflammatory and autoimmune diseases and cancer.

References

1. Hsu HC, Wu Y, Mountz JD. Tumor necrosis factor ligand-receptor superfamily and arthritis. Curr Dir Autoimmun 2006; 9:37-54.
2. Nash PT, Florin TH. Tumour necrosis factor inhibitors. Med J Aust 2005; 183:205-8.

3. Tanaka S, Nakamura K, Takahasi N et al. Role of RANKL in physiological and pathological bone resorption and therapeutics targeting the RANKL-RANK signaling system. Immunol Rev 2005; 208:30-49.
4. van Horssen R, ten Hagen TL, Eggermont AM. TNF-alpha in cancer treatment: molecular insights, antitumor effects and clinical utility. Oncologist 2006; 11:397-408.
5. Lejeune FJ, Lienard D, Matter M et al. Efficiency of recombinant human TNF in human cancer therapy. Cancer Immun 2002; 6:6-22.
6. Locksley RM, Killeen N, Lenardo MJ. The TNF and TNF receptor superfamilies: integrating mammalian biology. Cell 2001; 104:487-501.
7. Pan G, Bauer JH, Haridas V et al. Identification and functional characterization of DR6, a novel death domain-containing TNF receptor. FEBS Lett 1998; 431:351-6.
8. Kasof GM, Lu JJ, Liu D et al. Tumor necrosis factor-alpha induces the expression of DR6, a member of the TNF receptor family, through activation of NF-kappaB. Oncogene 2001; 20:7965-75.
9. Liu J, Na S, Glasebrook A et al. Enhanced CD4+ T-cell proliferation and Th2 cytokine production in DR6-deficient mice. Immunity 2001; 15:23-34.
10. Schmidt CS, Liu J, Zhang T et al. Enhanced B-cell expansion, survival and humoral responses by targeting death receptor 6. J Exp Med 2003; 197:51-62.
11. Zhao H, Yan M, Wang H et al. Impaired c-Jun amino terminal kinase activity and T-cell differentiation in death receptor 6-deficient mice. J Exp Med 2001; 194:1441-8.
12. Chow CW, Dong C, Flavell RA et al. c-Jun NH(2)-terminal kinase inhibits targeting of the protein phosphotase calcineurin to NFATc1. Mol Cell Biol 2000; 20:5227-34.
13. Liu J, Heuer JG, Na S et al. Accelerated onset and increased severity of acute graft-versus-host disease following adoptive transfer of DR6-deficient T-cells. J Immunol 2002; 169:3993-8.
14. Schmidt CS, Zhao J, Chain J et al. Resistance to myelin oligodendrocyte glycoprotein-induced experimental autoimmune encephalomyelitis by death receptor 6-deficient mice. J Immunol 2005; 175:2286-92.
15. Kikly K, Liu L, Na S et al. The IL-23/Th(17) axis: therapeutic targets for autoimmune inflammation. Curr Opin Immunol 2006; 18:670-5. Review.
16. Touil T, Fitzgerald D, Zhang GX et al. Pathophysiology of interleukin-23 in experimental autoimmune encephalomyelitis. Drug News Perspect 2006; 19:77-83. Review.
17. Langrish CL, McKenzie BS, Wilson NJ et al. IL-12 and IL-23: master regulators of innate and adaptive immunity. Immunol Rev 2004; 202:96-105. Review.
18. Zhang-Hoover J, Finn P, Stein-Streilein J. Modulation of ovalbumin-induced airway inflammation and hyperreactivity by tolerogenic APC. J Immunol 2005; 175:7117-24.
19. Venkataraman C, Justen K, Zhao J et al. Death receptor-6 regulates the development of pulmonary eosinophilia and airway inflammation in a mouse model of asthma. Immunol Lett 2006; 106:42-7.
20. Tam EM, Morrison CJ, Wu YI et al. Membrane protease proteomics: isotope-coded affinity tag MS identification of undescribed MT1-matrix metalloproteinase substrates. PNAS 2004; 101:6917-22.
21. Enright AJ, Van Dongen S, Ouzounis CA. An efficient algorithm for large-scale detection of protein families. Nucl Acids Res 2002; 30:1575-84.
22. Krogh A, Larsson B, von Heijne G et al. Predicting transmembrane protein topology with a hidden Markov model: Application to complete genomes. J Mol Biol 2001; 305:567-80.

CHAPTER 14

TRAIL and Other TRAIL Receptor Agonists as Novel Cancer Therapeutics

Christina Falschlehner, Tom M. Ganten, Ronald Koschny, Uta Schaefer and Henning Walczak*

Abstract

Tumor necrosis factor (TNF)-related apoptosis-inducing ligand (TRAIL), also known as Apo2L, is a member of the TNF superfamily (TNFSF) of cytokines. TRAIL gained much attention during the past decade due to the demonstration of its therapeutic potential as a tumor-specific apoptosis inducer. TRAIL was identified as a protein with high homology to other members of the TNF cytokine family, especially to the ligand of Fas/Apo-1 (CD95), CD95L (FasL/APO-1L). TRAIL has been shown to induce apoptosis selectively in many tumor cell lines without affecting normal cells and tissues, making TRAIL itself as well as agonists of the two human receptors of TRAIL which can submit an apoptotic signal, TRAIL-R1 (DR4) and TRAIL-R2 (DR5), promising novel biotherapeutics for cancer therapy. An increasing number of publications now shows that TRAIL resistance in primary human tumor cells will have to be overcome and that sensitization to TRAIL-induced apoptosis will be required in many cases. Therefore, it will also be instrumental to develop suitable diagnostic tests to identify patients who will benefit from TRAIL-based novel anticancer therapeutics and those who will not. Interestingly, the first clinical results even in monotherapy with TRAIL as well as various agonistic TRAIL receptor-specific antibodies have shown encouraging results. This chapter provides a compact overview on the biochemistry of the TRAIL/TRAIL-R system, the physiological role of TRAIL and its receptors and the results of clinical trials with TRAIL and various TRAIL-R agonistic antibodies.

The TRAIL/TRAIL-R System

The TNF-related apoptosis inducing ligand (TRAIL) can bind two apoptosis-inducing receptors, TRAIL-R1 (DR4) and TRAIL-R2 (DR5), two additional cell-bound receptors incapable of transmitting an apoptotic signal, TRAIL-R3 (LIT, DcR1) and TRAIL-R4 (TRUNDD, DcR2), also called decoy receptors and lastly, a soluble receptor called osteoprotegerin (OPG) (Fig. 1).

TRAIL-R1 and TRAIL-R2 were both identified in 1997.[1-4] Both receptors share a sequence homology of 58% and so far clearly distinct functions were not shown. The cytoplasmic domains of the death-inducing TRAIL receptors share significant homology to a cytoplasmic domain found in CD95 and TNF-R1. This domain is characteristic for all apoptosis-inducing members of the TNFR superfamily (SF) and is called the death domain (DD). The extracellular part of all TNFRSF members is characterized by the presence of cysteine-rich domains (CRD). TRAIL-R1 and TRAIL-R2 contain two complete CRDs which are important for ligand binding. TRAIL-R2 can be expressed in two different splice variants that differ by presence or absence of 23 amino

*Corresponding Author: Henning Walczak—Div. of Apoptosis Regulation (D040), Tumor Immunology Program, German Cancer Research Center (DKFZ), Im Neuenheimer Feld 580, 69120 Heidelberg, Germany. Email: h.walczak@dkfz.de

Therapeutic Targets of the TNF Superfamily, edited by Iqbal S. Grewal.
©2009 Landes Bioscience and Springer Science+Business Media.

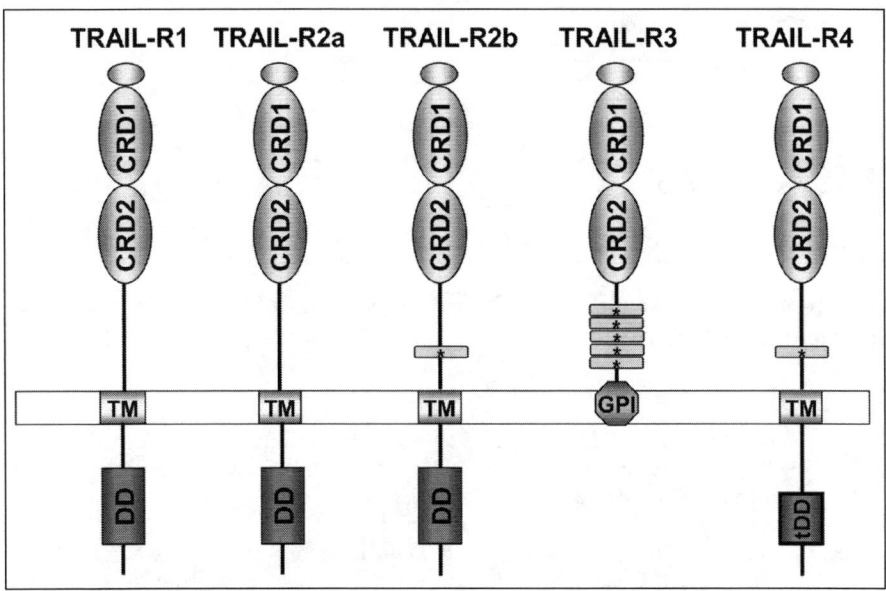

Figure 1. Structure of human TRAIL receptors 1-4. CRD = cysteine rich domain, * = pseudo-repeat, TM = transmembrane domain, GPI = Glycosylphosphatidylinositol anchor, DD = death domain, tDD = truncated death domain.

acids in the extracellular domain located between the CRDs and the transmembrane domain. A distinct role for these two variants has so far not been identified.

Almost all tissues express mRNA for all four TRAIL receptors. However mRNA expression levels do not correspond to cell surface expression of these proteins which is thought to be necessary for their function. It has also been shown that the expression pattern of TRAIL and its receptors differs between normal and tumor tissue.[5] A polymorphism within the ligand-binding domain has been associated with a higher incidence of bladder cancer and other mutations within TRAIL-R1 have been linked to several cancers.[6]

Apoptosis Signaling via TRAIL-R1 and TRAIL-R2

TRAIL signaling for induction of cell death by apoptosis occurs via the DD-containing TRAIL receptors TRAIL-R1 and TRAIL R2. On binding of TRAIL, the so called death inducing signalling complex, the DISC, is formed. Thereby, the so-called "extrinsic" pathway of apoptosis induction is triggered. The trimerization of the receptor leads to recruitment of FADD (Mort1), another DD-containing molecule. The interaction between FADD and the receptor results in a conformational change in FADD which allows its second functional domain, the death effector domain (DED), to interact with other DED-containing proteins. These are Caspase-8, Caspase-10, cFLIP (cellular FLICE-like inhibitory protein; FLICE is the old name for Caspase-8) and PED/PEA-15.[7-10]

Caspases are cysteine-dependent, aspartate-specific proteases which are able to cleave several distinct substrates once they are activated. Initiator caspases are present in the cell as inactive proenzymes to ensure that they are only activated when appropriately stimulated. Inactive pro-caspases consist of a long prodomain, a small subunit and a large subunit. Once recruited to their activation platforms, the DISC (in case of Caspase -8 and -10) or the apoptosome (in case of Caspase-9), these initiator caspases are autocatalytically activated and a caspase cascade is started.[11,12] However, effective transmission of apoptosis signaling depends on the proper expression of all necessary constituents of the apoptotic pathway and the concomitant absence of inhibitors of this pathway.

Hence, the decision between life and death of a cell crucially depends on its receptiveness for the apoptosis-inducing stimulus which can but does not have to be triggered when TRAIL-R1 and/or TRAIL-R2 are agonistically targeted.

Depending on whether mitochondrial apoptotic events are needed for apoptosis to occur following the triggering of CD95 or the TRAIL death receptors cells can be classified as belonging to one of two different classes. In so-called type I cells, the caspase cascade initiated at the DISC is sufficient to kill the cells independent of a mitochondrial pro-apoptotic stimulus. In contrast, type II cells need the apoptotic activation of mitochondria.

The mitochondrial apoptosis gateway is controlled by interaction of proteins belonging to different subgroups of the Bcl-2 superfamily.[13] All members of this superfamily share one or more of the so called Bcl-2 homology (BH) domains, BH1 to BH4 and can be divided in pro-apoptotic and pro-survival proteins. The pro-survival members, e.g., Bcl-2, Bcl-X_L and Mcl-1, contain all four BH domains. These proteins are associated with the mitochondrial outer membrane and prevent apoptosis. The pro-apoptotic members like Bax, Bak and Bok, associate with the outer mitochondrial membrane during apoptosis, thereby destabilising its integrity leading to release of pro-apoptotic factors from the mitochondrial inter-membrane space. They in turn are activated by members of the "BH3-only" Bcl-2 subfamily. BH3-only proteins, e.g., Bid, Bim, Bmf, Puma and Noxa, are characterized by the fact that they only contain the third BH domain. BH3-only proteins are activated in a number of different ways including triggering of CD95 or TRAIL death receptors, DNA damage or different cellular stresses.[14-16] Following ligand or agonistic antibody-mediated crosslinking of TRAIL-R1, TRAIL-R2 or CD95, Bid is cleaved to truncated Bid (tBid) by DISC-activated Caspase-8 and -10 connecting the extrinsic and the intrinsic, mitochondria-dependent apoptosis pathway (Fig. 2). Binding of tBid to mitochondria initiates mitochondrial apoptotic events which result in the release of cytochrome C, Smac/DIABLO and other pro-apoptotic factors from the mitochondrial inter-membrane space.[17,18] Upon release of cytochrome C and association with Apaf-1, the "apoptosome" is formed which serves as an activation platform of Caspase-9.[19] Smac/DIABLO in turn inhibits the action of inhibitor of apoptosis proteins (IAPs). DISC-activation also results in cleavage of Caspase-3. However, cleavage of Caspase-3 by Caspase-8 or -10 does not lead to its full activation. Therefore, an autocatalytic step has to occur which can be inhibited by IAPs.[20] The X-linked inhibitor of apoptosis protein (XIAP) has been shown to be the most potent inhibitor of activated caspases 3, 7 and 9.[21] Type II cells often express high levels of IAPs which can be counteracted by Smac/DIABLO. This high expression of IAPs in type II cells, rather than (or in addition to) the suggested stronger initiator caspase activation in type I versus type II cells, may explain the need for mitochondrial apoptotic events in type II but not in type I cells.

Physiological Role of the TRAIL/TRAIL-R System

To date, knockout mice for both, TRAIL and TRAIL-R (MK, mDR5), the only apoptosis-inducing receptor in mice, have been generated. These mice do not show an overt phenotype.[22-25] However, a role of the TRAIL/TRAIL-R system in tumor suppression was identified. When different syngeneic TRAIL sensitive tumor lines were transferred into TRAIL[-/-] mice increased tumor growth and increased formation of experimental metastasis could be observed.[22,25] In addition, fibrosarcomas induced by the carcinogen MCA grew more rapidly in the absence of TRAIL.[22] However, in autochthonous tumor models, the role of the TRAIL/TRAIL-R system is less clear. In several tumor-prone mice, e.g., in APC[min] mice, p53[-/-] mice[26] and Her2/neu transgenic mice,[27] tumor development was not affected by absence or presence of TRAIL or TRAIL-R. By contrast, aged TRAIL-deficient mice spontaneously develop lymphomas, which is also accelerated in TRAIL[-/-] p53[+/-] mice.[27] Thus, further studies are needed to clarify the role of the TRAIL/TRAIL-R system in tumorigenesis. It will be especially interesting to use autochthonous tumor models in which tumorigenesis can be followed through all stages up to the ultimate level which is the formation of metastasis.

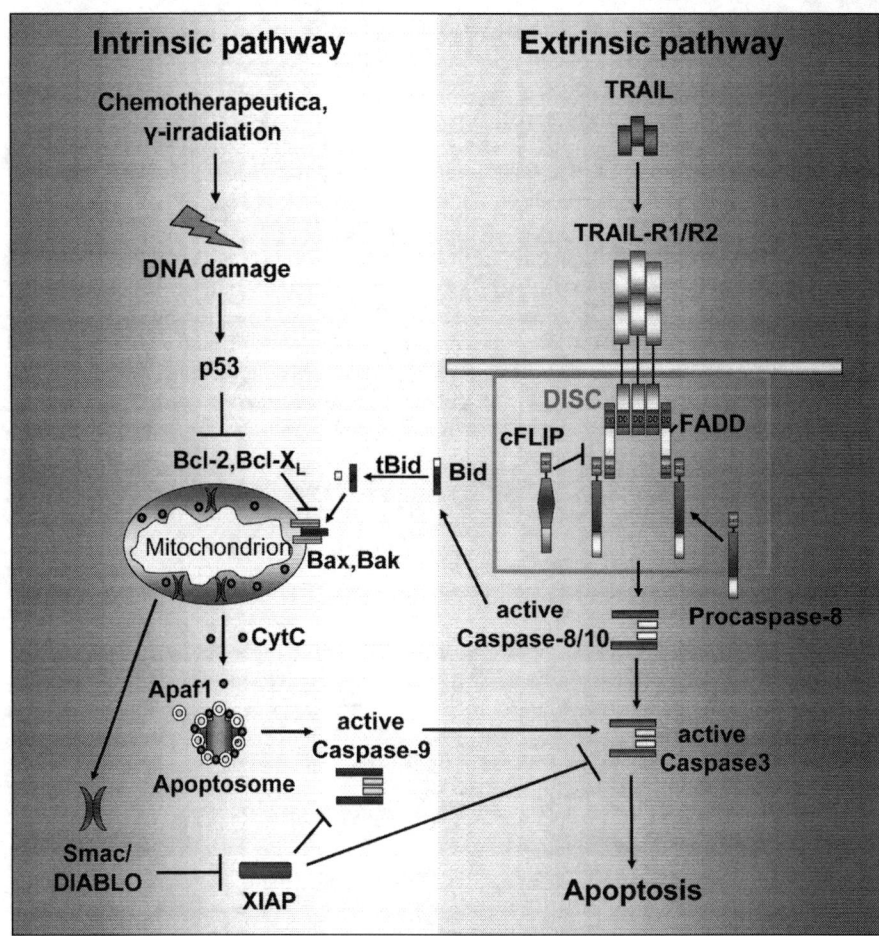

Figure 2. Interplay between intrinsic and extrinsic apoptosis signalling.

Expression of TRAIL is mainly found on different cells of both, the innate and adaptive immune response. TRAIL expression can be induced by appropriate stimulatory agents on NK cells, cytotoxic T-cells (CTLs) and dendritic cells (DCs).[28,29] Interestingly, liver NK cells constitutively express TRAIL.[30] TRAIL-deficient mice are not autoimmune-prone, even when aged.[31] However, in several models of autoimmune diseases the TRAIL/TRAIL-R system has been shown to be involved in the regulation of auto-reactive T-cells. When TRAIL is absent, collagen-induced arthritis, streptozotocin-induced diabetes,[32,33] experimental thyroiditis[34] and experimental autoimmune encephalitis (EAE)[35] were increased. In contrast, when TRAIL blocking reagents were not administered systemically but directly into the CNS, the disease was nearly blocked.[36] Thus, in EAE the killing of cells by TRAIL in the central nervous system exacerbates the disease whereas TRAIL-mediated effects in the periphery are involved in its prevention. In this context it is noteworthy that TRAIL has been implicated in the regulation of memory CTLs. CD8+ T-cells which have been primed in the absence of CD4+ T-cell help, so called "helpless" CD8+ T-cells, can only undergo a second round of clonal expansion when TRAIL is blocked or when TRAIL is absent as is the case in T-cells obtained from TRAIL-deficient mice.[37,38] In addition, it has recently been shown in a provocative study that TRAIL derived from helpless CD8[+] T-cells can suppress the activity of CD4[+] T-cells, hence eliminating help.[39]

TRAIL Receptor Agonists as Novel Biotherapeutics in Cancer Therapy

As shown in many preclinical studies, TRAIL as well as agonistic antibodies to TRAIL-R1 and TRAIL-R2 can efficiently induce apoptosis in numerous tumor cell lines but not in the majority of normal cells. Currently, an untagged recombinant form of TRAIL (Apo2L/TRAIL.0) and agonistic antibodies against TRAIL-R1 and TRAIL-R2 are in clinical trials for tumor therapy. We first summarize in vitro data on efficacy and toxicity of TRAIL, either alone or in combination with chemotherapeutic drugs, to kill primary cancer versus normal cells and then we provide an overview of the clinical studies performed so far with TRAIL receptor agonists.

Efficacy of TRAIL in Primary Tumor Cells versus Toxicity in Normal Cells

In contrast to the vast amount of preclinical data on apoptosis induction by TRAIL in cancer cell lines, little is known about the therapeutic potential of recombinant TRAIL in primary human tumor cells. TRAIL induces apoptosis in otherwise chemotherapy-resistant freshly isolated human multiple myeloma cells[40,41] but neither in primary B-cell acute or chronic lymphoblastic leukemia cells[42,43] nor in most of the investigated acute lymphoblastic leukemia, acute myelogenous leukemia, acute promyelocytic leukemia, or chronic lymphocytic leukemia cells.[44] Three of 6 isolated primary glioblastoma multiforme specimens,[45] all 13 analyzed astrocytoma and oligoastrocytoma cells of all 4 WHO grades of malignancy, isolated tumor cells from medulloblastoma, meningeoma, esthesioneuroblastoma[46] and soft tissue sarcoma patients[47] were also resistant to TRAIL.

Thus, an increasing number of studies demonstrates TRAIL resistance in primary human tumor cells especially in those of solid tumor entities which may dampen the expectations of clinical trials which are currently performed with TRAIL as a monotherapeutic agent.[48,49] Considering that TRAIL treatment of TRAIL-resistant pancreatic cancer and cholangiocarcinoma cells even increased tumor cell migration and metastatic spread in vitro and in vivo,[50,51] the unselected treatment of tumor patients with TRAIL may not only result in the lack of a clinical benefit but may even harm cancer patients. Consequently, there is a need for an in vitro sensitivity test of isolated tumor cells from individual patients and/or a set of predictive diagnostic markers which could differentiate between patients who would and patients who would not benefit from TRAIL-based (mono-)therapies. Independently, however, it seems that in most cases of primary tumors sensitizing regimens, i.e., via combinations with other bio- or chemotherapeutics and/or radiation therapy are needed for a broad and successful application of TRAIL in cancer patients.

As shown in Table 1, primary tumor cells from numerous different tumor entities could be sensitized to TRAIL-induced apoptosis by a plethora of chemotherapeutic drugs. Importantly, most of these combinatorial regiments lacked in vitro toxicity on normal tissues (Table 2).

Revealing the mechanism of TRAIL sensitization of tumor cells versus normal cells by these different chemotherapeutics will provide criteria to select the appropriate sensitizing protocol for a given kind of tumor in individual cancer patients. Examples of sensitizing mechanisms in tumor cells are provided in Table 1.

Clinically Used TRAIL-Based Therapies

TRAIL-receptor-targeted therapies currently pursued in Phase I and Phase II clinical studies include application of the untagged recombinant Apo2L/TRAIL as well as different humanized or human agonistic monoclonal antibodies (mAbs) targeting TRAIL-R1 and TRAIL-R2, either alone or in combination with chemotherapeutics. Table 3 summarizes the TRAIL receptor agonists currently investigated in clinical trials.

On basis of the identification and cloning of TRAIL-R2 and its ligand,[4,52,53] Apo2L/TRAIL is being codeveloped by Genentech and Amgen as a targeted therapy for solid tumors and hematological malignancies. The phase IB safety and pharmacokinetic study of recombinant human Apo2L/TRAIL alone and in combination with rituximab in patients with low-grade nonHodgkin's lymphoma (NHL) showed that administration of Apo2/TRAIL (8 mg/kg) and Rituximab (375

Table 1. Preclinical studies of sensitization of primary tumor cells for TRAIL-induced apoptosis

Primary Tumor Cells	TRAIL in Combination With	Proposed Mechanism	Reference
AML	HDAC inhibitors		56
CLL	HDAC inhibitors (Depsipeptide, valproic acid)	signal via TRAIL-R1	57,58
B-CLL	Cycloheximide	cFLIP$_L$ downregulation	59
MM	NF-κB inhibitor SN50	downregulation of Bcl-2, Bfl-1, IAPs upregulation of Bax	60
Erythroleukemic cells	irradiation	TRAIL-R1 upregulation	61
Colon cancer	irinotecan, 5-FU	TRAIL-R2 upregulation	62
Pancreatic cancer	gemcitabine		63
Renal cell carcinoma	doxorubicin	(in combination with Lexatumumab)	75
Soft tissue sarcoma	doxorubicine, cisplatin, etoposide, methotrexat, cyclophosphamid		47
Melanoma	tunicamycin	TRAIL-R1/R2 upregulation	76
Astrocytoma, Oligoastrocytoma	Bortezomib	TRAIL-R1/R2 upregulation, cFLIP$_L$ downregulation, Bax/Bak upregulation	46

mg/m^2) intravenously over 1 hour for 5 consecutive days every three weeks up to 4 cycles is safe and shows evidence of activity. So far, five patients have undergone tumor response assessment whereby two showed complete response, one a partial response and two did not respond to the therapy. Thus, although in vitro the apoptosis-inducing capacity of TRAIL on primary tumor cells appeared to be limited, the in vivo response of monotherapy with Apo2L/TRAIL at least in patients with low-grade nonHodgkin lymphoma looks quite promising. It will be very interesting to see the results of future studies which will include more patients. Importantly, this study clearly showed that no dose-limiting toxicity (DLT) or severe adverse effects (SAEs) were observed. Currently these studies are continued to test Apo2L/TRAIL and rituximab for expanded safety data and further dose optimization.

Human Genome Sciences (HGS) was the first company to test TRAIL receptor agonists in clinical trials. HGS is currently investigating fully humanized agonistic antibodies against TRAIL-R1 (HGS-ETR1/Mapatumab) and TRAIL-R2 (HGS-ETR2/Lexatumumab) as a therapy for NHL, colorectal cancer, nonsmall cell lung cancer (NSCLC) and advanced solid tumors. HGS has already completed three Phase II clinical trials of HGS-ETR1 as monotherapy in heavily pre-treated patients with NHL, colorectal cancer and NSCLC. The results of these trials show that HGS-ETR1 is well tolerated and HGS-ETR1 could be administered safely and repetitively. No dose-limiting toxicities up to the highest dose tested (10 mg/kg) were observed. Stable disease was observed in 29% of the patients that participated in the NSCLC study and in 32% of the patients that participated in the colorectal cancer study. Clinical response or stable disease could be observed in 14/17 patients with NHL diagnosed with follicular lymphomas.

HGS has currently initiated two Phase Ib trials evaluating the safety and tolerability of HGS-ETR1 in combination with chemotherapeutic agents (Paclitaxel + Carboplatin and Gemcitabine + Cisplatin) in the treatment of patients with advanced solid tumors including NSCLC, pancreatic cancer, cancer of unknown primary (CUP), biliary tract cancer and head and neck cancer.

Table 2. Preclinical toxicity studies of combinatorial TRAIL therapies in normal cells

Normal Tissue	TRAIL in Combination With	Outcome	Reference
Hepatocytes	5-FU, gemcitabine, irinotecan, oxaliplatin, Bortezomib (low dose)	not toxic	64,65
Hepatocytes	Cisplatin, Bortezomib (high dose)	toxic	65,66
Hepatocytes	HDAC inhibitors (valproic acid, ITF2357)	not toxic	67
Hepatocytes	Steatosis hepatis, Hepatisis C infection	toxic	77
Keratinocytes	Proteasome inhibtor (MG115)	toxic	68
Peripheral blood	HDAC inhibitors	not toxic	57,69
Resting lymphocytes mononuclear cells	Cisplatin	toxic	78
CD34(+) Progenitor cells	HDAC inhibitor	not toxic	56
Erythroblasts	irradiation	not toxic	61
Osteoblasts	etoposide, cisplatin, doxorubicin, methotrexat*, cyclophosphamid*	not toxic	70*
Osteoblasts	etoposide	not toxic	71
Osteoblasts	cisplatin, doxorubicin	toxic	71
Prostate stromal cells	doxorubicin	not toxic	72

First results of the Phase Ib studies demonstrate that the combination of HGS-ETR1 + chemotherapeutics was well tolerated and HGS-ETR1 can be administered safely and repetitively at doses up to 20 mg/kg intravenously. The maximum tolerated dose of HGS-ETR1 has, however, still not been reached. As the best overall response to HGS-ETR1 + gemcitabine + cisplatin 9/32 patients showed a partial response and 14/32 stable disease. Most of the observed adverse effects of the combinatorial regimens most likely reflect the toxicity profile of the used concomitant chemotherapeutics. In the phase Ib study of HGS-ETR1 + paclitaxel + carboplatin 4/20 patients showed partial response and 10/20 stable disease. However, combinatorial treatment with HGS-ETR1 + carboplatin + paclitaxel was not superior to HGS-ETR1 or paclitaxel + carboplatin alone. One patient showed dose-limiting toxicity due to HGS-ETR1. Furthermore HGS is currently performing a clinical phase II trial with advanced multiple myeloma (MM) to evaluate the efficacy and safety of HGS-ETR1 in combination with the proteasome inhibitor bortezomib (study number: HGS1012-C1055).

The safety of the TRAIL-R2-targeting fully humanized mAb HGS-ETR2 (Lexatumumab) in combination with gemcitabine, pemetrexed, doxorubicin or FOLFIRI has been investigated in a phase Ib study. Patients received one of the full-dose chemotherapy regimens and lexatumumab (5 mg/kg) every two weeks (for gemcitabine and FOLFIRI) or every three weeks (for pemetrexed and doxorubicin). Four to 6 patients were treated with 5 mg/kg lexatumumab in each chemotherapy cohort prior to dose escalation to 10 mg/kg. So far, 41 patients with a wide range of cancer types have received 164 courses of lexatumumab over the 2 dose levels. As lexatumumab was well-tolerated, no dose reductions of lexatumumab were required. Severe adverse events considered at least possibly related to lexatumumab included anemia, fatigue and dehydration. Tumor shrinkage has been observed, including confirmed partial responses (PRs) in the FOLFIRI and doxorubicin arms.

Daiichi Sankyo is developing TRA-8 (CS-1008), a humanized antiTRAIL-R2 monoclonal antibody for the treatment of advanced solid tumors and lymphomas. Preclinical studies showed an anti-cancer effect against human cancer cell lines in vitro and in tumor-bearing mice in vivo.

Apomab, a fully human affinity-matured IgG1 monoclonal antibody targeting TRAIL-R2 developed by Genentech is currently evaluated in phase I and II clinical trials.

Table 3. Therapeutic approaches targeting the TRAIL receptors in cancer therapy

Single Agent

HGS-ETR1 (Mapatumumab)	Human Genome Sciences	humanized anti-TRAIL-R1 agonistic mAb	Phase II completed: colorectal cancer, NHL, NSCLC
HGS-ETR2 (Lexatumumab)	Human Genome Sciences	humanized anti-TRAIL-R2 agonistic mAb	Phase I: advanced solid tumors
HGS-TR2J	Human Genome Sciences	humanized anti-TRAIL-R2 agonistic mAb	Phase I: advanced solid tumors
TRA-8 (CS-1008)	Daiichi Sankyo Inc.	humanized anti-TRAIL-R2 mAb	Phase I: advanced solid tumors and lymphomas (not yet recruiting)
Apo2L/TRAIL (AMG 951)	Genentech/ Amgen	soluble TRAIL, activates TRAIL-R1 and TRAIL-R2	Phase Ib
Apomab	Genentech	humanized anti-TRAIL-R2 mAb	Phase I/II: advanced solid tumors
AMG 655	Amgen	humanized anti-TRAIL-R2 agonistic mAb	Phase I: (initiated in 2005)
LBY135	Novartis	chimeric anti-TRAIL-R2 agonistic antibody	Phase I/II: advanced solid tumors

Combination with Chemotherapy

HGS-ETR1 + Paclitaxel + Carboplatin	Human Genome Sciences	humanized anti-TRAIL-R1 agonistic mAb + chemotherapy	Phase Ib: advanced solid tumors
HGS-ETR1 + Gemcitabine + Cisplatin	Human Genome Sciences	humanized anti-TRAIL-R1 agonistic mAb + chemotherapy	Phase Ib: advanced solid tumors
HGS-ETR1 + Bortezombib (Velcade®)	Human Genome Sciences	humanized anti-TRAIL-R1 mAb + proteasomeinhibitor	Phase II: advanced MM (recruiting since Oct. 2006)
HGS-ETR2 + Gemcitabine + Pemetrexed + Doxorubicin + FOLFIRI	Human Genome Sciences	humanized anti-TRAIL-R2 agonistic mAb + chemotherapy	Phase Ib: advanced solid tumors
Apo2L/TRAIL + Rituximab	Genentech/ Amgen	soluble TRAIL that activates TRAIL-R1 and TRAIL-R2 + anti-C20	Phase Ib/II: NHL (recruiting since June 2006)
Apomab + Avastin	Genentech	humanized anti-TRAIL-R2 agonistic mAb + anti-VEGF	Phase II: advanced solid tumors (initiated Q2 2007)
LBY135 + capecitabine	Novartis	chimeric anti-TRAIL-R2 agonistic mAb	Phase I/II: advanced solid tumors, (recruiting since 2006)

First pharmacokinetics studies showed that Apomab was well tolerated in patients treated with doses up to 20 mg/kg (<33% dose limiting (Grade 3 drug-related) toxicities in the first 2 doses + 24 hours). However, 2 disparate DLTs occurred among 11 patients treated at 10 mg/kg including asymptomatic transaminitis and pulmonary embolism C1D4. One patient out of six who received at least 4 cycles of Apomab showed 28% shrinkage of target lesions and symptomatic improvement after 4 cycles.[54] Phase II studies with Apomab in first-line nonsmall cell lung cancer in combination with Avastin and in sarcoma as a single agent were initiated in 2007. Furthermore, a Phase II study in indolent nonHodgkin's lymphoma in combination with Rituxan is planned.

AMG655, a fully human mAB targeting TRAIL-R2 developed by Amgen, is currently investigated in a phase Ib clinical study in adult patients with advanced solid tumors.

Three to nine patients were enrolled into 1 of 5 sequential dose cohorts (0.3, 1, 3, 10, or 20 mg/kg) of AMG655 administered intravenously every two weeks (Q2W). AMG655 administered up at doses of up to 20 mg/kg Q2W appears to be well tolerated in these patients. No DLTs or SAEs related to AMG655 treatment have been reported. No anti-AMG655 antibodies have been detected. However, nine patients reported adverse effects after AMG655 administration including pyrexia, fatigue and hypomagnesaemia. AMG655 demonstrated dose-linear kinetics with a half-life of ~10 days. The anti-tumor activity of AMG655 was confirmed with observation of a partial response in NSCLC and a metabolic partial response in colorectal cancer.

LBY135, an agonistic chimeric monoclonal antibody against TRAIL-R2, is developed by Novartis. In first in vitro studies, 50% of a panel of 40 human colon cancer cell lines were killed by LBY135 with an IC50 of 10 nM or less. This result is in line with the observed effects of other TRAIL receptor agonists. The in vivo anti-tumor efficacy of LBY135 was evaluated in human colorectal tumor xenograft models in mice.[55] Since 2006, Novartis is recruiting patients for an open-label, multi-center, 2-arm Phase I/II trial of LBY135 alone and in combination with capecitabine in advanced solid tumors (Nevada Cancer Institute).

In summary, the clinical trials performed so far demonstrate that Apo2L/TRAIL as well as mAbs against TRAIL-R1 or TRAIL-R2 are well tolerated when applied in humans and induce partial response and stable disease in a high percentage of patients. Considering that most if not all of the tumor patients enrolled in these clinical studies had been heavily pretreated and were mostly chemo-refractory at the time when TRAIL receptor agonists were given for the first time, it now seems safe to state that the clinical results obtained so far suggest that the concept of using TRAIL receptor agonists in cancer therapy[52,53] represents a promising therapeutic option for cancer patients.

References

1. Pan G, O'Rourke K, Chinnaiyan AM et al. The receptor for the cytotoxic ligand TRAIL. Science 1997; 276:111-113.
2. Screaton GR, Mongkolsapaya J, Xu XN et al. TRICK2, a new alternatively spliced receptor that transduces the cytotoxic signal from TRAIL. Curr Biol 1997; 7:693-696.
3. Sheridan JP, Marsters SA, Pitti RM et al. Control of TRAIL-induced apoptosis by a family of signaling and decoy receptors. Science 1997; 277:818-821.
4. Walczak H, Degli-Esposti MA, Johnson RS et al. TRAIL-R2: a novel apoptosis-mediating receptor for TRAIL. EMBO J 1997; 16:5386-5397.
5. Daniel PT, Wieder T, et al. The kiss of death: promises and failures of death receptors and ligands in cancer therapy. Leukemia 2001; 15(7):1022-32.
6. Kimberley FC, Screaton GR. Following a TRAIL: update on a ligand and its five receptors. Cell Res 2004; 14(5):359-372.
7. Walczak H, Sprick MR. Biochemistry and function of the DISC. Trends Biochem Sci 2001; 26(7):452-3.
8. Chen M, Orozco A et al. Activation of initiator caspases through a stable dimeric intermediate. J Biol Chem 2002; 277(52):50761-7.
9. Sprick MR, Rieser E et al. Caspase-10 is recruited to and activated at the native TRAIL and CD95 death-inducing signalling complexes in a FADD-dependent manner but can not functionally substitute caspase-8. EMBO J 2002; 21(17):4520-30.
10. Xiao C, Yang BF et al. Tumor necrosis factor-related apoptosis-inducing ligand-induced death-inducing signaling complex and its modulation by c-FLIP and PED/PEA-15 in glioma cells. J Biol Chem 2002; 277(28):25020-5.

11. Creagh EM, Martin SJ. Caspases: cellular demolition experts. Biochem Soc Trans 2001; 29(Pt 6):696-702.
12. Baliga, B, Kumar S. Apaf-1/cytochrome c apoptosome: an essential initiator of caspase activation or just a sideshow? Cell Death Differ 2003; 10(1):16-8.
13. Strasser A, The role of BH3-only proteins in the immune system. Nature reviews 2005; 5:189-200.
14. Wei MC, Lindsten T et al. tBID, a membrane-targeted death ligand, oligomerizes BAK to release cytochrome c. Genes Dev 2000; 14(16):2060-71.
15. Villunger A, Michalak EM et al. p53- and drug-induced apoptotic responses mediated by BH3-only proteins puma and noxa. Science 2003; 302(5647):1036-8.
16. Puthalakath H, O'Reilly LA et al. ER stress triggers apoptosis by activating BH3-only protein Bim. Cell 2007; 129(7):1337-49.
17. Verhagen AM, Ekert PG et al. Identification of DIABLO, a mammalian protein that promotes apoptosis by binding to and antagonizing IAP proteins. Cell 2000; 102(1):43-53.
18. Suzuki Y, Imai Y et al. A serine protease, HtrA2, is released from the mitochondria and interacts with XIAP, inducing cell death. Mol Cell 2001a; 8(3):613-21.
19. Riedl SJ, Salvesen GS. The apoptosome: signalling platform of cell death. Nat Rev Mol Cell Biol 2007; 8(5):405-13.
20. Eckelman BP, Salvesen GS et al. Human inhibitor of apoptosis proteins: why XIAP is the black sheep of the family. EMBO Rep 2006; 7(10):988-94.
21. Suzuki Y, Nakabayashi Y et al. X-linked inhibitor of apoptosis protein (XIAP) inhibits caspase-3 and -7 in distinct modes. J Biol Chem 2001b; 276(29):27058-63.
22. Cretney E, Takeda K, Yagita H et al. Increased susceptibility to tumor initiation and metastasis in TNF-related apoptosis-inducing ligand-deficient mice. J Immunol 2002; 168:1356-1361.
23. Diehl GE, Yue HH, Hsieh K et al. TRAIL-R as a negative regulator of innate immune cell responses. Immunity 2004; 21:877-889.
24. Finnberg N, Gruber JJ, Fei P et al. DR5 knockout mice are compromised in radiation-induced apoptosis. Mol Cell Biol 2005; 25:2000-2013.
25. Sedger LM, Glaccum MB, Schuh JC et al. Characterization of the in vivo function of TNF-alpha-related apoptosis-inducing ligand, TRAIL/Apo2L, using TRAIL/Apo2L gene-deficient mice. Eur J Immunol 2002; 32:2246-2254.
26. Yue HH, Diehl GE, Winoto A. Loss of TRAIL-R does not affect thymic or intestinal tumor development in p53 and adenomatous polyposis coli mutant mice. Cell Death Differ 2005; 12:94-97.
27. Zerafa N, Westwood JA, Cretney E et al. Cutting edge: TRAIL deficiency accelerates hematological malignancies. J Immunol 2005; 175:5586-5590.
28. Ehrlich S, Infante-Duarte C et al. Regulation of soluble and surface-bound TRAIL in human T-cells, B-cells and monocytes. Cytokine 2003; 24(6):244-53.
29. Halaas O, Vik R et al. Lipopolysaccharide induces expression of APO2 ligand/TRAIL in human monocytes and macrophages. Scand J Immunol 2000; 51(3):244-50.
30. Takeda K, Smyth MJ et al. Involvement of tumor necrosis factor-related apoptosis-inducing ligand in NK cell-mediated and IFN-gamma-dependent suppression of subcutaneous tumor growth. Cell Immunol 2001; 214(2):194-200.
31. Cretney E, Uldrich AP, Berzins SP et al. Normal thymocyte negative selection in TRAIL-deficient mice. J Exp Med 2003; 198:491-496.
32. Lamhamedi-Cherradi SE, Zheng S, Tisch RM et al. Critical roles of tumor necrosis factor-related apoptosis-inducing ligand in type 1 diabetes. Diabetes 2003a; 52:2274-2278.
33. Lamhamedi-Cherradi SE, Zheng SJ, Maguschak KA et al. Defective thymocyte apoptosis and accelerated autoimmune diseases in TRAIL-/- mice. Nat Immunol 2003b; 4:255-260.
34. Wang SH, Cao Z et al. Death ligand tumor necrosis factor-related apoptosis-inducing ligand inhibits experimental autoimmune thyroiditis. Endocrinology 2005; 146(11):4721-6.
35. Cretney E, McQualter JL. Kayagaki N et al. TNF-related apoptosis-inducing ligand (TRAIL)/Apo2L suppresses experimental autoimmune encephalomyelitis in mice. Immunol Cell Biol 2005a; 83:511-519.
36. Aktas O, Smorodchenko A et al. Neuronal damage in autoimmune neuroinflammation mediated by the death ligand TRAIL. Neuron 2005; 46(3):421-32.
37. Janssen EM, Droin NM et al. CD4+ T-cell help controls CD8+ T-cell memory via TRAIL-mediated activation-induced cell death. Nature 2005; 434(7029):88-93.
38. Hamilton SE, Wolkers MC et al. The generation of protective memory-like CD8+ T-cells during homeostatic proliferation requires CD4+ T-cells. Nat Immunol 2006; 7(5):475-81.
39. Griffith TS, Kazama H et al. Apoptotic cells induce tolerance by generating helpless CD8+ T-cells that produce TRAIL. J Immunol 2007; 178(5):2679-87.
40. Gazitt Y, TRAIL is a potent inducer of apoptosis in myeloma cells derived from multiple myeloma patients and is not cytotoxic to hematopoietic stem cells. Leukemia 1999; 13:1817-1824.

41. Mitsiades CS, Treon SP, Mitsiades N et al. TRAIL/Apo2L ligand selectively induces apoptosis and overcomes drug resistance in multiple myeloma: therapeutic applications. Blood 2001; 98:795-804.
42. Clodi K, Wimmer D, Li Y et al. Expression of tumour necrosis factor (TNF)-related apoptosis-inducing ligand (TRAIL) receptors and sensitivity to TRAIL-induced apoptosis in primary B-cell acute lymphoblastic leukaemia cells. British journal of haematology 2000; 111:580-586.
43. MacFarlane M, Harper N, Snowden RT et al. Mechanisms of resistance to TRAIL-induced apoptosis in primary B cell chronic lymphocytic leukaemia. Oncogene 2002; 21:6809-6818.
44. Snell V, Clodi K, Zhao S et al. Activity of TNF-related apoptosis-inducing ligand (TRAIL) in haematological malignancies. British journal of haematology 1997; 99:618-624.
45. Panner A, James CD, Berger MS et al. mTOR controls FLIPS translation and TRAIL sensitivity in glioblastoma multiforme cells. Mol Cell Biol 2005; 25:8809-8823.
46. Koschny R, Holland H et al. Bortezomib sensitizes primary human astrocytoma cells of WHO grades I to IV for tumor necrosis factor-related apoptosis-inducing ligand-induced apoptosis. Clin Cancer Res 2007b; 13(11):3403-12.
47. Clayer M, Bouralexis S, Evdokiou A et al. Enhanced apoptosis of soft tissue sarcoma cells with chemotherapy: A potential new approach using TRAIL. J Orthop Surg (Hong Kong) 2001; 9:19-22.
48. Hayakawa Y, Screpanti V, Yagita H et al. NK cell TRAIL eliminates immature dendritic cells in vivo and limits dendritic cell vaccination efficacy. J Immunol 2004; 172:123-129.
49. Secchiero P, Zerbinati C, Rimondi E et al. TRAIL promotes the survival, migration and proliferation of vascular smooth muscle cells. Cell Mol Life Sci 2004; 61:1965-1974.
50. Ishimura N, Isomoto H, Bronk SF et al. Trail induces cell migration and invasion in apoptosis-resistant cholangiocarcinoma cells. Am J Physiol Gastrointest Liver Physiol 2006; 290:G129-136.
51. Trauzold A, Siegmund D, Schniewind B et al. TRAIL promotes metastasis of human pancreatic ductal adenocarcinoma. Oncogene 2006; 25:7434-7439.
52. Ashkenazi A, Pai RC et al. Safety and antitumor activity of recombinant soluble Apo2 ligand. J Clin Invest 1999; 104(2):155-62.
53. Walczak H, Miller RE, Ariail K et al. Tumoricidal activity of tumor necrosis factor-related apoptosis-inducing ligand in vivo. Nat Med 1999; 5:157-163.
54. Camidge D, Herbst RS, Gordon M et al. Mendelson; Journal of Clinical Oncology, 2007 ASCO Annual Meeting Proceedings Part I. Vol 25, No. 18S (Supplement) 2007:3582.
55. Jing Li, Betty Tang, Cheng Jean et al. Novartis Inst. for BioMed. Research, Inc., Cambridge, MA, Genomics Institute of the Novartis Research Foundation, San Diego, CA; Poster; AACR Meeting 2007, Los Angeles, CA.
56. Nebbioso A, Clarke N, Voltz E et al. Tumor-selective action of HDAC inhibitors involves TRAIL induction in acute myeloid leukemia cells. Nat Med 2005; 11:77-84.
57. Inoue S, MacFarlane M, Harper N et al. Histone deacetylase inhibitors potentiate TNF-related apoptosis-inducing ligand (TRAIL)-induced apoptosis in lymphoid malignancies. Cell Death Differ 2004; 11 Suppl 2:S193-206.
58. MacFarlane M, Kohlhaas SL, Sutcliffe MJ et al. TRAIL receptor-selective mutants signal to apoptosis via TRAIL-R1 in primary lymphoid malignancies. Cancer Res 2005; 65:11265-11270.
59. Olsson A, Diaz T, Aguilar-Santelises M et al. Sensitization to TRAIL-induced apoptosis and modulation of FLICE-inhibitory protein in B chronic lymphocytic leukemia by actinomycin D. Leukemia 2001; 15:1868-1877.
60. Mitsiades N, Mitsiades CS, Poulaki V et al. Biologic sequelae of nuclear factor-kappaB blockade in multiple myeloma: therapeutic applications. Blood 2002; 99:4079-4086.
61. Di Pietro R, Secchiero P, Rana R et al. Ionizing radiation sensitizes erythroleukemic cells but not normal erythroblasts to tumor necrosis factor-related apoptosis-inducing ligand (TRAIL)—mediated cytotoxicity by selective up-regulation of TRAIL-R1. Blood 2001; 97:2596-2603.
62. Naka T, Sugamura K, Hylander BL et al. Effects of tumor necrosis factor-related apoptosis-inducing ligand alone and in combination with chemotherapeutic agents on patients' colon tumors grown in SCID mice. Cancer Res 2002; 62:5800-5806.
63. Hylander BL, Pitoniak R, Penetrante RB et al. The anti-tumor effect of Apo2L/TRAIL on patient pancreatic adenocarcinomas grown as xenografts in SCID mice. J Transl Med, 2005; 3:22.
64. Ganten TM, Koschny R, Haas TL et al. Proteasome inhibition sensitizes hepatocellular carcinoma cells, but not human hepatocytes, to TRAIL. Hepatology 2005; 42:588-597.
65. Ganten TM, Koschny R, Sykora J et al. Preclinical differentiation between apparently safe and potentially hepatotoxic applications of TRAIL either alone or in combination with chemotherapeutic drugs. Clin Cancer Res 2006; 12:2640-2646.
66. Koschny R, Ganten TM et al. TRAIL/bortezomib cotreatment is potentially hepatotoxic but induces cancer-specific apoptosis within a therapeutic window. Hepatology 2007a; 45(3):649-58.

67. Pathil A, Armeanu S, Venturelli S et al. HDAC inhibitor treatment of hepatoma cells induces both TRAIL-independent apoptosis and restoration of sensitivity to TRAIL. Hepatology 2006; 43:425-434.
68. Leverkus M, Sprick MR, Wachter T et al. Proteasome inhibition results in TRAIL sensitization of primary keratinocytes by removing the resistance-mediating block of effector caspase maturation. Mol Cell Biol 2003; 23:777-790.
69. Nakata S, Yoshida T, Horinaka M et al. Histone deacetylase inhibitors upregulate death receptor 5/TRAIL-R2 and sensitize apoptosis induced by TRAIL/APO2-L in human malignant tumor cells. Oncogene 2004; 23:6261-6271.
70. Atkins GJ, Bouralexis S, Evdokiou A et al. Human osteoblasts are resistant to Apo2L/TRAIL-mediated apoptosis. Bone 2002; 31:448-456.
71. Van Valen F, Fulda S, Schafer KL et al. Selective and nonselective toxicity of TRAIL/Apo2L combined with chemotherapy in human bone tumour cells vs. normal human cells. International journal of cancer 2003; 107:929-940.
72. Wu XX, Kakehi Y, Mizutani Y et al. Doxorubicin enhances TRAIL-induced apoptosis in prostate cancer. Int J Oncol 2002; 20:949-954.
73. Cretney E, Uldrich AP, Berzins SP et al. Are we really on the right TRAIL? Immunol Res 2005b; 31:161-164.
74. Koschny R, Walczak H, Ganten TM. The promise of TRAIL- potential and risks of a novel anti-cancer therapy. J Mol Med 2007.
75. Jin X, Wu XX, et al. Enhancement of death receptor 4 mediated apoptosis and cytotoxicity in renal cell carinoma cells by subtoxic concentrations of doxorubicin. J Urol 2007; 177(5):1894-1899.
76. Jiang CC, Chen LH, et al. Tunicamycin sensitizes human melanoma cells to tumor necrosis factor-related apoptosis-inducing ligand-induced apoptosis by up-regulation of TRAIL-R2 via the unfolded protein response. Cancer Res 2007; 67(12):5880-8.
77. Volkmann X, Fischer U, et al. Increased hepatotoxicity of tumor necrosis factor-related apoptosis-inducing ligand in diseased human liver. Hepatology. 2007. (published online in advance of print)
78. Meurette O, Fontaine A, et al. Cytotoxicity of TRAIL/anticancer drug combinations in human normal cells. Ann N Y Acad Sci 2006; 1090:209-16.

CHAPTER 15

Therapeutic Potential of VEGI/TL1A in Autoimmunity and Cancer

Gautam Sethi, Bokyung Sung and Bharat B. Aggarwal*

Abstract

Vascular endothelial growth inhibitor (VEGI, TNFSF-15) is a novel member of the tumor necrosis factor (TNF) superfamily that consists of 174 amino acids and exhibits a 20% to 30% sequence homology to other members of the TNF superfamily. The VEGI gene is expressed as a transmembrane protein predominantly in endothelial cells and induced generally in response to inflammatory stimuli. It mediates most of its cellular responses through the interaction of the death receptor-3. VEGI activates multiple cell signaling pathways including NF-κB, STAT3, JNK, p38 MAPK and p42/p44 MAPK. VEGI suppresses the proliferation of endothelial cells and tumor cells, induces maturation of dendritic cells and induces osteoclastogenesis. How VEGI mediates its effects in autoimmune diseases and tumorigenesis is the focus of this review.

Introduction

The TNF family of cytokines consists of type II transmembrane proteins (except TNF) and includes TNF, FasL, CD40L, CD30L, CD27L, 4-1BBL, OX40L,[1,2] TRAIL/APO-2L,[3] TRANCE,[4] TWEAK/DR3L,[5] APRIL,[6] LIGHT[7] and THANK.[8] These proteins have roles in diverse biological functions such as proliferation, differentiation and gene activation.[2,9] Binding to their cognate receptors initiates several signal transduction pathways that activate NF-κB[10] and c-*jun* N-terminal protein kinase, a member of the mitogen-activated protein kinase family.[11] Also activated is a cascade of caspases, ultimately resulting in apoptosis.[12] Recently a new member of the TNF family was identified and named as vascular endothelial cell growth inhibitor (VEGI).[13, 14] VEGI has recently received the HGMW-approved designation of TNF super family member 15 (TNFSF15). Although its transcript was found in many human tissues, including placenta, lung, kidney, skeletal muscle, pancreas, spleen, prostate, small intestine and colon, VEGI was expressed most abundantly in endoethelial cells.[13,15] It was established that the VEGI gene encodes a type II transmembrane protein with a molecular mass of 13 kD and that it exhibits a 20-30% overall sequence homology to human TNF and the Fas ligand.

The human VEGI gene spans about 17 kb and consists of four exons. Multiple VEGI transcripts generated by the use of cryptic splice sites and alternate exons have been described.[16] All known VEG1 isoforms exhibit a carboxyl terminal domain of 151 amino acid residues, which is encoded by part of the fourth exon, termed IVb. The initially characterized VEGI isoform, designated VEGI-174, is encoded by the fourth exon (parts IVa and IVb) alone, which includes both the putative transmembrane domain and the conserved extracellular domain. Two new isoforms, VEGI-251 and VEGI-192, were identified subsequently.[16] The VEGI-251 isoform is also known

*Corresponding Author: Bharat B. Aggarwal—Cytokine Research Laboratory, Department of Experimental Therapeutics, The University of Texas MD Anderson Cancer Center, Box 143, 1515 Holcombe Boulevard, Houston, Texas 77030, USA. Email: aggarwal@mdanderson.org

Therapeutic Targets of the TNF Superfamily, edited by Iqbal S. Grewal.
©2009 Landes Bioscience and Springer Science+Business Media.

as TNF-like ligand 1 (TLIA).[17] The VEGI-251 and 192 isoforms differ in their amino terminal regions, but share the conserved 151-amino acid residue carboxyl terminal domain. VEGI-251 possesses a putative secretory signal peptide and its overexpression causes apoptosis of endothelial cells and inhibition of tumor growth.[17] The salient features and functions of this cytokine are summarized in Table 1.

Signaling Mechanism(s) of VEGI/TL1A

VEGI/TL1A has been shown to exert its effects through activation of multiple signaling pathways including NF-κB, JNK, p38 MAPK and p42/p44 MAPK (Fig. 1). Our group showed for the first time that VEGI activated the transcription factor NF-κB as determined by the electrophoretic mobility shift assay, induced degradation of IκBα and nuclear translocation of p65 subunit of NF-κB. In addition, VEGI activated c-Jun N-terminal kinase.[18] Yu et al reported that VEGI mediates two distinct activities in endothelial cells: early G_1 arrest in G_0/G_1 cells responding to growth stimuli and programmed death in proliferating cells. When the cells were stimulated with growth conditions but treated simultaneously with VEGI, a reversible, early-G_1 growth arrest occurred, as evident by the lack of late G_1 markers such as hyperphosphorylation of the retinoblastoma gene product and upregulation of the *c-myc* gene. Additionally, VEGI treatment led to inhibition of the activities of cyclin-dependent kinases CDK2, CDK4 and CDK6. In contrast, VEGI treatment of cells that had entered the growth cycle resulted in apoptotic cell death, but not in nonproliferating cells treated with this cytokine. Additionally, stress-signaling proteins p38 and JNK were not as fully activated by VEGI in quiescent as compared with proliferating populations. These findings suggest a dual role for VEGI, the maintenance of growth arrest and induction of apoptosis, in the modulation of the endothelial cell cycle.[19] Migone and coworkers reported that TL1A, is a ligand for DR3 and decoy receptor TR6/DcR3 and that its expression is inducible by TNF and IL-1α. TL1A induced NF-κB activation and apoptosis in DR3-expressing cell lines, while TR6-Fc protein antagonizes these signaling events. This data suggests that interaction of TL1A with DR3 promotes T-cell expansion during an immune response, whereas TR6 has an opposing effect.[17] Yue and colleagues further examined whether TL1 induces apoptosis in endothelial cells and, its mechanism of action. Cultured bovine pulmonary artery endothelial cells (BPAEC) exposed to TL1A showed morphological and biochemical features characteristic of apoptosis. TL1A-induced apoptosis in BPAEC was a time- and concentration-dependent process. TL1A increased Fas expression in BPAEC and significantly activated stress-activated protein kinase (SAPK) and p38 mitogen-activated protein kinase (p38 MAPK). This cytokine also activated caspases in BPAEC and TL1A-induced apoptosis in BPAEC was significantly attenuated by the caspase inhibitor. The major component activated by TL1A in BPAEC was caspase-3, which was based on substrate specificity and immunocytochemical analysis. These findings suggested that TL1A may act as an autocrine factor to induce apoptosis in endothelial cells via activation of multiple signaling pathways, including stress protein kinases as well as certain caspases.[19] Wen and coworkers investigated the effect of TL1A and an agonistic DR3 monoclonal antibody in human erythroleukemic TF-1 cells, which express DR3 endogenously. TL1A induced the formation of a DR3 signaling complex containing TRADD, TRAF2 and RIP and activated the NF-κB and the ERK, JNK and p38 MAPK pathways.[20] However, TL1A or an agonistic DR3 monoclonal antibody did not induce apoptosis in these cells nor were there detectable levels of FADD or procaspase-8 seen in the signaling complex. Interestingly, DR3-mediated apoptosis was induced in TF-1 cells in the presence of a NF-κB pathway-specific inhibitor but not in the presence of mitogen-activated protein kinase inhibitors, either alone or in combination, suggesting that DR3-induced NF-κB activation was responsible for resistance to apoptosis in these cells. Consistent with this, it was found that TL1A significantly increased the production of c-IAP2, a known NF-κB -dependent anti-apoptotic protein and that the NF-κB inhibitor or cycloheximide prevented its synthesis. Furthermore, inhibition of c-IAP2 production by RNA interference significantly sensitized TF-1 cells to TL1A-induced apoptosis.[20]

Table 1. A list of salient features of VEGI

- VEGI is a type II transmembrane protein with a molecular mass of 22kD.
- The amino acid sequence has 20-30% sequence homology to other members of TNF superfamily.
- Residues 26-174 constitute an extracellular domain analogous to domains found in other members of TNF superfamily.
- The human VEGI gene spans about 17kb and consists of four exons.
- All known VEG1 isoforms exhibit a carboxyl terminal domain of 151 amino acid residues, which is encoded by part of the fourth exon, termed IVb.
- Three different isoforms of VEGI has been characterized so far.
- The initially characterized VEGI isoform, designated VEGI-174, is encoded by the fourth exon (parts IVa and IVb) alone, which includes both the putative transmembrane domain and the conserved extracellular domain.
- Two new isoforms, VEGI-251 and VEGI-192, were identified subsequently.
- The VEGI-251 isoform is also known as TNF-like ligand 1 (TL1A).
- The VEGI-251 and 192 isoforms differ in their amino terminal regions, but share the conserved 151-amino acid residue carboxyl terminal domain.
- VEGI-251 also possesses a putative secretory signal peptide.
- TL1A exerts its effect by binding to death domain-containing receptor-3 (DR3, TNFRSF12, TNFRSF25).
- Is also found in many adult human tissues and foam cells in atherosclerotic plaques.
- FcγR stimulation induces TL1A mRNA in both monocytes and dendritic cells.
- Inhibits the proliferation of endothelial and tumor cells.
- Antiangiogenic.
- Induces dendritic cell maturation.
- Induces activation of transcription factors such as NF-κB and STAT3.
- Induces activation of p38, JNK and ERK MAP kinases.
- Induces the expression of TNF, MMPs, MCP-1 and IL-8.
- TL1A up-regulates OX40L on neonatal CD4+ CD3-cells.
- DcR3 induces osteoclastogenesis from the cultures of monocyte, macrophage and bone marrow cells.
- TL1A/DR3 pathway plays a dominant role in the ultimate level of IL-12/IL-18-induced IFN-γ production by CCR9+ mucosal and gut-homing T-cells.
- Recombinant VEGI 192 suppresses the growth of Lewis lung cancer tumor model.
- Recombinant VEGI 251 suppresses the growth of xenograft breast and colon cancer tumors.
- TL1A is expressed in either synovial fluids or synovial tissue of rheumatoid factor (RF)-seropositive RA patients, but not RF-/RA patients.
- TL1A-DR3 interaction is of particular importance in Th1-mediated intestinal diseases, such as ulcerative colitis and Crohn's disease.
- Up-regulation of mRNA and protein levels of TL1A has been found in macrophages and CD4+/CD8+ lymphocytes of the intestinal lamina propria of patients with Crohn's disease.
- Single gene polymorphisms in TL1A also confer susceptibility to Crohn's disease.
- VEGI displays prognostic relevance as breast cancer patients with an overall poor prognosis express significantly lower levels of this cytokine as compared to those with a favorable prognosis.

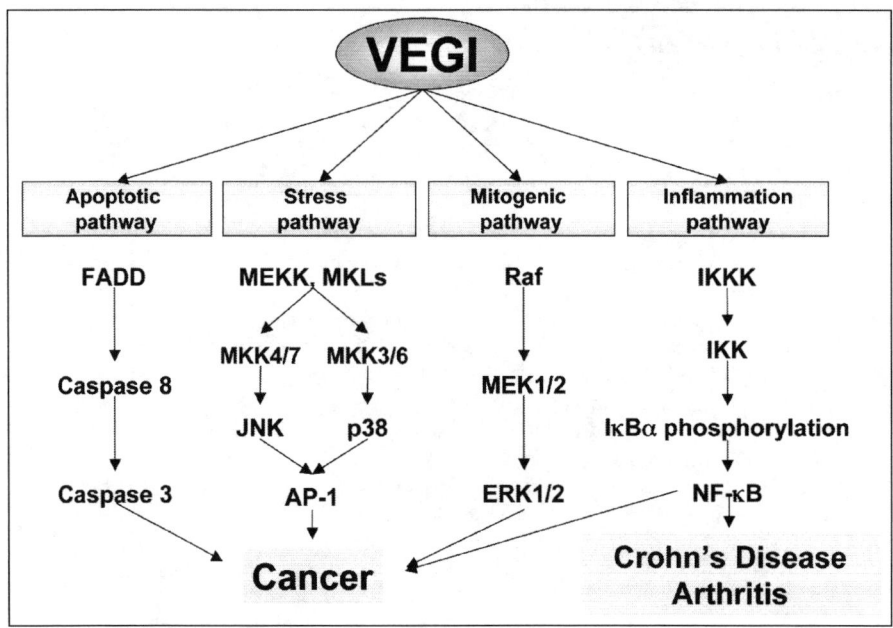

Figure 1. Signaling pathways activated by VEGI.

Role of VEGI/TL1A in Autoimmunity

Following identification of the VEGI isoform, it was found that it could bind to and activate TNF receptor family member known as Death Receptor 3 (DR3). Since DR3 is upregulated in activated T-cells, this group analyzed TLIA activity on T-cells. While TL1A alone or with anti-CD3 aor anti-CD28 costimulation did not induce proliferation of T-cells, it was found that pretreatment with TL1A enhances T-cell proliferation in response to IL-2, elevates expression of IL2Rα and β and induces secretion of both interferon-γ (IFN-γ) and granulocyte-macrophage colony stimulating factor (GM-CSF). They also showed that while resting T-cells, B-cells, NK cells, DC and monocytes did not express TL1A mRNA, transcript was induced by TNF, IL-1a, or PMA in human umbilical vein endothelial cells (HUVEC). Moreover, using a graft-versus-host-response (GVHR) model in which C57BL/6 splenocytes were injected intravenously into BALB/c X C57BL/6 mice, it was found that TL1A could increase GVHR in vivo, suggesting a role for this cytokine in immune response.[17,21]

Papadakis et al showed that TL1A or an agonistic anti-DR3 mAb can synergize with IL-12/IL-18 to augment IFN-γ production in human peripheral blood T-cells and NK cells. TL1A also enhanced IFN-γ production by IL-12/IL-18 stimulated CD56+ T-cells. When expressed as fold change, the synergistic effect of TL1A on cytokine-induced IFN- production was more pronounced on CD4+ and CD8+ T-cells than on CD56+ T-cells or NK cells. Intracellular cytokine staining showed that TL1A significantly enhanced both the percentage and the mean fluorescence intensity of IFN-γ producing T-cells in response to IL-12/IL-18. The combination of IL-12 and IL-18 markedly up-regulated DR3 expression in NK cells, whereas it had minimal effect in T-cells.[22] Thus, TL1A could be involved in initiating or promoting Th1 responses because—its receptor (DR3) is induced on most T-cells by activation;[2] TL1A, induced on T-cells or other immune system cells, could act by direct cell-to-cell surface ligand—receptor interaction, or more widely after release in a soluble form;[3] the TL1A/DR3 interaction potently costimulates IFN-γ production by DR3+ T-cells and is anti-apoptotic.

Kim and coworkers[23] recently showed that both neonatal and adult CD4+ CD3- cells express the TNF family member, death receptor 3 (TNFRSF25) and that addition of TL1A the ligand for death receptor 3, up-regulates OX40L on neonatal CD4+ CD3- cells. They further demonstrated that this differentiation occurs in vivo: neonatal CD4+ CD3- cells up-regulate both CD30L and OX40L after adoptive transfer into an adult recipient. Prehn et al[24] recently investigated TL1A expression by antigen presenting cells (APCs), such as blood monocytes and in vitro-derived dendritic cells (DC) following activation of several types of known activating pathways, including TLR ligands, IFN-γ and FcγR activation. They demonstrated that FcγR activation induces a strong up-regulation of TL1A mRNA in monocytes as well as DC and that FcγR activation resulted in the appearance of TL1A in supernatants and on the surface of a fraction of monocytes and DC. In contrast, TLR ligands did not up-regulate TL1A substantially while inducing strong TNF-α and IL-6 secretion in monocytes and DC. Furthermore, in monocyte-T-cell cocultures, FcγR activation resulted in enhanced IFN-γ production by T-cells that could be blocked by anti-TL1A Abs. Substantial TL1A production following FcγR activation, perhaps by contact with opsonized bacteria, defines a new mechanism by which monocytes and DC, by producing TL1A, can drive DR3+ cells, such as NK and activated T-cells, to very highly activated functional states by either direct contact of APCs with T-cells or via soluble TL1A.

Tian et al[25] reported that VEGI induces DCs maturation, a critical event in inflammation-initiated immunity. VEGI-stimulated bone marrow-derived immature DCs display early activation of maturation signaling molecules NF-κB, STAT3, p38 and JNK and cytoskeleton reorganization and dendrite formation. The activation signals were partially inhibited by using a neutralizing Ab against death domain-containing receptor-3 (DR3) or a truncated form of DR3 consisting of the extracellular domain, indicating an involvement of DR3 in the transmission of VEGI activity. A VEGI isoform, TL1A, did not induce similar activities under otherwise identical experimental conditions. Additionally, the cells reveal significantly enhanced expression of mature DC-specific marker CD83, secondary lymphoid tissue-directing chemokine receptor CCR7, the MHC class-II protein (MHC-II) and costimulatory molecules CD40, CD80 and CD86. Functionally, the cells exhibit decreased Ag endocytosis, increased cell surface distribution of MHC-II and increased secretion of IL-12 and TNF. Moreover, VEGI-stimulated DCs were able to facilitate the differentiation of CD4+ naive T-cells in cocultures.

Furthermore, TL1A expression has been detected in T-cells in intestinal lamina propria of inflammatory bowel disease (IBD), such as Crohn's disease (CD) and ulcerative colitis, thus indicating that TL1A might play a role in IBD acting as a Th1 polarizing cytokine.[26-29] Bamias and colleagues[30] investigated the role of TL1A in IBD by functioning as a Th1-polarizing cytokine. The expression, cellular localization and functional activity of TL1A and DR3 were studied in intestinal tissue specimens as well as isolated lamina propria mononuclear cells from IBD patients and controls. TL1A mRNA and protein expression was up-regulated in IBD, particularly in involved areas of Crohn's disease. TL1A production was localized to the intestinal lamina propria in macrophages and CD4+ and CD8+ lymphocytes from CD patients as well as in plasma cells from ulcerative colitis patients. The amount of TL1A protein and the number of TL1A-positive cells correlated with the severity of inflammation, most significantly in CD. Increased numbers of immunoreactive DR3-positive T-lymphocytes were detected in the intestinal lamina propria from IBD patients. Addition of recombinant human TL1A to cultures of PHA-stimulated lamina propria mononuclear from CD patients significantly augmented IFN-gamma production by 4-fold, whereas a minimal effect was observed in control patients. While resting peripheral blood (PB) T-cells did not express TL1A, activating stimuli induced cell membrane-associated TL1A (mb-TL1A) on some T-cells. In contrast, a fraction LP T-cells, especially CD4+, constitutively expressed mb-TL1A and DR3, with higher fractions detected in ulcerative colitis and Crohn's disease.[31] Thus, TL1A could be involved as co-initiator and/or amplifier of a dysregulated Th1 response in Crohn's disease. A recent study has provided a genetic perspective on the role of TL1A in the human Th1 mucosal response in Crohn's disease. This genome-wide association study revealed a highly significant association of single nucleotide polymorphism haplotypes of the *tl1a* gene with Crohn's disease in a large cohort of Japanese patients as well as in two separate, smaller European cohorts.[32] Recently, Bamias et al[33] demonstrated that TL1A and its receptor DR3 are up-regulated in inflamed gut mucosa in two distinct murine models of ileal inflammation. TL1A seems to be primarily expressed by lamina propria dendritic cells (DC).

Cassatella and coworkers[34] reported that mononuclear phagocytes appear to be a major source of TL1A in rheumatoid arthritis (RA), as revealed by their strong TL1A expression in either synovial fluids or synovial tissue of rheumatoid factor (RF)-seropositive RA patients, but not RF-/RA patients. Accordingly, in vitro experiments revealed that human monocytes express and release significant amounts of soluble TL1A when stimulated with insoluble immune complexes (IC), polyethylene glycol precipitates from the serum of RF+/RA patients, or with insoluble ICs purified from RA synovial fluids. Monocyte-derived soluble TL1A was biologically active as determined by its capacity to induce apoptosis of the human erythroleukemic cell line TF-1, as well as to cooperate with IL-12 and IL-18 in inducing the production of IFN-gamma by CD4+ T-cells. Because RA is a chronic inflammatory disease with autoimmune etiology, in which ICs, autoantibodies (including RF) and various cytokines contribute to its pathology, this report indicates TL1A could be involved in its pathogenesis and contribute to the severity of RA disease that is typical of RF+/RA patients.

Yang et al[35] showed that DcR3 could induce osteoclast formation from human monocytes, murine RAW264.7 macrophages and bone marrow cells. DcR3-differentiated cells exhibit characteristics unique for osteoclasts, including polynuclear giant morphology, bone resorption, TRAP, CD51/61 and MMP-9 expression. Consistent with the abrogation of osteoclastogenic effect of DcR3 by TNFR-Fc, DcR3 treatment can induce osteoclastogenic cytokine TNF-α release through ERK and p38 MAPK signaling pathways. This report indicated that DcR3 via coupling reverse signaling of ERK and p38 MAPK and stimulating TNF-α synthesis is a critical regulator of osteoclast formation. Tang and coworkers recently found that DcR3 transgenic mice show a decrease of bone mineral density (BMD), bone mineral content (BMC) and bone volume, accompanied by an increase of osteoclast formation, thereby establishing that in vivo effect of DcR3 may play an important role in osteolytic bone diseases.[36]

Role of VEGI/TL1A as Negative Regulator of Angiogenesis

Several lines of evidence indicate that VEGI acts as a negative regulator of angiogenesis. VEGI is differentially expressed in proliferating and quiescent endothelial cells. When examined by Northern blot using total RNA preparations from cultured HUVEC, VEGI mRNA levels increases in cell number.[19] Low levels of VEGI mRNA were detected in newly seeded cells and the levels of VEGI increased with increasing cell number until a plateau was reached as the cultures became confluent. Moreover, the up-regulation of VEGI in endothelial cells following treatment with anti-angiogenic doses of TNF-α emphasizes the potential role of VEGI in inhibiting angiogenesis. TNF-α modulates angiogenesis in a dose-dependent manner, with low levels stimulating, but high levels inhibiting endothelial cell growth in vitro.[37] Yu et al reported that high, inhibitory doses of TNF-α resulted in up-regulation of VEGI in a variety of endothelial cell types.[19] Interestingly, all three isoforms were coordinately upregulated in a dose- and time-dependent manner.[16] The cytostatic profile of VEGI, along with its upregulation by TNF-α, suggests that VEGI may mediate some of the effects of TNF-α on endothelial cells. Indeed, TNF-α inhibits both VEGF and bFGF-induced endothelial proliferation[38,39] and induces regression of tumors in mice.[40] Interestingly, TL1A can also be transiently up-regulated by IL-1α, PMA and bFGF[17] and down-regulated by IFN-γ.[16]

DcR3 has been used experimentally to establish that VEGI acts as an endogenous negative regulator of angiogenesis. TL1A can bind to DcR3, which results in neutralization of VEGI activity.[17] A recent study suggests that overexpression of DcR3 augments in vitro HUVEC proliferation, migration and tube formation on Matrigel, whereas DcR3 did not affect these activities in human aortic endothelial cells (HAEC), which do not express VEGI. In addition, DcR3 accelerates vessel formation in vivo in the Matrigel plug assay and the CAM assay.[41] These activities result from inhibition of endogenous VEGI-251, as the other known ligands of DcR3, FasL and LIGHT, are not expressed by HUVEC.[41] DcR3 is often upregulated in cancer and its levels are elevated in sera of cancer patients.[45-48]

Overexpression of DcR3 may allow cancers to escape immune detection and neutralize an important endogenous negative regulator of angiogenesis,[41] thereby facilitating the angiogenic switch.

Role of VEGI/TL1A in Cancer

The anticancer activity of VEGI has been investigated using several models both in vitro as well as in vivo. Our group reported for the first time that VEGI could inhibit the proliferation of breast carcinoma, epithelial and myeloid tumor cells; and activated caspase-3 leading to PARP cleavage. The activity of VEGI could neither be neutralized by antibodies against TNF, nor could it compete with TNF binding, indicating that the activity of VEGI is not due to TNF and it binds to a distinct receptor.[18] In a sygenic mouse colon cancer model, murine colon carcinoma cells (MC-38) were stably transfected with either the VEGI-174 or sVEGI, where the transmembrane domain was replaced by a secretion signal. VEGI overexpression did not affect T-cell growth in culture. The cells were intra-dermally implanted in syngeneic C57BL6 mice. Vector-transfected and VEGI-174 transfected cells grew into tumors at a rate comparable to wild type MC38 cells. In contrast, overexpressing sVEGI suppressed the growth of the implanted cells accompanied by decreased vascularization.[15]

The anticancer potential of VEGI was also examined in a breast cancer xenograft tumor model in which the cancer cells were co-injected with Chinese hamster ovary cells (CHO) overexpressing a secreted form of the VEGI protein. The co-injection resulted in potent inhibition of xenograft tumor growth.[42] Since VEGI did not inhibit the growth of breast cancer cells in culture in this study, the anticancer activity of the cytokine most likely arises from its antiangiogenic activity. Zhai et al[42] also examined the anticancer activity of VEGI-overexpressing CHO cells in a prostate cancer animal model. The CHO cells were mixed with prostate cancer cells (PC3) at various different ratios. The cell mixtures were then injected subcutaneously in athymic nude mice and the growth of the xenograft tumors was monitored. The tumors initially grew, but in a few weeks almost all of the tumors disappeared in groups with higher CHO: PC3 ratios. PC3 cells implanted alone exhibited progressive tumor growth. These results indicate that high levels of VEGI may cause the eradication of established tumors. In a different approach, Pan and coworkers constructed an adenovirus expressing a fusion protein composed of endostatin and a VEGI protein containing the C-terminal 151 residues, which was termed as AdhENDO-VEGI151. Subcutaneous injection of this fusion protein inhibited tumor growth by 88% in a liver xenograft model that was associ-ated with decreased microvessel density.[43] Hou and colleagues examined the anticancer activity of VEGI-192 with a Lewis lung cancer murine tumor model. Systemic administration of VEGI-192 gave rise to a marked inhibition of tumor growth. As much as 50% inhibition of the tumor growth rate was achieved with treatment initiated when the tumor volumes reached nearly 5% of the body weight. Inhibition of tumor formation was also observed when VEGI-192 was given at the time of tumor inoculation. Consistently, an increase in survival time of the treated animals was found. The VEGI-192-treated animals showed no liver or kidney toxicity.[44]

Chew et al found that overexpression of full-length VEGI-174 by cancer cells had little effect on the growth of the xenograft breast tumors. However, an overexpression of the intact VEGI-251, as well as the sVEGI fusion protein, retarded tumor growth significantly.[16] Parr and coworkers recently analyzed the VEGI expression in relation to breast cancer patient clinical parameters. The VEGI ex-pression profile was assessed qualitatively (RT-PCR), quantitatively (real-time Quantitative-PCR) and immuno-histochemically (IHC), in a panel of 24 human normal and cancer cell lines and in a cohort of 151 mammary tissue samples with a 6-year median follow-up. Patients who had died of breast cancer or had local recurrence of the disease expressed significantly lower levels of VEGI in comparison to the elevated levels in the disease free patients. High levels of VEGI were associated with an increased chance of patient survival. Importantly, patients with breast tumors expressing reduced levels of VEGI had a poorer prognosis than those patients expressing high levels of VEGI. However, no significant correlations were observed between VEGI expression and tumor grade, TNM classification, or nodal involvement. This report confirmed that VEGI displays prognostic relevance as breast cancer patients with an overall poor prognosis express significantly lower levels of VEGI compared to those with a favorable prognosis.[45]

Conclusion

VEGI/TL1A is one of the primitive members of the TNFR superfamily. TNF itself has not been found in chickens, but recently the cloning of TL1A from chickens has been reported.[54] The finding implies that TL1A is a part of the early immune system and raises the question of what are the endogenous triggers of TL1A expression. Although it has been reported that TNF and IL-1β can induce TL1A expression, whether it is through the nucleotide-binding oligomerization domain (NOD) pathway, is not clear. TL1A expression is tightly regulated under physiological conditions and it will be of importance to understand the ways by which TL1A expression is triggered and whether differences in TL1A expression between individuals can account for increased susceptibility to development of various autoimmune disorders. Targeting TL1A now constitutes an important therapy for patients suffering with Crohn's disease and RA. Many approaches including the use of blocking antibodies to DR3, soluble DcR3 receptor, or neutralizing monoclonal antibodies specific for TL1A are being employed. The outcome of clinical trials using these agents could revolutionize the treatment modalities associated with these diseases.

Acknowledgement

Dr. Aggarwal is a Ransom Horne Jr, Professor of Cancer Research. This work was supported by a grant from the Clayton Foundation for Research (to BBA).

References

1. Smith CA, Farrah T, Goodwin RG. The TNF receptor superfamily of cellular and viral proteins: activation, costimulation and death. Cell 1994; 76:959-962.
2. Aggarwal BB. 2003. Signalling pathways of the TNF superfamily: a double-edged sword. Nat Rev Immunol 3:745-756.
3. Pitti RM, Marsters SA, Ruppert S et al. Induction of apoptosis by Apo-2 ligand, a new member of the tumor necrosis factor cytokine family. J Biol Chem 1996; 271:12687-12690.
4. Wong BR, Rho J, Arron J et al. TRANCE is a novel ligand of the tumor necrosis factor receptor family that activates c-Jun N-terminal kinase in T-cells. J Biol Chem 1997; 272:25190-25194.
5. Chicheportiche Y, Bourdon PR, Xu H et al. APRIL TWEAK, a new secreted ligand in the tumor necrosis factor family that weakly induces apoptosis. J Biol Chem 1997; 272:32401-32410.
6. Hahne M, Kataoka T, Schroter M et al. A new ligand of the tumor necrosis factor family, stimulates tumor cell growth. J Exp Med 1998; 188:1185-1190.
7. Mauri DN, Ebner R, Montgomery RI et al. LIGHT, a new member of the TNF superfamily and lymphotoxin alpha are ligands for herpesvirus entry mediator. Immunity 1998; 8:21-30.
8. Mukhopadhyay A, Ni J, Zhai Y et al. Identification and characterization of a novel cytokine, THANK, a TNF homologue that activates apoptosis, nuclear factor-kappaB and c-Jun NH2-terminal kinase. J Biol Chem 1999; 274:15978-15981.
9. Bhardwaj A, Aggarwal BB. Receptor-mediated choreography of life and death. J Clin Immunol 2003; 23:317-332.
10. Aggarwal BB. Nuclear factor-kappaB: the enemy within. Cancer Cell 2004; 6:203-208.
11. Westwick JK, Weitzel C, Minden A et al. Tumor necrosis factor alpha stimulates AP-1 activity through prolonged activation of the c-Jun kinase. J Biol Chem 1994; 269:26396-26401.
12. Darnay BG, Aggarwal BB. Early events in TNF signaling: a story of associations and dissociations. J Leukoc Biol 1997; 61:559-566.
13. Tan KB, Harrop J, Reddy M et al. Characterization of a novel TNF-like ligand and recently described TNF ligand and TNF receptor superfamily genes and their constitutive and inducible expression in hematopoietic and nonhematopoietic cells. Gene 1997; 204:35-46.
14. Yue TL, Ni J, Romanic AM et al. TL1, a novel tumor necrosis factor-like cytokine, induces apoptosis in endothelial cells. Involvement of activation of stress protein kinases (stress-activated protein kinase and p38 mitogen-activated protein kinase) and caspase-3-like protease. J Biol Chem 1999; 274:1479-1486.
15. Zhai Y, Ni J, Jiang GW et al. VEGI, a novel cytokine of the tumor necrosis factor family, is an angiogenesis inhibitor that suppresses the growth of colon carcinomas in vivo. FASEB J 1999; 13:181-189.
16. Chew LJ, Pan H, Yu J et al. A novel secreted splice variant of vascular endothelial cell growth inhibitor. FASEB J 2002; 16:742-744.

17. Migone TS, Zhang J, Luo X et al. TL1A is a TNF-like ligand for DR3 and TR6/DcR3 and functions as a T-cell costimulator. Immunity 2002; 16:479-492.
18. Haridas V, Shrivastava A, Su J et al. VEGI, a new member of the TNF family activates nuclear factor-kappa B and c-Jun N-terminal kinase and modulates cell growth. Oncogene 1999; 18:6496-6504.
19. Yu J, Tian S, Metheny-Barlow L et al. Modulation of endothelial cell growth arrest and apoptosis by vascular endothelial growth inhibitor. Circ Res 2001; 89:1161-1167.
20. Wen L, Zhuang L, Luo X et al. TL1A-induced NF-kappaB activation and c-IAP2 production prevent DR3-mediated apoptosis in TF-1 cells. J Biol Chem 2003; 278:39251-39258.
21. Metheny-Barlow LJ, Li LY. Vascular endothelial growth inhibitor (VEGI), an endogenous negative regulator of angiogenesis. Semin Ophthalmol 2006; 21:49-58.
22. Papadakis KA, Prehn JL, Landers C et al. TL1A synergizes with IL-12 and IL-18 to enhance IFN-gamma production in human T-cells and NK cells. J Immunol 2004; 172:7002-7007.
23. Kim MY, Toellner KM, White A et al. Neonatal and adult CD4+ CD3- cells share similar gene expression profile and neonatal cells up-regulate OX40 ligand in response to TL1A (TNFSF15). J Immunol 2006; 177:3074-3081.
24. Prehn JL, Thomas LS, Landers CJ et al. The T-cell costimulator TL1A is induced by FcgammaR signaling in human monocytes and dendritic cells. J Immunol 2007; 178:4033-4038.
25. Tian F, Grimaldo S, Fugita M et al. The endothelial cell-produced antiangiogenic cytokine vascular endothelial growth inhibitor induces dendritic cell maturation. J Immunol 2007; 179:3742-3751.
26. Picornell Y, Mei L, Taylor K et al. TNFSF15 is an ethnic-specific IBD gene. Inflamm Bowel Dis 2007;
27. Kim S, Fotiadu A, Kotoula V. Increased expression of soluble decoy receptor 3 in acutely inflamed intestinal epithelia. Clin Immunol 2005; 115:286-294.
28. Young HA, Tovey MG. TL1A: a mediator of gut inflammation. Proc Natl Acad Sci USA 2006; 103:8303-8304.
29. Cobrin GM, Abreu MT. Defects in mucosal immunity leading to Crohn's disease. Immunol Rev 2005; 206:277-295.
30. Bamias G, Martin C, Marini 3rd M et al. Expression, localization and functional activity of TL1A, a novel Th1-polarizing cytokine in inflammatory bowel disease. J Immunol 2003; 171:4868-4874.
31. Prehn JL, Mehdizadeh S, Landers CJ et al. Potential role for TL1A, the new TNF-family member and potent costimulator of IFN-gamma, in mucosal inflammation. Clin Immunol 2004; 112:66-77.
32. Yamazaki K, McGovern D, Ragoussis J et al. Single nucleotide polymorphisms in TNFSF15 confer susceptibility to Crohn's disease. Hum Mol Genet 2005; 14:3499-3506.
33. Bamias G, Mishina M, Nyce M et al. Role of TL1A and its receptor DR3 in two models of chronic murine ileitis. Proc Natl Acad Sci USA 2006; 103:8441-8446.
34. Cassatella MA, Pereira-da-Silva G, Tinazzi I et al. Soluble TNF-like cytokine (TL1A) production by immune complexes stimulated monocytes in rheumatoid arthritis. J Immunol 2007; 178:7325-7333.
35. Yang CR, Wang JH, Hsieh SL et al. Decoy receptor 3 (DcR3) induces osteoclast formation from monocyte/macrophage lineage precursor cells. Cell Death Differ 2004; 11 Suppl 1:S97-107.
36. Tang CH, Hsu TL, Lin WW et al. Attenuation of bone mass and increase of osteoclast formation in decoy receptor 3 transgenic mice. J Biol Chem 2007; 282:2346-2354.
37. Leek RD, Harris AL, Lewis CE. Cytokine networks in solid human tumors: regulation of angiogenesis. J Leukoc Biol 1994; 56:423-435.
38. Frater-Schroder M, Risau W, Hallmann R et al. Tumor necrosis factor type alpha, a potent inhibitor of endothelial cell growth in vitro, is angiogenic in vivo. Proc Natl Acad Sci USA 1987; 84:5277-5281.
39. Patterson C, Perrella MA, Endege WO et al. Downregulation of vascular endothelial growth factor receptors by tumor necrosis factor-alpha in cultured human vascular endothelial cells. J Clin Invest 1996; 98:490-496.
40. Wright P, Braun R, Babiuk L et al. Adenovirus-mediated TNF-alpha gene transfer induces significant tumor regression in mice. Cancer Biother Radiopharm 1999; 14:49-57.
41. Yang CR, Hsieh SL, Teng CM et al. Soluble decoy receptor 3 induces angiogenesis by neutralization of TL1A, a cytokine belonging to tumor necrosis factor superfamily and exhibiting angiostatic action. Cancer Res 2004; 64:1122-1129.
42. Zhai Y, Yu J, Iruela-Arispe L et al. Inhibition of angiogenesis and breast cancer xenograft tumor growth by VEGI, a novel cytokine of the TNF superfamily. Int J Cancer 1999; 82:131-136.
43. Pan X, Wang Y, Zhang M et al. Effects of endostatin-vascular endothelial growth inhibitor chimeric recombinant adenoviruses on antiangiogenesis. World J Gastroenterol 2004; 10:1409-1414.
44. Hou W, Medynski D, Wu S et al. VEGI-192, a new isoform of TNFSF15, specifically eliminates tumor vascular endothelial cells and suppresses tumor growth. Clin Cancer Res 2005; 11:5595-5602.
45. Parr C, Gan CH, Watkins G et al. Reduced vascular endothelial growth inhibitor (VEGI) expression is associated with poor prognosis in breast cancer patients. Angiogenesis 2006; 9:73-81.

INDEX